Helen R Bryce

Developing Occupation-Centered Programs for the Community

A Workbook for Students and Professionals

Linda S. Fazio, Ph.D., OTR, FAOTA

Professor of Clinical Occupational Therapy
Department of Occupational Science and Occupational Therapy
University of Southern California
Los Angeles, California

Prentice
Hall

Upper Saddle River, New Jersey

Library of Congress Cataloging-in-Publication Data

Fazio, Linda S.
  Developing occupation-centered programs for the community: a workbook for students and professionals/Linda Stoll Fazio.
    p. cm.
  Includes bibliographical references and index.
  ISBN 0-13-083332-0
  1. Occupational therapy services—Planning. 2. Community mental health services—Planning. I. Title

RC487 .F39 2000
362.2'2—dc21   00-044136

To my daughters, April and Holly, who are always at the center of my community, sharing in many of my occupations, and untiring in their contributions to the meaning in my life.

Publisher: *Julie Alexander*
Acquisitions Editor: *Mark Cohen*
Director of Production and Manufacturing: *Bruce Johnson*
Managing Production Editor: *Patrick Walsh*
Manufacturing Manager: *Ilene Sanford*
Production Liaison: *Julie Boddorf*
Production Editor: *Larry Goldberg*
Creative Director: *Marianne Frasco*
Cover Design Coordinator: *Maria Guglielmo*
Cover Designer: *Ruta Fiorino*
Interior Designer: *Carlisle Communications*
Director of Marketing: *Leslie Cavaliere*
Marketing Coordinator: *Cindy Frederick*
Editorial Assistant: *Melissa Kerian*
Composition: *Carlisle Communications*
Printing and Binding: *R. R. Donnelley & Sons*

Prentice-Hall International (UK) Limited, *London*
Prentice-Hall of Australia Pty. Limited, *Sydney*
Prentice-Hall Canada Inc., *Toronto*
Prentice-Hall Hispanoamericana, S. A., *Mexico*
Prentice-Hall of India Private Limited, *New Delhi*
Prentice-Hall of Japan, Inc., *Tokyo*
Prentice-Hall Singapore Pte. Ltd.
Editora Prentice-Hall do Brasil, Ltda., *Rio de Janeiro*

10 9 8 7 6 5 4 3 2 1
ISBN 0-13-083332-0

Contents

Preface

Developing Occupation-Centered Programs for the Community: A Workbook for Students and Professionals is a practical guide to mark the way for the return of occupational therapy to community practice. Some practitioners, of course, have never left. Rather, they have remained at the center of their patients'/clients' communities throughout their practice, and their models for intervention always have been inclusive of the context and dynamics of community.

For others who have aligned themselves with the medical/institutional models for treatment—the models that in some cases may have created a dependent community of the ill and disabled—returning to community practice may be a reawakening or at least a reminder of the power of the human spirit to forge ahead and to be independent. We can inspire our *communities* through skill building and coaching via occupation. We can recognize the intricacy involved in the simplicity of meaning and help our clients to achieve it. We can guide those who embrace wellness and autonomy in achieving that status regardless of the presence of illness or differing abilities. We can advocate for a strong and optimistic future for our clients and for our profession. We can create and build positive communities as well as contribute to existing ones.

For the occupational therapy practitioner of one, five, or twenty-five years, the world of practice may have been enlightening, satisfying, disappointing, or all of these things, but it has seldom been without challenge. Practice today and in the future represents yet another challenge—or better, an opportunity. It represents a crossroads where we have many potential choices to make. We can learn the language of managed care, and we can hone our administrative, managerial, and political skills to become leaders as we advocate for ourselves as practitioners and for our patients/clients as consumers within that more traditional environment. Although the path of managed care may be uncertain, some of us will and should choose that arena for the "good fight."

For others, though, who may not see their future taking the direction of managed care, the path to alternative or community-based practice is by no means any easier, although it can offer immeasurable personal rewards. Beyond the entry-level skills that must be exceptional to practice in the community, the practitioner must have creativity, ingenuity, and resourcefulness. In addition, he or she must have the accompanying commitment to the rights of everyone to have the opportunity, knowledge, and skills to lead a self-assessed and productive life with dignity and quality.

There has never been a time when our return to community as our context for practice is more appropriate or more needed. And for the student, it is a place to begin. As Margaret Mead has said:

> Never doubt that a small group of thoughtful committed citizens can change the world. Indeed it's the only thing that ever has.
>
> Lecture, University of Wisconsin-Milwaukee (1973)

When I first heard these words during graduate school, they inspired me. Although I had "given up" on occupational therapy for a time, her words encouraged me to return—and to return with a vengeance. I knew that occupational therapy could change the world, even if for only one patient. Later I discovered that neither occupational therapy nor one patient could change the world. In fact, it was *occupation* and the impact of *occupation-centered interventions* within the context of *community* that held this power to bring about change.

I have shared this belief with students for some time and have, with their help, devised ways to bridge their admission into community practice. It is time to write it down and to describe how to get started. It is my expectation that this book will guide you in the process of developing occupation-centered community programming. It will help you begin. The spirit and energy that is required to create change is up to you.

I am reminded of a story told by the potter Paul Soldner as he demonstrated his techniques during a student workshop in Colorado during the 1960s. As a student he had observed a photo of a clay pot in an artist's journal. He was enamored with the form and the stature of the pot and tried for years to raise a similar example from his potter's wheel. Finally successful, he raised the pot of his dreams, just like the photo, to a striking four feet in height. It was some time before he discovered that the pot in the photo, his dream for years, was only four inches high. This is what I would like you to do with my community programming examples— take them from four inches to four feet!

The glue that holds the world together is community—in place, in spirit, and in meaning. This new millennium is the time for us as occupation-centered practitioners to again return to the community.

Linda S. Fazio

Acknowledgments

The programming described in this text represents the ideas and work of many over a number of years. Most of the examples do not exist as they are described but, in fact, have been collapsed and redesigned into "best practice" scenarios. Not all of them have been tried, and some of the ones that have did not always happen in the way they are presented; you are benefitting from the experiences of many. Nothing happens just right the first time and sometimes not even the second or third times.

Although they have been modified, many of the programming examples were very much influenced by the work of colleagues and students. I have been privileged to enjoy the company of students for most of my professional life. My students have been instrumental in teaching me that the world is not flat; perhaps it cannot even be described in any terms with which we have become comfortable because the world changes with our perceptions. To most students, occupational therapy is a very small window on reality based on a few observations that are most likely made in the hospital or institutional setting. To others, occupational therapy is a fairly unknown commodity and is little more than a blank canvas of opportunity upon which one is preparing to paint a future. I am always amazed by the creativity of students and their hard work and most of all by their untiring "goodness" and trust in the buoyancy of the human spirit. If practice is changed, they will be the ones to do it.

I would like to thank all of my colleagues, first at Texas Woman's University and now at the University of Southern California and Mount St. Mary's College. They have contributed to my thoughts and ideas, some reflected in this book and some not.

I specifically would like to thank Carolyn Snyder, Renee Soderlund, and Deborah Pitts, my colleagues in the Department of Occupational Science and Occupational Therapy at the University of Southern California, for their contributions to the success of student involvement in community-centered program design, development, and implementation. Also, through her leadership, Florence A. Clark, Chair of the Department of Occupational Science and Occupational Therapy at the University of Southern California, has created an environment that is rich with ideas and opportunities—an environment that fosters creativity, excitement, and exploration.

I would also like to thank Lynn Whitley, Education Program Coordinator for the Sea Grant Program at the University of Southern California, who so generously shared information and cooperation as we worked together in the development of the Sea Grant/Parent-Child Education Program. In addition, I would like to thank

Dyanne Van Peter, Research and Development Coordinator for the Social Science Research Institute and Project Coordinator of the Parent-Child Education Program, who provided many of the photographs.

I would like to thank the following reviewers for their helpful comments and suggestions: S. Kay Ashworth, Sinclair Community College; Shirley J. Jackson, Howard University; Deane B. McCraith, Boston University; and Judith A. Melvin, Arizona School of Health Sciences.

I most certainly wish to thank my students both at the University of Southern California and at Mount St. Mary's College in Los Angeles. Specifically, I would like to thank the following former students for their ideas and work that are represented in this book: Aileen Agcaoili, Leslie Ann Ambrosius, Allison Anodide, Madeleine Arel-Davis, Amy Beneck, Bridget Brown, Lisa Broze, Yvonne Bueno, Christine Carlson, Della Chaffe, Lauren Cosgrove, Jennifer Cukingnan, Jan Daimaru, Tegan DaRe, Heather Pyle-De Renne, Mary Dockter, Shawn Donovan, Hilary Dorinson, Jennifer Doyle, Holly Eck, Julie Faldmo, Lisa Feldman, Sharon Fritz, April Furlong, Ilene Fuson, Dina Gagliano, Denise Goddeyne, Mary Graddon, Karen Green, Melissa Gutierrez, April Haller, Mark Harrison, Angelina Herridge, Junie Hong, Joanie Hooper, Lindsay Hughes, Theodore Johnson, Kazumi Kasuya, Harpreet Khandpur, Lydia Kim, Kelly Koelbel, John Kriege, Teri Ladwig, Kelly Lenti, Tricia Lo, Maria Lopez, Diana Martin, Tracey Martin, Yoko Masuda, Laura Matsumoto, Carol McAlister, Patricia Harmon-Mills, Marsha Mitchell, Amy Muhlenpoh-Armstrong, Stacy Neill, Brigette Nisly, Suzanna Oses, Amy Peacock-McClennan, Terry Peralta, Shawn Phipps, Michelle Plasch, Shellie Reeder, Jennifer Reimer, Sheila Ruiz, Deborah Ryan, Nora Serelis-Garunketis, Rekha Shastry, Randy Siegel, Carrie Spalding, Stephanie Staley, Elly Steese, Teresa Sullivan, Kristin Sutliff, Maria Tan, George Toth-Fejel, Joelle Tran, Sarah Turner, Dyanne Van Peter, Jacy Ver Maas-Lee, Audra Wagner, Ava Wang, Karen Wong, Marcia Wang, Tina Wong, Leslie Wooten, Erin Wyman, and Jeannie Yee.

Linda S. Fazio

Introduction

In the practice environment of "the community," we are no longer limited to the traditional definitions of occupational therapy but are invited, as occupational therapy practitioners, to expand our thinking to *occupation-centered interventions*. We must educate ourselves and our students to understand *occupation* and occupation as it is practiced in the *community*. We must come to know other professionals, organizations, and agencies who work in tandem to support the meanings and functions associated with community; alongside them, we must offer our unique occupation-centered perspective.

In the community we can provide remediation, prevention, and maintenance. Payment structures are reimbursing for all of these practice arenas; whether or not they will reimburse occupational therapy practitioners for these services, however, will be up to us. We must work to develop our thinking regarding occupation as the foundation for intervention and to insist that all of our practices reflect occupation-centered approaches. Only in this way will we have a unique service to offer the consumer. To remain viable, these occupation-centered interventions must be effective, efficient, and offered at a reasonable cost.

Of course, the opportunity to develop programming in the community while still a student and then to extend one's experience through service-learning in that same environment is what this text is about. If one wishes to initiate a community-based program without either of these "bridges," then the task is more formidable but certainly not impossible. It is the way many of us have initiated such an experience, and this text should help one avoid some of the potential frustrations. There are ways to create "bridges," including finding a mentor and/or selecting an advisory group to assist in the development and programming process, and these will be discussed in the text.

For students this may be one of the most meaningful and relevant projects in which they will have the opportunity to engage, and for practicing therapists it may be the portal to one of the most satisfying adventures of their professional life.

How to Use This Workbook

FOR THE PRACTICING PROFESSIONAL

If you are an occupational therapist or an occupational therapy assistant who has decided to explore the possibilities and potential of practice, I commend you. By making this decision, you already are halfway there. You are a bit of a risk taker and certainly a leader.

Perhaps the decision was not entirely your own. Your supervisor may have decided to branch out from a more conventional practice in an attempt to stay afloat in the managed care environment. Your supervisor or your patients, clients, or their caregivers may have asked you for a new program. Perhaps your significant other is planning to take up residence in a location where there appears to be little opportunity for occupational therapy practice. Or maybe you are just tired of what your practice experience has become or is becoming, and you need a new challenge.

Whatever the reason, I am glad you bought this book, and I hope it will give you the information you are seeking. Certainly it does not provide all of the answers, for every situation is different, but the challenge is what you are looking for, right? This book will help make the challenge less overwhelming. You should start the workbook at the beginning and complete all of the exercises, while tailoring them to the program you are considering. Even if the populations described in the Part III programming examples are nothing like what you are contemplating, you may wish to read them anyway. There may be an idea waiting for your discovery.

FOR THE INSTRUCTOR AND THE STUDENT

Although appropriate for the experienced occupational therapy practitioner, information and exercises provided in this book are intended for use in the classroom to assist instructors and students in the process of learning how to develop occupation-centered community programs. The content can stand alone as a course in program development or as an interactive experience attached to administrative lecture content. Depending on the structure of your curriculum and your community, you may wish to expand some of the exercises with additions of your own. You can also minimize or adapt others to be compatible with what your students have learned or are learning in other courses.

I would recommend the following two directives for students who wish to engage in the learning experience:

1. Completion of the step-by-step *process* as outlined in this text, which results in a design for a community program

2. Drafting a *proposal* to market the program to consumers and/or funding sources

THE RECOMMENDED PROCESS
What You Will Do in the Classroom
1. Selection of a Working Group

Developing even a "mock" program is too much work for one student to accomplish in the course of a quarter or a semester. But even if this were possible, working in a small group is a learning experience by itself and most appropriate to the content and exercises described in the chapters to follow. Although an instructor should be available to mentor students through the process, students should be allowed to self-select groups so that the responsibility of managing emerging dynamics as tasks are delegated is their own. Groups of five or six are able to accomplish the task without overwhelming individual members.

2. Selection of a Site/Population

Of course, the selection of a site and population is a bit different when structured for the classroom as opposed to the therapist who has a site and population in mind. However, it is most useful to work with actual situations rather than mythical ones. Instructors may wish to develop a system whereby clinical fieldwork educators are invited to provide ideas for new programs that they might wish to develop (but nothing too prescriptive). The students will require some structure but also flexibility in order to develop their own ideas. In the Department of Occupational Science and Occupational Therapy at the University of Southern California, we have developed and have continued to provide programming for sites in our University community for our service-learning courses, Level 1 fieldworks, and our faculty practice. With several years of "history" in our surrounding communities, we receive many requests for programs by word of mouth from local Boys and Girls Clubs, after-school programs, City Parks and Recreation Departments, Churches, YMCAs and YWCAs, shelters, and numerous crime-prevention and delinquency-prevention programs around the city. Alumni also provide ideas for programming.

When agencies or therapists offer suggestions for community programs, there is an expectation that they be willing to meet with the student group on-site to provide assistance in the students' process of (1) obtaining and understanding the mission and philosophy of the institution/agency, (2) assessing the need for services, (3) developing a profile of the service community, and (4) providing any other information that must come directly from the site. For their contributions they are invited to the presentation of the proposals and in some cases are given copies of the proposal. In addition, through service learning and independent study courses, the programs may be implemented by and receive continuing development from students. Service learning and independent study are defined as follows:

Service learning is defined as those experiences where the student's academic learning process is enhanced by providing necessary and needed services to individuals and/or groups in the University community.

Independent study requires a contractual agreement between student and faculty member that is structured around goals and objectives for an individualized and creative learning experience.

In the classroom the student groups are provided with a list of potential sites and a brief description of the populations served by those sites. Through group interest and consensus, a site/population is selected for program development.

3. Generate Ideas for Potential Programs (Chapter 5)

We can describe the generation of "ideas" in this context as simple and unrestricted brainstorming. Students should think about what they could do if they did not have the restrictions of finances, space, and skills. Of course, compromises must be made in the continued process of planning, but if thinking is too limited at the outset, students will come away from the process with very little of their original plan. The process of brainstorming generates energy, enthusiasm, creativity, and commitment to an ideal. Students are often much better at this than the experienced therapist who can be too restricted by *what won't work, what's just too expensive,* and perceived boundaries such as *what can't be done* and a too narrow or limited view of occupational therapy. Generating ideas for community programs is empowering and is great fun.

4. Visit the Community and the Site and Begin the Process of Assessing the Need for Occupation-Centered Programs (Chapter 6)

Opportunity to meet with the site manager, coordinator, or director is critical at this early stage of planning. Prior to this meeting, the students must generate a list of questions to be asked, which will constitute the Phase I assessment of need and will structure the Phase II assessment of need that will occur later. The initial questions will include the following:

1. What is the mission and the philosophy of the facility or the agency?
2. What population does the facility/agency serve?
3. What programs currently exist, and what are the manager's perspectives on needed programming?
4. What specific portion of the population would require the suggested program? This is the population that the students will "target."
5. What are the manager's suggestions for the most meaningful and efficient methods the students might use to assess the specific needs from the targeted population?

6. Any other questions the students might think of to facilitate the early planning process.

The answers to these questions will be used to structure continued group discussion, "brainstorming" of potential ideas for programs, and a list of questions/concerns where additional information will be needed to continue the process.

5. Develop the Community Profile, the Service Profile, and Trends Analysis (Chapter 6 and Chapter 3)

Based on the responses to the questions asked on-site and the information provided through the mission and philosophy statements and perhaps through program brochures or annual reports, the students can complete a brief profile (description) of the facility/agency and the community in which it is located. In addition, a profile is developed of the targeted population for which services will be provided. Expanded research into the community where the program will be offered coupled with a brief analysis of trends that may impact the demographics of the community and the population served and a discussion of how best to respond to these trends will further strengthen the developing plan.

6. Research the Target Population and Develop Phase II of the Needs Assessment (Chapter 6)

Further research will likely be required to enhance the information already received concerning the targeted population. This will help to prepare a solid, occupation-centered foundation from which to fully develop the design of the program. In this stage, students refer to their textbooks and other resources to learn as much as they can about the targeted population. This information along with the information received in the on-site visit (Phase I assessment of need) will structure the development of a Phase II needs assessment of the population that will be receiving services. In some cases this second assessment of need may be directed to the potential clients/patients, to the parents/caregivers, or sometimes to other professionals. At each stage of the process, the students revisit their original ideas for programming to determine fit with the additional information.

7. Develop Program Goals and Objectives (Chapter 7)

All of the work accomplished thus far is now beginning to come together. The Phase I and Phase II needs assessments have provided the information necessary to develop specific goals for the program, and measurable objectives are drafted for each program goal. The ability to measure the objectives will be revisited in the evaluation of program effectiveness.

8. Develop the Scope of the Program (Chapter 7)

Working from the goals and objectives and the frame of reference, the program is developed fully to include specific patients/clients/members, range of services to be provided, and volume of services that can/will be provided.

9. Determine Resources Needed to Accomplish the Program Goals and Objectives (Chapters 8, 9, and 10)

Students will now identify the resources needed, which may include staff, space, supplies, and equipment.

10. Determine Costs (Chapter 11)

Based on a review of all of the information collected to this point, the students will determine direct and indirect costs, salaries and benefits, supplies, and equipment. A table of start-up, one-year costs, and three-year costs will be developed.

11. Revenue Projections and Identification of Potential Funding Sources (Chapter 11)

The students will now determine if the proposed program will be for-profit, not-for-profit, or perhaps designed for service learning. Costs will be compared to revenue required, and (depending on the structure of the program) funding sources will be identified and considered. If monies must be obtained to start the program, then potential granting/funding agencies would be identified along with their time lines and protocols for obtaining funds.

12. Evaluating Effectiveness (Chapter 12)

An evaluation plan must be developed from the goals and objectives that have been established for the program. The evaluation plan may include formative and summative measures. Individual patient/client/member plans may be evaluated and can contribute to the evaluation process, but the purpose here is to evaluate the outcomes of the program.

13. Develop Marketing Strategies and a Time Line (Chapters 13 and 14)

Strategies will be developed for the best ways to let the community, including other professionals and the targeted population, know about the program. A start-up time line will include events such as when and how staff will be identified and hired, building renovations or new construction, inspections or accreditations that may be necessary, acquisition of funding, development of policies and procedures, ordering and arrival of supplies and equipment, and how and when the program will be marketed and promoted.

Also included on the time line will be periodic evaluation of the program (if funding is obtained from a gift/granting agency, then the agency's time lines for reporting and reapplication will be included as well).

THE PROPOSAL
What You Will Write

The proposal is the actual document gleaned from the above process. It is the initial marketing/business plan. It is short and to the point and is designed to "sell" the organization or funding agency on the programming idea. Students present the proposal in a 10- to 15-minute time frame, aided by whatever visuals they wish. The agency representatives are invited to the presentations, and the atmosphere is professional and efficient but not withholding enthusiasm. In some cases the student presentations are given at the facility rather than on the campus, and in some cases the presentations are given at both sites.

For the professional, the presentation will almost always be conducted at the site/facility, sometimes before the administration of the facility, the administration and staff, or a board of directors. If independent funding is being sought, then the proposal might be presented to that group as well.

The following outline is used to summarize the information in the body of the proposal. If substantial information has been collected through the needs assessment, if numerous granting resources have been identified, if an elaborate evaluation plan has been designed, or if any other information is obtained that is potentially useful in convincing the agency of the program planners' expertise and thoroughness, then it is placed in the appendices.

1. Statement(s) summarizing the mission and philosophy of the sponsoring institution/agency, the community profile, and the trends analysis
2. Summary statements to describe the client population, the service profile, the findings of the needs assessment(s), goals and objectives for the program, the frame of reference and rationale to support the services to be provided and a description of the services
3. Financial/economic considerations to include:
   (a) Projections of expenses
   (b) Proposed start-up costs
   (c) Identification of amount of funds needed to support the program
   (d) First-year operating budget
   (e) Anticipated fluctuations in first three budget years
      If the plan includes seeking funding for start-up, then potential funding sources would be provided. If the program will be marketed to the consumer, then a plan for how this will be done is included.
4. The evaluation plan (how and when it will be conducted and how it will be used)
5. The time line
6. Appendices that include any materials from your process that you believe will strengthen the proposal (such as your actual needs assessment, your program-evaluation process, your marketing plan/materials, and so on)

Again, the proposal constitutes the business plan that is usually presented to the site or agency. It is targeted, fairly brief (body of five to six pages), has a cover page and table of contents (including appendices), and is paginated. The "in-person" short presentation may be made to one individual or to several people. The verbal presentation may utilize over-head transparencies, slides, or computer-assisted materials. It should always be professional (no skits, songs, or dances) and is followed by receipt of the written proposal.

The presentation should generate enthusiasm and incentive for the recipient individual or group to read the lengthier written proposal that is submitted following the verbal presentation. The planner(s) must "believe" in the proposal and, further, must support this belief by evidence of hard, detailed, accurate work. The proposal should be neat and completely free from distracting spelling, grammar, or information errors.

You now have the outline, so let's begin.

CHAPTER

Defining Community

Learning Objectives

1. To appreciate the many definitions and meanings associated with *community*
2. To understand the distinction between *community* and *the community*
3. To understand *community* as an organizing theme in our development of occupation-centered programs

Key Terms

1. Community
2. Locale

As we begin a new century, it would appear that the pendulum of patient/client care is again swinging away from the institution to the community. This is true not only for occupational therapy but also for many health care providers. Just as mental health and illness and the concerns of humane care established our origins as occupational therapists, these same concerns have ushered our return to the community as a favored site for practice—and we are not alone. In recent years those traditional disciplines providing psychiatric services have begun to embrace the community as a desired and necessary context for intervention. It is difficult to know whether this move into the community was in response to the sweeping socioeconomic pressures and resulting deinstitutionalization or whether it was selected as the best mode of care. Oseroff, Longo, and Joseph (1998) suggest that these choices to establish practices in the community were proactive, not reactive. According to these authors, the system reform that has taken place over the last decade in psychiatric service delivery has challenged institutional models to suggest that the natural setting may be the most effective arena for service delivery. They are particularly supportive of natural treatment environments for children and young adults. This view has been echoed most recently by many pediatric practitioners, including occupational therapists, who suggest that the environment of family, the home, and the school are the most conducive environments to affecting change in the child (Agrin, 1987; England, 1992; Hanft, Burke, Cahil, Swenson-Miller, & Humphry, 1992; Henggeler, 1996; Hyde and Woodworth, 1994; Nelson & Landsman, 1992; Noonan & McCormick, 1993; Schaaf & Mulrooney, 1989; Schultz, 1992). This renewed attention to context in establishing the parameters for the most successful interventions for all ages has returned us to the community. If we are to use this context of community within which to place our programs, then we must understand its intricacies and variability.

Just what is this phenomenon that we are so liberally describing as community? Webster defines community as the "state of being held in common; . . . life in association with others; . . . a number of individuals associated together by the fact of residence in the same locality; . . . a number of persons having common ties or interests" (1975, p. 204). Community, then, can be an associated group of persons, a family, a group of colleagues, and neighbors who reside in a *neighborhood*. Sometimes we hear people refer to *community spirit*, meaning a shared feeling of optimism and hope; this can be experienced, for example, by a group setting out to clean up graffiti or by a group wishing the team to victory. In fact, community can exist within an institutional care setting and is often encouraged, particularly for those who will spend their lives in that setting. Community, then, can be affixed to a place (locale) in combination with a spirit of sharing, membership, and commitment, or it can simply *be* a spirit of sharing, membership, and commitment.

COMMUNITY AS A PAST AND PRESENT FOCUS FOR RESEARCH AND INVESTIGATION

Community with its accompanying definitions and scope of investigation has long been a central theme in the study of sociology. When we review the sociological literature, we find that this discipline has established a number of definitions for the term. Lyon (1987, p. 5) noted some ninety-four in the sociological literature of 1955. Although there were many definitions noted in his review of the literature at the time, he was able to establish three common characteristics: locale, common ties, and social interactions. Other sociological researchers, including Park (1936) and Bernard (1973), concur with these common characteristics. In general, though, the use of locale as a central definition for community has been widely accepted across disciplines.

Anthropologists have also long shared an interest in *community*, particularly as defined by **locale.** Although Hillery (1955) supports the view that locale is a central characteristic of community, he proposed that groups of people differing in place and time may also differ in their interpretations of meaning surrounding locale. In his examples, which are based on modes of subsistence, agricultural peoples attach a fixed settlement to their meaning of locale, while hunters/gatherers who subsist by traveling over large geographic areas define locale as a less identifiable place.

It is likely that even hunters and gatherers along with nomadic groups who also travel over wide areas designate locales and attach some significance to them (that is, sources of water, ceremonial/burial sites, and so on). These locales may be designated sites where nomadic bands or groups join together to form communities, albeit a looser definition of community than that of an agricultural group. Those who have studied the transitions from hunter/gatherer to agriculturist have noted that when groups begin to first tend plants and then grow them, they become locked to a site, or locale (Childe, 1953; Heiser, 1973). Perhaps these groups then become locked to a community as well.

Also discussing community from an anthropological perspective, Moore (1996) reminds us that in biology, community refers to a breeding population. His discussions center around bands as the elemental human communities of hunters and gatherers (p. 105). As biological creatures humans also have breeding-population communities. But community means a good deal more to humans than a group with which one may breed. According to Moore, community is "the unit that orchestrates individual movements in space over time," and in our cultural world, "community is the setting in which, from one generation to the next, human beings learn how to be fully human" (p. 96). In fact, the unit is also where cultural creativity and innovation take place.

WHAT DOES COMMUNITY MEAN TODAY?

The previous discussions may shed light on our understanding of the present-day metropolitan and urban communities in which we will want to establish programs. Many people today frequently relocate during their lives; most reside far from their communities (locales) of origin. It is likely that more transient attachments may be formed for those who move from one locale to another in pursuit of career and economic opportunity, and a sense of *community* with accompanying commitments and responsibilities may be more tenuous. Of course, any privileges or rights attached to *community* might also be forfeited—at least those that are offered following a period of investment, or tenure. This view of community would appear to place more responsibility for the attributes of community as described by Moore (1996) on the family and/or the individual. Do these individuals and families have the information and skills to establish communities for themselves? Metropolitan communities where many cultures come together may also redefine our interpretations of community; will these communities provide stress and disengagement, or will they offer us new definitions of cultural creativity and innovation? Will we evolve new ways of learning to be "human"? If so, will occupation-centered practitioners have a role in facilitating this new learning? How will we identify what kinds of services a community might need, want, and value? It is likely that desired services may vary considerably from one locale to another and from one constituency to another. Cognizant of this potential dilemma, Warren (1987) has proposed that we must understand and appreciate that *community*, particularly the urban community, represents a "local web of relationships around the locality-relevant functions" (p. ii). In his interpretation, various formal and informal networks within a community are connected to others outside the locality. When one seeks to establish a program in and/or for a community, it will be necessary to appreciate and understand what likely will be an intricate and complex series of relationships "between" communities. Even if we may be planning a program that appears fairly isolated in locale or in conceptualization, we must consider extended and overlapping communities and systems, particularly in the present era of heightened communication and access to information. Parsons (1951) would remind us that even *within* a community there may be substantial complexity displayed by the interplay between cultures and the varied levels of society. In fact, by establishing a program within a community, we are introducing yet another layer of complexity that may cause temporary shifts in balance. These potential shifts can be tempered by establishing the program in developmental increments, as we will describe in Part II.

The foregoing is important information as we are designing relevant and meaningful programs for our service populations. And what can we learn about the community itself? Is the community one that appears well established? Or is it one that is in process? What is the nature of common ties, and what are the patterns of social interaction? Are children part of the community of families? In fact, do we know how the presence of children impacts on *community*? Are the interactions, communications, and expectations influenced by the presence of children? By the presence of elders? These are provocative questions to be investigated, and they may influence and impact our understanding of so-called specialized communities: older adults; young, childless adults; and institutions serving specific populations.

Hillery (1955) makes a distinction between *community* and *the community*. His distinction separates the idea of common ties and social interactions from locale. In his view, *community* is the most powerful of the two concepts, emphasizing moral commitment, social cohesion, and continuity in time, or what might be described by the German term *Gemeinschaft*. In fact, a community may be represented by no fixed locale at all, and yet the presence of a strong sense of unity may still be apparent (Nisbet, 1967). This may be a significant point of understanding in what we have described as the transient world of today.

Nisbet's interpretation of community may help us understand such questions as how and why retirees who move from their long-established homes to high-rise senior residences can either feel that they are part of a community, or feel that they are not. And his interpretation can further help us, as care providers, encourage the building of community for those who feel excluded.

Shifting paradigms responsive to the fluidity of attachment to locale by present-day populations heavily invested in technology may, in fact, define a new, more global sense of community. Does the *information highway* take us *home*? Does it establish the boundaries of community in a way that we find comforting and satisfying? Or does this global thinking and loss of attachment to locale prompt individuals today, more than ever before, to lust more for the real and assumed benefits of *community*. Nisbet (1953, 1967) suggested this to be the case decades ago. Perhaps we are simply redefining and reframing locale to be without boundaries (and restraints), and perhaps we are placing our emphasis on other aspects of community that we deem to be more significant.

Community may also be conceptualized in a way that negates both locale and emotional investment; this refers to those communities defined by common interests, intellectual bonds, and/or professional bonds (Goode, 1957; Nisbet, 1953). The *community* of occupational therapists, the medical community, and the community of women/men are all examples.

COMMUNITY AND OCCUPATION-CENTERED PRACTICE

With the words *community* and *occupation-centered practice*, we bring together the elements of a theme that will organize our return to the community in the new millennium. Certainly occupational therapy practitioners have been in the community before (perhaps always), but this time *occupation* will be at the center of our practices. Centering our practice in occupation frees us to utilize our knowledge and skills in many new, creative, and marketable venues. By locating our programs in the community defined by locale or spirit, we are accepting the challenge of responding to that community's need with what must be new and innovative *ways of being*. Yearly vast populations are excluded from access to health care; therefore, it is imperative that we do more than ever before to help prevent illness and trauma and that we provide information, access, skills, and caring to "even out the odds" and to empower those who are at risk for becoming new members of the disenfranchised.

Spurred by a desire to extend democracy beyond what she described as its political expression and sensitive to a strong need to extend humanitarian values and concerns, Jane Addams (1893/1990) was dedicated to the community represented by the evolving Chicago location of Hull House. Her commitment and resulting work, which was followed by Julia Lathrop and Eleanor Clark Slagle (1922, 1933), established our legacy by placing occupation strongly at the center of community. Their combined philosophies and commitment to the community they served provide the cognitive and emotional map that will guide us as we reestablish our presence in service to our communities.

REFERENCES

Addams, J. (1990). The subjective necessity for social settlements. In *Twenty years at hull house*. Urbana: University of Illinois Press. (Original work published 1893)

Agrin, A. (1987). Occupational therapy with emotionally disturbed children in a public elementary school. *Occupational Therapy in Mental Health, 7*, 105–113.

Bernard, J. (1973). *The sociology of community*. Glenview, IL: Scott Foresman.

Childe, V. G. (1953). *New light on the most ancient East*. New York: W. W. Norton.

England, M. J. (1992). Building systems of care for youth with mental illness. *Hospital and Community Psychiatry, 43,* 630–633.

Goode, W. J. (1957, April). Community within a community: The professions. *American Sociological Review, 22,* 194–200.

Hanft, B., Burke, J. P., Cahill, M., Swenson-Miller, K., & Humphry, R. (1992). *Working with families: A curriculum guide for pediatric occupational therapists*. Chapel Hill, NC: Frank Porter Graham Child Development Center.

Heiser, C. (1973). *Seed to civilization*. San Francisco: W. H. Freeman.

Henggeler, S. W. (1996). Eliminating (almost) treatment dropout of substance abusing or dependent delinquents through home-based multisystemic therapy. *American Journal of Psychiatry, 153*(3), 427–428.

Hillery, G. (1955). Definitions of community: Areas of agreement. *Rural Sociology, 20,* 194–204.

Hyde, K., & Woodworth, K. (1994). Reforming services to children and families. *The Family Preservation Initiative of Baltimore City, Inc., FY 1994 annual report*. Baltimore: Family Preservation Initiative.

International Webster New Encyclopedic Dictionary of the English Language. (1975). Chicago: The English Language Institute of America.

Lyon, L. (1987). *The community in urban society*. Chicago: The Dorsey Press.

Moore, A. (1996). The band community: Synchronizing human activity cycles for group cooperation. In R. Zemke & F. Clark (Eds.), *Occupational science: The evolving discipline* (pp. 95–106). Philadelphia: F. A. Davis.

Nelson, K. E., & Landsman, M. J. (1992). *Alternative models of family preservation: Family-based services in context*. Springfield, IL: Charles C. Thomas.

Nisbet, R. (1953). *The quest for community*. New York: Oxford University Press.

Nisbet, R. (1967). *The sociological tradition*. New York: Basic Books.

Noonan, M. J., & McCormick, L. (1993). *Early intervention in natural environments: Methods and procedures*. Pacific Grove, CA: Brooks/Cole.

Oseroff, C., Longo, M., & Joseph, I. (1998). Finding our way home: Home- and community-based care. In H. Ghuman & R. Sarles (Eds.), *Handbook of child and adolescent outpatient, day treatment and community psychiatry* (pp. 359–368). Philadelphia: Brunner/Mazel.

Park, R. (1936). Human ecology. *American Journal of Sociology, 17*(1), 1–15.

Parsons, T. (1951). *The social system*. Glencoe, IL: Free Press.

Schaaf, R. C., & Mulrooney, L. (1989). Occupational therapy in early intervention: A family-centered approach. *American Journal of Occupational Therapy, 43,* 745–754.

Schultz, S. (1992). School based occupational therapy for students with behavior disorders. *Occupational Therapy in Health Care, 8,* 173–196.

Slagle, E. C. (1922). Training aides for mental patients. *Papers on Occupational Therapy*. Utica, NY: State Hospital Press.

Slagle, E. C., and Robeson, H. A. (1933). Syllabus for training of nurses in occupational therapy. Utica, NY: State Hospital Press.

Warren, R. (1987). Foreword. In L. Lyon, *The community in urban society*. Chicago: The Dorsey Press.

Occupation: A History

Learning Objectives

1. To explore the development of *occupation* as a unifying concept for occupational therapy practice
2. To identify elements of occupation appropriate for guiding community practice
3. To understand the practice environment of community as a system
4. To appreciate the diversity of occupation-centered practice available in the context of community.

Key Terms

1. Occupation
2. Moral Treatment
3. Purposeful Activity
4. Systems Model

The second key concept that accompanies *community* in helping us to define the theme for this text is **occupation.** When discussing occupation from her perspective as a craftswoman, Erickson (1976) noted the shift in thinking from occupation/work to occupation/activity as the beginning of what would become the developing ideas to support the discipline of *occupational therapy*. She saw this perspective taking shape as it was expressed in the first courses to train nurses and aides in the practice of "occupation" at the Chicago School of Civics and Philanthropy in 1908. Erikson's interests centered around the role of planned activities in the development of institutional communities. She was particularly interested in the shift to occupation as therapy for the patient as opposed to keeping a patient occupied with work for the support and management of the institution. However, long before the shift from occupation as work to occupation as activity described by Erickson became apparent, there were forces already at work to establish the premise from which this shift would later occur.

BELIEF IN OCCUPATION AND THE DEVELOPMENT OF A PROFESSION

What would be described as **moral treatment** sheltered the seeds of an idea that stemmed from the view that the disordered thinking of the "insane" was, in fact, in response to the disordered society of which these so-called insane people were a part. Institutional care was developed as a respite that would not only protect the insane with care that was supported by moral beliefs but would also create a positive environment that would exact a cure for this state of disordered thinking (and, for the individual patient, would return order to chaos).

As this introduction would indicate, the roots of occupational therapy and many other caregiving disciplines are strongly interconnected with the evolving history of mental illness, including the causes of such a state favored at the time and how to mediate those perceived causes. Until the biophysical model became the one favored by medical practitioners, it was virtually impossible to consider the causes of mental illness outside the context of the community. In the first communities, those who were perceived to be mentally ill were placed in strategic roles (such as shaman, healer, and medicine man) to enhance and strengthen the group or community by establishing an acceptable order for behavior and ritual. Moore (1992) referred to these persons as shamans, and perhaps some could be called prophets. According to Moore, both prophets and shamans may have been "once-troubled individuals" who found their own restorative myths and rituals and then became curers of others (p. 316). These practices have continued into fairly recent times for tribal-band peoples. It can be supported that the early witch trials of the Puritans may also have been ways to deal with those persons perceived to be mentally ill in an effort to protect, strengthen, and bring order to the community. By the 18th century, there were new factors threatening the structure and function of established communities. The demands of a restless society that was growing in numbers, in beliefs, and in ideas certainly posed a threat. Cultures and ethnicities were colliding, particularly in the new "America." Communities were forming and reforming daily in response to new and potential threats that would either destroy them or strengthen them. With family members seeking new beginnings, the European communities certainly were feeling the brunt of this new social mobility. For whatever reasons, clearly there were those who were unequipped to deal with the demands of such a social climate. Assuredly it was first the family's responsibility to care for these victims of chaos, who became known in thoughtful circles as the insane. But the family was a part of the larger community, and the limits of order were likely first ascribed by this community; the demands on family were perhaps too great. The insane were often locked away—also a way to encourage order and to ensure a continuing place for the family within the community. But is it fair, right, or honorable, to lock a family member away or even to send a family member to an institution to be chained? Is this morality? There were those who said no. Probably many did, but the history of occupational therapy remembers only a few, including Phillippe Pinel, William Tuke, Thomas Fowler, and Benjamin Rush (Bing, 1981, 1993; Bockoven, 1971, 1972). Greatly influenced by the moral principles of the Quakers both in England and the United States, the families of the insane were provided with an option. The early 19th century brought a wave of social justice that would not only provide care for the insane but would rehabilitate them as well. The respite—the asylum—would provide order, daily routine, and consistency, often in pastoral environments (Rothman, 1971). Perhaps these isolative asylums were an altruistic gesture to rehabilitate the insane, and perhaps they were also a way to remove them from the evolving communities where they lacked an acceptable role. Regardless of the motives of the physicians and administrators, these asylums served to establish new communities based on order and balance.

Because order is established through a balance of rest and work, constructive work became central to this new community of those who were insane. Erikson (1976) recounts an 1840 quote from Luther Bell of the McLean Hospital in Boston: "Systematic, regular employment in useful body labor . . . is one appliance of moral treatment, which has proved immeasurably superior to all others" (p. 16). Certainly the Puritan and Calvinist ethics offered strong support for this belief in the goodness of "work." As evidenced by the way both children and adults define themselves by their work-related occupations, this legacy is with us today.

Near the end of the 1800s, the asylum communities were far less than their earliest conceptions had hoped for (Peloquin, 1989). They, too, had become extensions of the existing society—they were disordered. In many ways, the ideal community had proved an unreliable experiment. However, times were changing. Medicine was approaching the belief that mental illness was not a reaction to social chaos but was rather physiological in nature. Diagnosis and professional caregivers who were trained specifically for the care of the mentally ill became important. Exploitative work in mental institutions was to be abolished.

Perhaps this is where we, as occupational therapists, came in and *occupation* as we have come to know it was conceived; this is not occupation as work but what became known as the *creative occupation* (Erikson, 1976, p. 18). As mentioned earlier, it was in 1908 at the Chicago School of Civics and Philanthropy that this new creative occupation became the grist of a curriculum; courses were developed in handicraft, exercise, and recreation, and those who worked with mental patients were trained in these vehicles of therapy (Peloquin, 1989; Tracy, 1910). Eleanor Clarke Slagle became a student of these curative occupations when she attended the course of study provided by Julia Lathrop of Hull House at the Chicago School, and she became a convincing proponent of the normalizing effect of occupations (Peloquin, 1991; Quiroga, 1995). Of course, balance in occupation was recognized as important; while these early proponents of creative, curative, and normalizing occupation also maintained an interest in work and rest, the balance now strongly included the recognition of leisure and play. Arts and crafts were often seen as offering not only a respite from the quickening pace of society, but they were also sometimes viewed as the transition between work and leisure. Many of the early *craft as therapy* programs quickly evolved into workshops where crafts were sold to benefit the continuation of programs. Artists and craftsmen of the times were also defining their roles and entertaining their futures both as individuals and as members of an evolving society (Levine, 1987; Wilcock, 1998). Many of these artists and craftsmen became the early hospital workshop teachers who worked alongside nurses and others. Certainly their ideologies became mixed with the proponents of "occupation." *Occupation* was in the process of maturation, layer by layer, to culminate in an ideology that would create a new society of caregivers.

There is more to this story, of course; the founders of what was to become a profession based on the belief in occupation brought with them an existing belief in one or more of the premises that would support *occupation* therapy. Herbert Hall extended the ideas of occupation beyond mental illness to include the multitude of problems that were threatening the physical and emotional well-being of the turn-of-the-century citizen by combining his foundation in medicine with his belief in the curative effects of arts and crafts (Licht, 1967; Quiroga, 1995). An architect and founder named George Barton was also greatly influenced by the arts and crafts movement; coupling these ideals with his own illness experiences, he became a strong advocate for the rehabilitative effects of occupation. Another of the founders, William R. Dunton, Jr., through his practice experiences as a psychiatrist became a strong proponent of the curative effects of occupation as well (Dunton, 1915, 1918). Because Eleanor Clarke Slagle's belief in the power of occupation and her work in "habit training" set the foundation for her many contributions to the organization of occupational therapy, she is sometimes referred to as "the mother of occupational therapy" (Sabonis-Chafee & Hussey, 1998). Susan Tracy had long been involved in both the arts and crafts movement and in the training of nurses to provide therapeutic occupations for patients. She is recognized as the first author of what was to become *occupational therapy*, as expressed in her 1910 book, *Studies in Invalid Occupations*. One other individual often grouped with the founders in descriptions of occupational therapy history is Adolf Meyer. Meyer (1977) brought yet another element to the mix—a commitment to holism. Meyer believed that the individual was far more than a series of anatomical parts to be studied, that the individual should be engaged in activity, and that the activity must be purposeful. For Meyer, **purposeful activity** promoted health; represented in a balance of work and play and rest and sleep, this became the philosophy of occupational therapy. Although different in many ways, all of these founders had a common commitment to the potential power of occupation in helping to establish an effective rehabilitative process. Though the trust in the curative effects of *occupation* was firmly established by the early 1900s, it would be some time before the growing profession of occupational therapy would again embrace these beliefs as strongly as it had in the founding years.

OCCUPATION: EMERGING AND GAINING STRENGTH

Through the years of the World Wars, the founding philosophies supporting a central, unifying belief in occupation were soundly tested. Of course, we must remember that no profession exists in a vacuum. Professions are established to meet the needs of society, however those needs may be translated. Occupational therapy has maintained the flexibility and adaptive resiliency to do just that and has maintained a viable position in the cadre of health care providers since the founding years. Kielhofner (1992) suggests that occupational therapy first emerged and continues to exist because "it has an implicit social contract to address the problems of those members of society who have limited capacity to perform in their everyday occupations" (p. 3). The years of epidemic illness (tuberculosis and polio) and the injuries resulting from the World Wars served to further establish that skillfully orchestrated therapy through the utilization of occupation could, in fact, influence an individual's ability to again function in and contribute to the world. This belief in occupation continues into the present and is now being utilized by practitioners to not only help individuals regain and maintain function but also to act on their worlds in ways that they find most meaningful and satisfying.

Through the 1900s occupational therapists continued to define and refine occupation as an organizing concept for the profession. As researchers investigated occupation as a unifying concept for organizing knowledge in occupational therapy and as they published their ideas, all occupational therapists were able to again explore the potential of occupation for providing the most effective change for our patients and for unifying our profession. The beliefs of the founders were not lost; they were only sleeping and waiting for the time when they could be further developed and matched to other areas of expanding knowledge in the disciplines of philosophy, sociology, biology, and anthropology. Mary Reilly (1962) united the past with the present when in her 1961 Eleanor Clarke Slagle lecture, she proposed that the original hypothesis of occupational therapy can be stated "that man through the use of his hands, as they are energized by mind and will, can influence the state of his own health" (pp. 1–9). This lecture and the writings to follow elaborated an occupational behavior paradigm of practice that renewed our beliefs in the philosophical principles established by the founders. Following Reilly, others continued to develop the tenets of occupation. Yerxa began to explore the development of a basic science of occupation. Her work and the work of her colleagues built on the foundations of many disciplines, and through that work she has reminded us that humans attach meaning to their occupations through their cultures (Clark, Wood, and Larson, 1998; Yerxa et al., 1990). Others remind us that humans are resourceful in mobilizing occupation to act on their world and to manipulate and transform their world (Engelhardt, 1977; Reilly, 1962; Rogers, 1983). And Hall (1969) establishes for us that in utilizing our occupations, we are responsive to time. In our continued investigations of occupation, we have also developed our knowledge of play, daily living tasks, and work (Kielhofner, 1985, 1995; Reilly, 1974; Shannon, 1970). Kielhofner (1995) has brought all of these ideas together in the definition of human occupation as "doing culturally meaningful work, play or daily living tasks in the stream of time and in the contexts of one's physical and social world" (p. 3).

A definition is useful and helps us to establish the parameters of this thing that we call occupation. Pierce (1999) reminds us that many definitions are a sign of a healthy discipline. Recent occupational therapy literature provides us with a few from which to select. Nelson (1977, 1988) defines occupation based on occupational form and occupational performance, and Gray (1998) defines occupation in response to occupation as ends and as means. Some of the most recent work in elaborating occupation is that of occupational science; the definition of occupation particular to this science is "the daily activities that can be named in the lexicon of the culture and that fill the stream of time" (Clark, Wood, and Larson, 1998; Yerxa et al., 1990). Undoubtedly there will be other definitions forthcoming as we continue to explore and elaborate occupation as the central unifying concept around which we will develop present and future practice.

Regardless of definition, there seems to be little doubt that the belief in occupation as well as the dedication to meaningful activity remains strong. Occupation-centered intervention unites us as practitioners.

PRACTICING OCCUPATION IN THE COMMUNITY

Our earlier discussions elaborated on the connection between society and the individual. Individuals act in and on the society and community of which they are members. Many practitioners today are casting a shadow on the organization of practice as we have come to know it. They suggest that practice will be in the school system, home health agencies, private practices, industry, and in an assortment of "community" facilities (Kielhofner, 1992; Kniepmann, 1997; Wilcock, 1998). Kielhofner (1992) suggests that this potential shift in practice environments will place an even greater pressure on occupational therapy to develop a knowledge base that will serve practitioners well in a variety of practice scenarios. There is no doubt that these present and potential community practice sites will place incredible demands on the practitioner. Autonomous decision making through access to a wide array of resources will be required. This decision making will be in response to the demands and expectations of a client population that may be well prepared to advocate for service needs within a community that not only supports services but may require them as well.

WHAT PRACTICE FRAMES WILL WE CHOOSE TO STRUCTURE OUR USE OF OCCUPATION?

A firm philosophical "seat" in occupation must be a prerequisite to any practice that we are describing as occupation centered. Occupation will provide the perspective for our practices in the community, regardless of their individual characteristics. In entering the community as our practice context, we will likely find ourselves resurrecting old models to fit the community practice environment; perhaps we will redesign some or invent new ones. Certainly we will retain those models that have served us well in other practice settings. We will continue to work with people of all ages; therefore, some of us may choose to integrate, for example, a sensory-integration model or the model of human occupation or other models into our community practices. But practice in the community presents us with a context filled with ambiguity and variability; this arena will likely require the use of more comprehensive, layered structures within which to seat those models we have found appropriate for our individual patients/clients in institutional settings.

Understanding Systems as a Way of Thinking About Community Practice

Most certainly in understanding the community as our context for intervention, we will use a **systems model** to initiate our thinking. *General systems theory (GST)* is the term used to describe the scientific efforts to identify the structural, behavioral, and developmental features of living organisms and how they influence each other (Boulding, 1956; von Bertalanffy, 1968). The use of systems thinking is a way to help us understand things that interact. Gray, Kennedy, and Zemke (1997) suggest to us ways that dynamic systems theory may be applied to occupation, thus blending key components of occupation-centered practice—the components of occupation and the multiplicity of systems that make up community. For our usage in community intervention, we are interested in how the human (an open system) receives and is influenced by information (input), the processing of this information, and the behavioral change that occurs as a result (output). Whether our role is prevention, promotion, or remediation, we are interested in the dynamics of this process within the larger system of environment/community.

If we wish to develop a new way to think about the practice of occupation in the community, then it would likely be from this dynamic systems perspective as a foundation of understanding. We might then adopt or perhaps develop a theory, frame of reference, or paradigm from which to view our practice in the community, that is, a way to think about the community and the relationship of individuals to each other and to the many layers of community. We are not suggesting that this is a simple process. The community is a complex open system with many interrelated levels of function. For our purposes, we would believe that these multiple systems must interrelate in such a way to produce meaningful occupation. As facilitators of this process, we are active participants and add to the complexity of this open system.

Once we have gained an appreciation of the complexity of the system within which we are practicing, we will want to choose a map or maps to best reach our destination. McColl, Gerein, and Valentine (1997) suggest that the occupational therapy practitioner who is able to assess a situation and choose between a number of models is perhaps best able to meet the challenges of practice (p. 526). These authors are speaking from a "response to disability" perspective, and we might assume that it is even more true in the complex "system" presented to us by the community. In the community we must not only respond to the needs of our clients with disability but also to the needs of those who may require prevention, or wellness services. To be eclectic in our choices means that we must have a thorough understanding of all those models or frames from which we may choose to ensure the appropriate and effective delivery of services.

Comprehensive Models for Community Intervention

McColl, Gerein, and Valentine (1997) discuss several models of practice from a disability perspective that we can expand for community use to include multiple roles of prevention, restoration, maintenance of function, and remediation (McColl, 1998). The first model, the client-centered rehabilitation model, is one in which clients engage therapists to help them solve the problems they encounter as they seek to achieve their goals (1997, pp. 511–513). The client is in charge of his or her life and only seeks the therapist's expertise in providing information and guidance. Of course, this is an oversimplification of the process, but it serves to emphasize the importance of a client-driven goal structure. This model recognizes and encourages autonomy and places the therapist in the critical role of facilitator, instructor, advocate, and guide. In the context of community, the therapist will provide the map that will assist the client in traversing his or her way to a meaningful, self-selected place in the community. The therapist helps "clear the way" and also provides the direction and instruction when it is needed. The therapist does not do the work of the client but guides and facilitates the work the client chooses to do.

The second model discussed by McColl, Gerein, and Valentine emphasizes the social origins of issues relating to disability (1997, pp. 513–515). The model defines community as geographical, referring to a particular area or locality, but it also recognizes community to be relational, referring to a group with shared interests and values, mutual obligations, a common history, or some other affinity. We are reminded by Kniepmann (1997) that community is always more than a geographic location for our practices; it also includes an "orientation to collective health, social priorities, and different modes for service provision" (1997, p. 540). For the community-based rehabilitation model the community is first that of persons who are disabled but secondly, persons who are disabled within the context of the larger community.

There are three assumptions associated with the community-based rehabilitation model that are important to our multiple community roles; these include but extend beyond the community of the disabled. The first assumption recognizes that people with disabilities do not exist in isolation; rather, they are an integral part of the larger community that also includes their families, friends, and neighbors. There is an assumed relationship; a "system is in place" that both supports clients in the community who are disabled and may also benefit from their contributions to the larger economic and social environment.

The second and important assumption is that individuals and communities have available to them the resources needed to influence and enhance their own health, and it may be the practitioners' role to assist these individuals and communities in first identifying and then accessing these resources. And the last assumption is that it is not only more possible but also perhaps more important to make small inroads of improvement to the quality of life for all people with disabilities in a community than to select out a few for the highest standard of care (1997, pp. 513–514). Together these assumptions provide us with an orientation for work in the community with all people whether or not they are disabled or at risk for the onset of disabling conditions.

Another model of interest to occupation-centered community-based practice is that of independent living. The origins of the independent-living model developed out of a collective political movement of persons with disabilities (Cole, 1979; DeJong, 1979, 1993; Lysack & Kaufert, 1994; McColl, Gerein, & Valentine, 1997). The politics and advocacy necessary to prevail and to achieve one's goals is central to occupation-centered practice in the community. Regardless of our client population or our clients' goals, we must be cognizant of the politics that influence the dissemination of resources, and we along with our clients must assume the role and responsibility of advocacy.

The Community Practitioner in the Roles of Prevention and Promotion

We have talked about prevention as one of the significant roles of community practice. Kniepmann (1997) discusses the prevention of disability and the maintenance of health from a number of perspectives. It is her contention that as a profession, we must use the knowledge we have to help maintain health—whether it be prevention, health promotion, or building those characteristics we associate with the condition of wellness. In community health today, there are several ways one might work toward prevention. These may be defined as primary, secondary, or tertiary (Kniepmann, 1997, pp. 532–534). A brief review of these potential options will be useful to expand our knowledge of practice in the community.

Primary prevention is directed toward the greater society. Efforts to avoid the onset of pathologies might be accomplished by reducing susceptibility in a number of ways, including minimizing environmental factors that increase risk of disease or injury (Tarlov & Pope, 1991). Spraying wetlands for mosquitoes is one example of primary prevention. Although perhaps not directly involved in efforts toward primary prevention, occupational therapy practitioners in the community are often instigators and promotors of such efforts. For example, they might consult to town planning boards about architectural barriers or suggest prevention and maintenance programs for persons who are mentally ill and homeless.

Tarlov and Pope (1991) describe secondary prevention as efforts to target groups in the community who are thought to be "at risk." This can involve early detection of a potential health problem, followed by appropriate interventions to halt, reverse, or slow down progression. Occupational therapy practitioners are certainly involved in secondary prevention, which can run the gamut from parenting classes for teens to the encouragement of condom use for those at risk for sexually transmitted diseases (STDs). Teaching the well elderly how to access public transportation in an effort to widen their options for accessing meaningful occupation and thus maintaining health would also be considered secondary prevention.

The focus of tertiary prevention is to maximize function and to minimize the detrimental effects of illness or injury (Kniepmann, 1997, pp. 532–533). Although this is an area already very familiar to occupational therapy practitioners, we also want to emphasize efforts toward a focus on function, advocacy for social policy as it can influence one's health and ability to be independent, and the direct intervention concerns of the individual.

Most of the programs we discuss in this text that deal with prevention fall under the category of secondary prevention; however, some of our programming assumes elements of tertiary prevention as well. Associated with prevention but with a different directive, health promotion has been the favored topic of many occupational therapists, including Madill, Townsend, and Schultz (1989) and McComas and Carswell (1994). For occupational therapy practitioners, health promotion or optimization is based in part on our basic belief that a balance of work, rest, self-care, and leisure/play is necessary for optimal health and well-being. Prompted by this belief, occupation is utilized to organize our daily rounds of activity that include this recommended balance. For many of our clients, guidance is needed in first recognizing deficits of balance; this is then followed by the offer of assistance in developing the skills, knowledge, and behaviors needed to engage in those self-selected activities that provide "meaningful" balance.

It is not realistic to think that we can separate prevention of illness or trauma and the promotion of health and wellness; one is implied within the other. By providing those aspects of promotion that include information and resources geared to individual needs and wants and through orchestrated changes in behavior and motivation, we will reduce risk and thus help to prevent illness and accidents. Fuhrer (1994) talks of the feelings of elevated health and subjective well-being experienced by people who are engaged in activities they feel are health promoting (p. 359). First, we must enlarge our own awareness of community resources that promote health, whether these be options for education, medical care, or perhaps exercise classes. Our awareness of programs is then followed by the sharing of these resources with the client through well-articulated programming that is intended to bring about the desired directive of either prevention or promotion (Dyck, 1993; Finlayson & Edwards, 1995; Jaffe, 1986; Kniepmann, 1997).

When we wish to promote the health and well-being of our clients, we cannot assume that they will all be equally engaged in the process, nor will all agree on the parameters of "health." Even though most people would support the idea of seeking better health, oftentimes working toward the goal is received less enthusiastically. A review of those characteristics that influence learning and resulting behavior change will be helpful as you prepare to work in prevention and promotion. If you have previous clinical experience, this kind of practice may not be unlike intervention work that you have already accomplished in the institutional environments of mental and physical rehabilitation. The teaching and acquisition of health-promoting behaviors is not simple, as anyone who has ever failed to maintain an exercise program can attest to. Understanding something of the building of self-efficacy and empowerment is critical to the success of this kind of programming. Kniepmann (1997) provides a useful summary of those constructs for behavioral change that will help in developing successful community programs to include the characteristics of social learning theory, self-efficacy, and perceptions of control as described in the research of Bandura (1977, 1982), Bandura and Walters (1963), and Rotter (1966).

THE FUTURE OF OCCUPATION-CENTERED PRACTICE IN THE COMMUNITY: 2000 AND BEYOND

There is little doubt that health care is changing and that in response occupational therapy is changing as well. In 1995 the American Occupational Therapy Association commissioned Health Policy Alternatives, Inc. to examine the future of health care and particularly occupational therapy's future within health care. It reported numerous markers of the rapid changes in America's health care system, most of them carrying negative implications, and it attributed these primarily to escalating costs and the lack of accompanying growth in the population or the underlying economy in order to maintain a balance (1996, p. 1).

It has now been a few years since this report was published, and we are witnessing some of the implications in our workplaces. First there were reductions in institutional administrative structures, particularly in middle management, and these were followed by reductions in treatment staff with resulting pressures in maintaining case loads. The social, economic, and political worlds in which we live and practice have always encouraged, discouraged, or sometimes prevented how and where we choose to practice. Historically, there appears to be cyclical and necessary reversals in exchange systems—fat years and lean years. Restraint is the counterbalance of excess.

Also, in 1996 the Pew Health Professions Commission predicted the pressures on physicians and nurses and also indicated that there would be pressures to consolidate the "allied" health professions. In its 1998 report, the commission asked that health professionals "continue to consider, in fundamental ways how they best add value to the delivery of health services" (p. i). It suggested that practitioners must contribute to the system in meaningful ways (that is, measure outcomes) or they would risk losing their autonomy. There were messages to educators of future health care professionals as well, which included recommendations to stop preparing students for "yesterday's health care system" and to start preparing students for "emerging systems" (1998, p. iii). It was further suggested that this preparation include broader education with regard to systems, organizational skills, and population skills. Occupational therapists have been articulating these same messages. Baum and Law in a special issue of the *American Journal of Occupational Therapy* called on the profession to be "responsive to the needs of our times" (1998, p. 7). There is little doubt that "the needs of our times" include all of society's ills: abuse, violence, joblessness, futility, and ignorance. In addition, there are new ills that result in increased stress, including competition for limited resources, pressure on family and other systems, and the loneliness and isolation that technology can produce. Baum and Law also remind us that in these troubled times, it is through engagement in occupation that people develop and maintain health (1998, p. 7). And, we might add, it is also through member-ship in a shared community.

Practice in the community that includes intervention, maintenance, and pre-vention is new for many health care providers, but for occupational therapy it is a reemerging practice arena. Appropriate to occupational therapy practitioners' renewed interests in community-based practice are other recommendations of the Pew Health Professions Commission to include: (1) the encouragement of diver-sity to reflect the nation's population (that is, our out-reach programs to inner-city and ethnic urban population "pockets"); (2) the inclusion of interdisciplinary team competence (that is, our expansion of "teams" to include both professional and layperson community members such as friends and neighbors); (3) efforts to con-tinue to move toward ambulatory practice (our extensions of ambulatory practice to include not only intervention but also maintenance of health and wellness and prevention of injury and illness); and (4) the encouragement of public service for all health professional students and graduates (that is, our service learning oppor-tunities in the community).

The Pew Health Professions Commission's fifth recommendation is particu-larly significant to this text, and pertinent quotes from it follow:

> . . . Health professional programs should require a significant amount of work in community settings as a requirement for graduation. This work should be integrated into the curriculum.

> . . . Students should assist in the design and development of such programs.

> . . . Communities and the health agencies that serve them should actively participate in the partnerships through which these service programs can be built.

> . . . Existing programs of national service tied to debt forgiveness should be expanded and enlarged in order to incorporate more health professional graduates.

> . . . Professional associations should actively incorporate the idea of public service into regulation and professional development activity. (1998, pp. iii–vi)

The Pew summary report "Healthy America: Practitioners for 2005" extends the above directives to include prevention in its set of recommendations to educa-tors. The report notes that the "largest share of our graduates will spend their ca-reers in home- and community-based settings. . . . " (Pew Commission, 1992, p. 5; Shugar, O'Neill, and Bader, 1991).

One of our emerging roles in today's society will be to build healthy communi-ties. Baum and Law (1997, 1998) suggest that occupational therapists must under-stand how people interpret and practice occupation, how they apply structure to their daily lives, and how they assign meaning. This can best be done in their natu-ral, self-selected environments—in other words, in their community. Community therapists, according to these authors, must not only be attuned to the intervention needs of their client, but they also must be equally attentive to the ecological, physical, social, cultural, and health environments of the community in order to improve the client's options for healthy living (1998, p. 8). Many of the program examples described in this text do just that; they are very responsive to environment. Some of them, such as the program embedded in the philosophies of the Jane Goodall "Roots and Shoots" Club, have preservation and protection of the environment as a central theme. Baum and Christiansen refer to a changing paradigm in medicine and health care from a biomedical, acute-centered, and provider-driven approach to one that places more responsibility on the consumer (1997, p. 31). And, we might conclude, this places more responsibility on us as occupational therapy practitioners to guide the consumer in how to facilitate healthy habits and behaviors and in how to navigate the community systems to obtain the information and services that they require.

Wilcock (1998) broadens our perspective of community to include global concerns in her call for occupational therapists to be responsive to the objectives of the World Health Organization and potential roles in what she describes as the "new public health" (p. 221). She advocates for a strong foundation in occupation that would prepare the therapist for practices in wellness, preventive medicine, social equity, community development, and ecological sustainability.

Since the above recommendations and directives target all health care practitioners, we are not alone in considering ways to practice in the community setting. However, occupational therapists have an ongoing history of practice in the community, with a body of published information to help those who may be new explore their options. You should review the extensive list of publications at the close of this chapter and examine those that interest you. Many occupational therapists have always practiced in the community, and those who have know that it can be a significantly rewarding practice. It is virtually impossible to practice in the direct environment of the client—in the community system—without being aware of the need for maintenance of health, wellness, and prevention. The community system invites, and likely demands, a comprehensive array of services that includes all that we know and more. We must be practitioners, educators, skill-builders, politicians, health promoters, and advocates.

Not only is our community practice history an advantage as we prepare for return to the community, but our unifying belief and dedication to occupation as a way to orchestrate our practices is also a substantial strength. Few professions have an agreed-upon belief system strong enough to organize their interventions without losing their sense of purpose in what can be a complex and demanding care environment—that of *the community*. It is our time to embrace the values and ideals of our founders and to meet the challenges of community head-on but with a safety net. That safety net is our belief in the power of *occupation*.

REFERENCES

Bandura, A. (1977). Self-efficacy: Toward a unifying theory of behavioral change. *Psychological Review, 84*, 191–215.

Bandura, A. (1982). Self-efficacy mechanism in human agency. *American Psychologist, 37*, 122–147.

Bandura, A., & Walters, R. H. (1963). *Social learning and personality development.* New York: Holt, Rinehart, and Winston.

Baum, C., & Christiansen, C. (1997). The occupational therapy context: philosophy, principles, practice. In C. Christiansen, and C. Baum (Eds.), *Occupational therapy enabling function and well-being* (pp. 28–43). Thorofare, NJ: Slack.

Baum, C., & Law, M. (1997). Occupational therapy practice: Focusing on occupational performance. *American Journal of Occupational Therapy, 51,* 277–288.

Baum, C., & Law, M. (1998, January). Nationally speaking: Community health: A responsibility, an opportunity, and a fit for occupational therapy. *American Journal of Occupational Therapy, 52*(1), 7–10.

Bing, R. (1981). Occupational therapy revisited: A paraphrastic journey. *American Journal of Occupational Therapy, 35,* 499–518.

Bing, R. (1993). Living forward, understanding backward. In S. Ryan (Ed.), *The certified occupational therapy assistant: Principles, concepts, and techniques.* Thorofare, NJ: Slack.

Bockoven, J. S. (1971). Legacy of moral treatment 1800s to 1910. *American Journal of Occupational Therapy, XXV*(5), 223–225.

Bockoven, J. S. (1972). Occupational therapy: A neglected source of community rehumanization. In J. S. Bockoven (Ed.) *Moral treatment in community mental health* (pp. 217–227). New York: Springer.

Boulding, K. E. (1956). General systems theory: The skeleton of science. *Management Science, 2*(3), 197–208.

Christiansen, C., & Baum, C. (1997). Understanding occupation, definitions and concepts. In C. Christiansen and C. Baum (Eds.), *Occupational therapy enabling function and well-being* (pp. 4–21). Thorofare, NJ: Slack.

Clark, F., Wood, W., and Larson, E. (1998). Occupational science: Occupational therapy's legacy for the 21st century. In M. Neistadt and E. Crepeau (Eds.), *Willard and Spackman's occupational therapy* (9th ed., pp. 13–21). Philadelphia: Lippincott.

Cole, J. A. (1979). What's new about independent living. *Archives of physical medicine and rehabilitation, 60,* 458–461.

DeJong, G. (1979). Independent living: From social movement to analytic paradigm. *Archives of physical medicine and rehabilitation, 60,* 435–446.

DeJong, G. (1993). Health care reform and disability: Affirming our commitment to the community. *Archives of physical medicine and rehabilitation, 74,* 1,017–1,024.

Dunton, W. R. (1915). *Occupational therapy: A manual for nurses.* Philadelphia: W. B. Saunders.

Dunton, W. R. (1918). The principles of occupational therapy. In *Proceedings of the National Society for the Promotion of Occupational Therapy: Second annual meeting.* Catonsville, MD: Spring Grove State Hospital Press.

Dyck, I. (1993). Health promotion, occupational therapy and multiculturalism: Lessons from research. *Canadian Journal of Occupational Therapy, 60,* 120–129.

Engelhardt, H. T. (1977). Defining occupational therapy: The meaning of therapy and the virtues of occupation. *American Journal of Occupational Therapy, 31*(10), 666–672.

Erikson, J. M. (1976). *Activity, recovery, and growth.* New York: W. W. Norton.

Finlayson, M., & Edwards, J. (1995). Integrating the concepts of health promotion and community into occupational therapy practice. *Canadian Journal of Occupational Therapy, 62,* 70–75.

Fuhrer, M. J. (1994). Subjective well-being: Implications for medical rehabilitation outcomes and models of disablement. *American Journal of Physical Medicine and Rehabilitation, 73,* 358–364.

Gray, J. M. (1998). Putting occupation into practice: Occupation as ends, occupation as means. *American Journal of Occupational Therapy, 52,* 354–364.

Gray, J. M., Kennedy, B. L., & Zemke, R. (1997). Application of dynamic systems theory to occupation. In R. Zemke, and F. Clark (Eds.), *Occupational science, The evolving discipline* (pp. 309–324). Philadelphia: F. A. Davis.

Hall, E. T. (1969). *The silent language.* Greenwich, CT: Fawcett Publications.

Health Policy Alternatives, Inc. (1996, November). *Health care and market reform: Workforce implications for occupational therapy.* Limited Publication: 444 No. Capitol St., N.W., Suite 821, Washington, DC.

Jaffe, E. G. (1986). Nationally Speaking: The role of occupational therapy in disease prevention and health promotion. *American Journal of Occupational Therapy, 40,* 749–752.

Kielhofner, G. (1985). *A Model of human occupation: Theory and application.* Baltimore: Williams and Wilkins.

Kielhofner, G. (1992). *Conceptual foundations of occupational therapy.* Philadelphia: F. A. Davis.

Kielhofner, G. (1995). *A model of human occupation: Theory and Application* (2nd ed.). Baltimore: Williams and Wilkins.

Kniepmann, K. (1997). Prevention of disability and maintenance of health. In C. Christiansen and C. Baum (Eds.), *Occupational therapy enabling function and well-being* (pp. 531–553). Thorofare, NJ: Slack.

Levine, R. E. (1987). The influence of the arts and crafts movement on the professional status of occupational therapy. *American Journal of Occupational Therapy, 41*(4), 248–254.

Licht, S. (1967). The founding and founders of the American Occupational Therapy Association. *American Journal of Occupational Therapy, 21,* 269.

Lysack, C., & Kaufert, J. (1994). Comparing the origins and ideologies of the independent living movement and community based rehabilitation. *International Journal of Rehabilitation Research, 17,* 231–240.

Madill, H., Townsend, E., & Schultz, P. (1989). Implementing a health promotion strategy in occupational therapy education and practice. *Canadian Journal of Occupational Therapy, 56,* 67–72.

McColl, M. A. (1998). What do we need to know to practice occupational therapy in the community. *American Journal of Occupational Therapy, 52*(1), 11–18.

McColl, M. A., Gerein, N., and Valentine, F. (1997). Meeting the challenges of disability: Models for enabling function and well-being. In C. Christiansen and C. Baum (Eds.), *Occupational therapy enabling function and well-being* (pp. 509–527). Thorofare, NJ: Slack.

McComas, J., & Carswell, A. (1994). A model for action in health promotion: A community experience. *Canadian Journal of Rehabilitation, 7*, 257–265.

Meyer, A. (1977). The philosophy of occupation therapy. *American Journal of Occupational Therapy, 31*(10). (Original work published in 1922, *Archives Occupational Therapy, 1*(1))

Moore, A. (1992). *Cultural anthropology.* San Diego, CA: Collegiate Press.

Nelson, D. (1977). Why the profession of occupational therapy will flourish in the 21st century, 1996 Eleanor Clarke Slagle lecture. *American Journal of Occupational Therapy, 51*, 11–24.

Nelson, D. (1988). Occupation: Form and performance. *American Journal of Occupational Therapy, 42*, 633–641.

Peloquin, S. (1989). Moral treatment: Contexts considered. *American Journal of Occupational Therapy, 43*(8), 537–544.

Peloquin, S. (1991). Occupational therapy service: Individual and collective understandings of the founders, part 2. *American Journal of Occupational Therapy, 45*(8), 733–744.

Pew Health Professions Commission. (1992). *Summary: Healthy America: Practitioners for 2005. A Beginning Dialogue for U.S. Schools of Allied Health.* San Francisco: The Center for the Health Professions, University of California.

Pew Health Professions Commission. (1996, November). *Critical Challenges: Revitalizing the Health Professions for the Twenty-First Century. Third Report, First Release.* San Francisco: The Center for the Health Professions, University of California.

Pew Health Professions Commission. (1998, December). *Recreating Health Professional Practice for a New Century. Fourth Report.* San Francisco: The Center for the Health Professions, University of California.

Pierce, D. (1999). Putting occupation to work in occupational therapy curricula. *Education Special Interest Section Quarterly, 9*(3). Bethesda, MD: American Occupational Therapy Association.

Quiroga, V. (1995). *Occupational therapy: The first 30 years 1900 to 1930.* Bethesda, MD: American Occupational Therapy Association.

Reilly, M. (1962). Occupational therapy can be one of the great ideas of 20th century medicine. *American Journal of Occupational Therapy, 16*, pp. 1–9.

Reilly, M. (1974). *Play as exploratory learning.* Beverly Hills, CA: Sage.

Rogers, J. (1983). The study of human occupation. In G. Kielhofner (Ed.), *Health through occupation: Theory and practice in occupational therapy.* Philadelphia: F. A. Davis.

Rothman, D. J. (1971). *The discovery of the asylum.* Boston: Little, Brown.

Rotter, J. B. (1966). Generalized expectancies for internal versus external control of reinforcement. *Psychological Monographs: General and Applied, 80*, 1–28.

Sabonis-Chafee, B., & Hussey, S. (1998). *Introduction to occupational therapy.* St. Louis, MO: Mosby.

Shannon, P. (1970). The work-play model: A basis for occupational therapy programming. *American Journal of Occupational Therapy, 24*, 215–218.

Shugar, D. A., O'Neill, E. H., and Bader, J. D. (Eds.). (1991). *Healthy America: Practitioners for 2005. An agenda for action for U.S. health professional schools.* Durham, NC: Pew Health Professions Commission.

Tarlov, A., & Pope, A. (1991). *Disability in America: Toward a national agenda for prevention.* Washington, DC: Institute of Medicine, National Academy Press.

Tracy, S. E. (1910). *Studies in invalid occupation.* Boston: Whitcomb and Barrows.

von Bertalanffy, L. (1968). *General systems theory.* New York: Braziller.

Wilcock, A. (1998). *An occupational perspective of health.* Thorofare, NJ: Slack.

Yerxa, E. J., Clark, F., Frank, G., Jackson, J., Parham, D., Pierce, D., Stein C., & Zemke, R. (1990). An introduction to occupational science: A foundation for occupational therapy in the 21st century. *Occupational Therapy in Health Care, 6*(4), 1–17.

You may wish to review the following recommended occupational therapy literature describing community-based programming of the 1960s, 1970s, and 1980s.

Auerbach, E. (1974, May–June). Community involvement: The Bernal. *The American Journal of Occupational Therapy, 28*(5), 272–273.

Bartlett, M. (1977, September). A community therapist in Alaska. *The American Journal of Occupational Therapy, 31*(8), 485–487.

Braun, K. L., & Wake, W. (1988). Community long term care: PT/OT involvement in patient rehabilitation and maintenance. In E. Taira (Ed.), *Community programs for the health impaired elderly* (pp. 5–19). New York: The Haworth Press.

Broekema, M. C., Danz, K. H., & Schloemer, C. U. (1975, January). Occupational therapy in a community aftercare program. *The American Journal of Occupational Therapy, 29*(1), 22–27.

Burnett, S., & Yerxa, E. (1980, March). Community-based and college-based needs assessment of physically disabled persons. *The American Journal of Occupational Therapy, 34*(3), 201–207.

Cantwell, J. L. (1970, November–December). The community-junior college: Challenges to occupational therapy education. *The American Journal of Occupational Therapy, XXIV*(8), 576–578.

Cermak, S. (1976, March). Community-based learning in occupational therapy, *The American Journal of Occupational Therapy, 30*(3), 157–161.

Christiansen, C. H., & Davidson, D. A. (1974, July). A community health program with low achieving adolescents. *The American Journal of Occupational Therapy, 28*(6), 346–350.

Coleman, W. (1975, August). Occupational therapy and child abuse. *The American Journal of Occupational Therapy, 29*(7), 412–417.

Covey, S. (1970, October). Occupational therapy in the community. *The American Journal of Occupational Therapy, XXIV*(7), 508–509.

Cromwell, F. S., & Kielhofner, G. (1976, November–December). An educational strategy for occupational therapy community service at the University of Southern California. *The American Journal of Occupational Therapy, 30*(10), 629–633.

DeMars, P. K. (1975, January). Training adult retardates for private enterprise. *The American Journal of Occupational Therapy, 29*(1), 39–42.

DePoy, E. (1987, July). Community-based occupational therapy with a head-injured adult. *The American Journal of Occupational Therapy, 41*(7), 461–464.

Fazio, L. S. (1988). Sexuality and aging: A community wellness program. In E. Taira (Ed.), *Community programs for the health impaired elderly* (pp. 59–70). New York: The Haworth Press.

Finn, G. L. (1972). The occupational therapist in prevention programs. *The American Journal of Occupational Therapy, 26,* 59–66.

Grossman, J. (1971, November–December). Community experience for students. *The American Journal of Occupational Therapy, 28*(1), 589–591.

Grossman, J. (1977, July). Preventive health care and community programming. *The American Journal of Occupational Therapy, 31*(6), 351–354.

Hasselkus, B. R., & Brown, M. (1983, February). Respite care for community elderly. *The American Journal of Occupational Therapy, 37*(2), 83–88.

Hightower, M. (1974, May–June). A part of the community—rehabilitation—or apart from the community. *The American Journal of Occupational Therapy, 28*(5), 296–298.

Hoff, S. (1988). The occupational therapist as case manager in an adult day healthcare setting. In E. Taira (Ed.), *Community programs for the health impaired elderly* (pp. 21–31). New York: The Haworth Press.

Holmes, C., & Bauer, W. (1970, April). Establishing an occupational therapy department in a community hospital. *The American Journal of Occupational Therapy, XXIV*(3), 219–221.

Howe, M., & Dippy, K. (1968). The role of occupational therapy in community mental health. *The American Journal of Occupational Therapy, XXII*(6), 521–524.

Howe, M., Weaver, C., & Dulay, J. (1981, November). The development of a work-oriented day center program. *The American Journal of Occupational Therapy, 35*(11), 711–718.

Hurff, J. M., Poulsen, M. K., Van Hoven, J., & Olson, S. (1985, April). A library skills program serving adults with mental retardation: An interdisciplinary approach. *The American Journal of Occupational Therapy, 39*(4), 233–239.

Johnson, J., & Smith, M. (1966). Changing concepts of occupational therapy in a community rehabilitation center. *The American Journal of Occupational Therapy, XX*(6), pp. 267–273.

Laukaran, V. H. (1977, February). Toward a model of occupational therapy for community health. *The American Journal of Occupational Therapy, 31*(2), 71–74.

Llorens, L. (1971, October). Occupational therapy in community child health. *The American Journal of Occupational Therapy, XXV*(7), 335–339.

Magrun, W. M., and Tigges, K. N. (1982, February). A transdisciplinary mobile intervention program for rural areas. *The American Journal of Occupational Therapy, 36*(2), 90–94.

Maguire, G. A. (1979, February). Volunteer program to assist the elderly to remain in home settings. *The American Journal of Occupational Therapy, 33*(2), 98–101.

Maynard, M. (1986, November). Health promotion through employee assistance programs: A role for occupational therapists. *The American Journal of Occupational Therapy, 40*(11), 771–776.

McColl, M., & Quinn, B. (1985, September). A quality assurance method for community occupational therapy. *The American Journal of Occupational Therapy, 39*(9), 570–577.

Neistadt, M., & Marques, K. (1984, October). An independent living skills training program. *The American Journal of Occupational Therapy, 38*(10), 671–676.

Neistadt, M., & O'Reilly, M. (1988). Independent living skills groups in a level 1 fieldwork experience. *The American Journal of Occupational Therapy, 42*(12), 782–786.

Nochajski, S. B., & Gordon, C. Y. (1987, January). The use of Trivial Pursuit in teaching community living skills to adults with developmental disabilities. *The American Journal of Occupational Therapy, 41*(1), 10–15.

Shalik, L. D., & Shalik, H. (1987, April). Cluster homes: A community for profoundly and severely retarded persons. *The American Journal of Occupational Therapy, 41*(4), 222–226.

Stein, F. (1972, September). Community rehabilitation of disadvantaged youth. *The American Journal of Occupational Therapy, 26* (6), 277–283.

Tickle, L. S., & Yerxa, E. (1981, October). Need satisfaction of older persons living in the community and in institutions, Part 1: the environment. *The American Journal of Occupational Therapy, 35*(10), 644–649.

Tickle, L. S., & Yerxa, E. (1981, October). Need satisfaction of older persons living in the community and in institutions, Part 2: role of activity. *The American Journal of Occupational Therapy, 35*(10), 650–655.

Walker, L. (1971, October). Occupational therapy in the well community. *The American Journal of Occupational Therapy, XXV*(7), 345–347.

West, W. A. (1967). The occupational therapist's changing responsibility to the community. *The American Journal of Occupational Therapy, XXI*(5), 312–316.

West, W. A. (1969). The growing importance of prevention. *The American Journal of Occupational Therapy, 23*, 226–231.

Wiemer, R. B. (1972, January–February). Some concepts of prevention as an aspect of community health. *The American Journal of Occupational Therapy, 26*(1), 1–9.

Wiemer, R. B., & West, W. A. (1970, July–August). Occupational therapy in community health care. *The American Journal of Occupational Therapy, 24*(5), 323–328.

You may wish to review the following recommended readings relative to community-centered occupational therapy practice published in the 1990s.

Brownson, C. A. (1998). Funding community practice: Stage 1. *American Journal of Occupational Therapy, 52*(1), 60–64.

Bumphrey, E. E. (1995). The role of occupational therapy in health promotion. In E. E. Bumphrey (Ed.), *Community practice: A text for occupational therapists and others involved in community care* (pp. 68–78). London: Prentice Hall.

Burkhardt, A. (1997, June). Occupational therapy and wellness. *O.T. Practice,* 28–35.

Camardese, M. B., & Youngman, D. (1996). H.O.P.E.: Education, employment, and people who are homeless and mentally ill. *Psychiatric Rehabilitation Journal, 19*(4), 45–56.

Collins, L. F. (1996, October). Perspectives on your private practice: Starting an individualized practice. *O.T. Practice,* 26–27.

Collins, L. F. (1996, October). Moving on when private practice no longer works for you. *O.T. Practice,* 28–29.

Collins, L. F. (1996, February). Thriving in a rural setting. *O.T. Practice,* 40–44.

Collins, L. F. (1997, April). Connecting the community: Shared housing of New Orleans, Inc. *O.T. Practice,* 40–47.

Crist, P., & Stoffel, V. (1992). *The Americans with Disabilities Act of 1990* and employees with mental impairments: personal efficacy and the environment. *American Journal of Occupational Therapy, 46*(5), 434–443.

DeMaus, P. (1992). An occupational therapy life skills curriculum model for a Native American tribe: A health promotion program based on ethnographic field research. *American Journal of Occupational Therapy, 46*(8), 727–736.

Devereaux, E. (1991). The Issue Is: Community-based practice. *American Journal of Occupational Therapy, 45*(10), 944–946.

Dunn, W., Brown, C., & McGuigan, A. (1994). The ecology of human performance: A framework for considering the effect of context. *American Journal of Occupational Therapy, 48,* 595–607.

Gage, M., & Polatajko, H. (1994). Enhancing occupational performance through an understanding of perceived self-efficacy. *American Journal of Occupational Therapy, 48*(5), 452–461.

Giles, G. (1994). Editorial: Why provide community support for persons with brain injury? *American Journal of Occupational Therapy, 48*(4), 255–296.

Grady, A. P. (1995). Building inclusive community: A challenge for occupational therapy: 1994 Eleanor Clarke Slagle Lecture. *American Journal of Occupational Therapy, 49,* 300–310.

Greene, D. (1997). The use of service learning in client environments to enhance ethical reasoning in students. *American Journal of Occupational Therapy, 51*(10), 844–852.

Hurff, J. M., Lowe, H. E., Ho, B. J., & Hoffman, N. M. (1990). Networking: A successful linkage for community occupational therapists. *American Journal of Occupational Therapy, 44*(5), 424–430.

Ingstad, B. (1990). The disabled person in the community: Social and cultural perspectives. *International Journal of Rehabilitation Research, 13,* 187–194.

Kari, N., & Michels, P. (1991). The Lazarus Project: The politics of empowerment. *American Journal of Occupational Therapy, 45*(8), 719–725.

Knis, L. L. (1997, March). O.T. and the community: Helping those with mental illness to transition. *O.T. Practice,* 36–41.

Lysack, C., Stadnyk, R., Paterson, M., McLeod, K., & Krefting, L. (1995). Professional expertise of occupational therapists in community practice: Results of an Ontario survey. *Canadian Journal of Occupational Therapy, 62,* 138–147.

Oliver, M. (1990). *The politics of disablement.* London: MacMillan.

Parker, M. G., & Thorslund, M. (1991). The use of technical aids among community-based elderly. *American Journal of Occupational Therapy, 45*(8), 712–718.

Pizzi, M. (1992). Hospice: The creation of meaning for people with life threatening illness. *O.T. Practice, 4*(1), 1–7.

Reitz, S. M. (1992). A historical review of occupational therapy's role in preventive health and wellness. *American Journal of Occupational Therapy, 46,* 50–55.

Robnett, R. (1997, May). Paradigms of community practice. *O.T. Practice,* 30–35.

Ryan, S. (1993). The role of the COTA as an activities director. In S. Ryan (Ed.), *Practice issues in occupational therapy education* (pp. 193–204). Thorofare, NJ: Slack.

Schelly, C., Sample, P., & Spencer, K. (1992). The Americans With Disabilities Act of 1990 expands employment opportunities for persons with developmental disabilities. *American Journal of Occupational Therapy, 46*(5), 457–460.

Siebert, C. (1997). A description of fieldwork in the home care setting. *American Journal of Occupational Therapy, 51*(6), 423–429.

Special issue on community health. (1998). *American Journal of Occupational Therapy, 52*(1).

Special issue on occupation. (1998). *American Journal of Occupational Therapy, 52*(6).

Special issue on occupation, spirituality, and life meaning. (1997). *American Journal of Occupational Therapy, 51*(3).

Spencer, J. (1991). An ethnographic study of independent living alternatives. *American Journal of Occupational Therapy, 45*(3), 243–250.

Vanier, C., & Hebert, M. (1995). An occupational therapy course on community practice. *Canadian Journal of Occupational Therapy, 62* 76–81.

Voas, R. (1997). Drinking and driving prevention in the community: Program planning and implementation. *Addiction, 92* (Supplement 2), S201–S219.

Welberding, D. (1991). The quarterway house: More than an alternative of care. *O.T. in Mental Health, 11*(1), 65–91.

The following may be a useful resource to community practitioners in rural settings.

Breaking New Ground Resource Center, Purdue University, 1146 Agricultural Engineering Building, West Lafayette, Indiana, 47907-1146 (assists people with disabilities who are employed in agriculture through written resources and contacts in the community)

Identifying Trends and Forecasting Futures

Learning Objectives

1. To learn how to identify current events reported in the media and in professional literature that may impact you and your potential program
2. To explore how historical events and eras have impacted health care and the occupational therapy profession
3. To analyze trends to make forecasts regarding the potential success of your planned program

Key Terms

1. Trends
2. Forecasts

Case Example

A community program can be designed to encourage positive parent-child communication through activities and experiences that focus on shared occupations. Such a program prepares the child for a successful academic future. The planning and funding of such a program may be greatly influenced by current trends in public sentiment prompted by recent school bombings. This results in a resurgence of parental concern regarding children's use of unstructured time and the lack of positive parent-child experiences.

Continued in the exercise on page 32

Strengthening the bonds between children and their parents through cooperation in meaningful activities creates partnerships for future change.

What is happening in the community, region, state, country, and world today that will impact us and our ideas and plans for the future? As we venture into the design and development of new programming, it becomes critical that the practice of following trends becomes a part of daily and weekly routines. This is not to suggest that each of us should construct a sophisticated statistical *trends analysis;* rather, we should use the existing information in the literature and the media to chart the direction in which things will likely go (*trends*). According to Celente, a "trend is a definite, predictable direction or sequence of events," and "tracking trends shows us how we got here, where we are, and where we're going" (1991, pp. 4–5). We then should use these *trends* to make *forecasts.* These **forecasts,** or scenarios of the probable future, will permit us to make more critical judgments regarding our own futures relative to practice and, particularly, to new or continued community programming.

Examples of shifting trends may include the change from "national economic systems (to) an international economy" and the shift from "the management of illness via the management of medication (to) the genetic treatment of illness" (Ramsey and Robertson, 1993, p. 28). In addition, computer technology and electronics, transportation systems, and educational technology have all experienced shifting trends.

In fact, today we really do not have much choice in the matter of considering and responding to trends. In the preface to the original edition of *The Temporary Society,* Bennis and Slater (1968) comment that to engage in the forecasting of social trends "in a world of unprecedented complexity during changes of unparalleled rapidity" is probably as absurd as it is necessary.

At least on a weekly basis (and preferably daily), major newspapers should be read to ferret out events that may impact us as we practice "occupation-centered" interventions. For example, what are the current political events at both the inter-national, national, and state levels? By perusing current events, we can determine where the public sentiments lie and where the state and federal dollars are going, and we may be able to forecast where these funds are likely to go in the future. Wars, political intrigues, and adolescent or young adult fads may appear to be vastly remote from our concerns for therapy, wellness, and health, but if we remain alert, these things can, and likely will, impact the programming we might propose and the funding available to make it possible.

ANALYZING TRENDS BY REVIEWING HISTORY

Our analysis of current and developing trends must also include our awareness of history. We all know of the tremendous impact World War I and World War II had on the history of occupational therapy. The first clinic-community program devel-oped by the author of this text was for veterans of Vietnam. Although this pro-gramming was in response to numbers and need, it unfortunately was initiated with inadequate preparation that an earlier event/trends review might have of-fered. The programming met the immediate need in something of a crisis mode, but it could have been more proactive had the insights and advanced preparation from (an) analysis of trends been utilized. An analysis or analyses of the social trends and the characteristics of the developing counterculture might have en-couraged the design of programming that would have helped Vietnam veterans reenter the community and avoid the emotional trauma that many encountered. This would be true of any programming designed to meet the needs of persons ex-periencing crisis situations and programming designed to assist in the process of cultural/environmental assimilation (such as for refugees).

Current best-selling books in the popular marketplace give us information re-garding the interests, needs, and wants of the public—the public that we, too, are a part of and seek to serve. Often novelists of both fiction and nonfiction, screen writers, song writers, and other representatives of popular culture can provide a window to trends or perhaps even set them.

FINDING TRENDS IN PROFESSIONAL LITERATURE

Certainly we must read our own professional literature and that of other health care practitioners, but program descriptions likely will be responding to trends rather than setting them. Those who are setting trends probably will not know it for some time, and even then they may not make a publishable record of such events. We must, however, remain aware of the actions our professional organiza-tion is taking at both the state and national levels with regard to the requirements for education and practice. Many of our leaders have been and are courageous trendsetters, but the profession of occupational therapy historically has been con-servative; it has moved toward the future tentatively, avoiding uncharted territo-ries. Whatever stance you prefer, our professional affiliations offer us both freedoms and restraints, and neither can be ignored.

Practice in the community does not mean practice outside of our discipline or our profession but in many ways requires an even closer relationship to our values and ethics than in the more institutional-based environments. We may find it difficult at first to open our thinking to entertain innovative arenas from which practice may originate. Certainly legislative decisions, public laws and reforms, and state and local budgeting are factors that may specifically influence our practices, but we most likely learn of these while we are feeling their effects. Often our reactions are prompted either by not being prepared (and "missing the boat" while another, more savvy, provider steps in) or, sadly, by preparing and investing in a rigid service model that is rapidly becoming obsolete.

QUESTIONS TO CONSIDER

Sometimes events, perhaps predictive of trends, appear to have little to do with us and are ignored. Certainly no one can doubt that health care in the United States is rapidly changing. Could these changes have been predicted? An analysis of the large expenditures incurred in the therapy provisions of the 1980s and 1990s likely would have at least partially predicted the inevitable downsizing we are presently experiencing. Even now there are regional changes that are predictive of changes that have occurred or will occur across the country. What are professionals doing to prepare for the changes that may occur? This prompts some interesting questions. Should health care providers seek more or less regulation? With what disciplines should we form alliances? Is it time for new liaisons?

THE IMPACT OF TRENDS—GENERATING MORE QUESTIONS TO CONSIDER

It would appear that people are becoming more responsible for the state of their health. Is this a trend? Did the changes in the perceived quality of health care prompted by the corporate entry into an arena thought to be humanistic cause us to become responsive to the need to care for ourselves? Are young adults learning to place their trust exclusively in their own actions? Will the next generation be even more internally controlled than the last one? How will they prepare for shrinking resources and diminished health care and retirement dollars? There is little doubt that they will live longer than their predecessors. Grasping control of your health and life without sacrificing quality and meaning requires skills. Who will provide those skills? Will the trend become a frenzied desire to protect your physical and emotional health and the health of your children in order not to use resources for illness? Or will there be a growing number of drug, alcohol, and accident victims? Will the rich expect to pay for their own services and everyone else will be without access to services?

Therapists entering the workforce in the 1950s, 1960s, and 1970s witnessed the ebb-flow cycling of reimbursement and salaries, programming styles, and resources; in response, they have had several turns at the reinvention of the profession. It would appear that the time is right for yet another such reinvention.

And what about the so-called Generation X? Apparently this group is already engaged in the quest for meaning outside the traditional domains of institutional prerogative. What better group is there to engage in the health care practices of tomorrow, both as giver and receiver? Will this group require new modes of skill and information provision?

The above discussion is a series of questions prompted by a cursory review of trends—trends that promote forecasts and trends that, assuming we listen, will help us to outline future practices.

The following exercises will help you learn the initial steps to the process of forecasting the direction of future practice.

▰▰▰ EXERCISE 1 ▰▰▰▰▰▰▰▰▰▰▰
Identifying Trends by Tracing History

1. To begin this exercise, review your knowledge of history, including occupational therapy history. Under the categories provided, note those things and occurrences that have impacted the nature of our profession today (think broadly, and add categories if you wish). You may also transfer this grid to a transparency or to the board to facilitate group work.

	Events	Philosophies	Attitudes	Technology
pre-1930				
1930–1950				
1950–1970				
1970–1990				
1990–2000				

From your position in the present, review the previous exercise, and highlight those things/events that have, in your observation, made a *positive* impact on the profession of occupational therapy and those things/events that may have had a *negative* impact.

Is there anything happening in the profession today that your analyses of events might have predicted with regard to practice, legislation, education, or reimbursement?

If you wish, discuss with your classmates, colleagues, or others, and note your comments below:

_____

_____

EXERCISE 2
Identifying Recent Trends

1. Since identifying trends may be a new process for you, it may be helpful to do a sorting activity to begin. Either by placing labels on a large table or by writing on a board, note the following categories of events that may be responsive to trends:

1. Events reflective of *public attitudes*
2. Events reflective of *economics*
3. Events (local, regional, national, international) reflective of *politics*
4. Events reflective of *public interests*
5. Events in *education*
6. Events in *medicine*
7. Events in *health*
8. Events in scientific *research*

   Can you think of other categories?

   Provide yourself with not only your local newspaper but also copies of such newspapers as *The Washington Post, The New York Times, The Wall Street Journal,* and any others that you believe will help you create a view of the future. What is happening in Europe, for example, may certainly be significant. (Look at the impact the English had on the history of American rock and roll!) However, the above-mentioned newspapers will likely highlight events for you that may be of significance. Watch local and national news programs for at least a week before you begin this exercise. Also use the Internet to determine what people are interested in and what they are chatting about. Remember that not everything you see on the Internet is factual. Although fiction can tell us a lot when we are looking for trends, we must learn early on to separate fact from fiction or conjecture, particularly when doing research (Garretson, 1997). (See the references at the end of this chapter for sources to help you evaluate Internet information.)

2. As you go through your newspapers, news journals, and notes gleaned from newscasts and the Internet, clip those you have selected and place them under the categories noted previously. If this is done as part of a class exercise, do it first without discussion. When everyone is finished, discuss your findings. Is there agreement? Disagreement? While this is an equally valid exercise when done alone, having other opinions and perspectives broadens your observations.

3. As a class or with colleagues, review your selections and separate out those you think may represent a trend that could impact occupation-centered intervention, either therapy-based or health-wellness promotion models. Remove all of the news items that you decide are *not* likely to impact occupation-centered programming.

4. Working with those items remaining, separate out your selections to make two categories—one category of those trend predictors that may have a *positive* impact on occupation-centered intervention and another category for those that may have a *negative* impact.

STEPS TO IDENTIFYING TRENDS AND FORECASTING FUTURES

The following list summarizes the steps to identifying trends and forecasting futures:

1. Find resources such as newspapers, Internet, television, and others.
2. Clip pertinent articles and notes, and place them under one of the identified eight categories.
3. Review your categories and clippings.
4. Remove any news item(s) that you feel *will not* likely impact the practice of occupation-centered interventions.
5. Make two categories of those items remaining—one category of those items that may have a *positive* impact and one category for those items that may have a *negative* impact on occupation-centered programs.
6. Review your categories, and try some forecasting. What is likely to happen next?

From the identification of *trends* come *forecasts*. Forecasts are what you might anticipate or predict will come of the reviewed trends. Forecasts can supply answers to questions such as: What impact will these apparent trends have on you professionally and personally?

From the work you have completed in the previous exercises, can you make forecasts or predictions as to how those things you have identified will likely have an impact on present and/or future occupation-centered interventions, either therapy-based or health maintenance/promotion/wellness practices? How will they impact you personally? How will they impact your professional expectations?

5. Note your forecast(s) or prediction(s) below.

_____

_____

_____

_____

_____

a. What do you anticipate will be the impact of your forecast(s) or prediction(s) on occupation-centered intervention in general?

_____

_____

_____

_____

_____

b. What do you anticipate will be the impact on you, personally and professionally?

_____

_____

_____

_____

_____

6. Considering what you have found, note below any identified trends/forecasts that may influence your interests in community programming (either positively or negatively).

a. Presently, my community programming interests are:

_____

_____

_____

_____

_____

b. Trends that *may* have a positive impact:

_____

_____

_____

_____

_____

c. Trends that *may* have a negative impact:

_____

_____

_____

_____

_____

Remember that even if you identify negative trends, this does not necessarily mean that you give up your ideas; rather, it means that you use the present information to make adaptations to your future plans or at least to develop contingency plans.

7. If you have identified negative trends in the previous exercise, how might you wish to adapt your planning, or what contingency plans will you adopt in order to be better prepared for your future?

_____

_____

_____

_____

_____

Continue to be aware of events and trends, and continue to make forecasts. You may wish to begin charting your forecasts to see how accurate you are. Organize a file that categorizes your interests; when you see something (such as a newspaper article or a news story), clip it and drop it in your file. Review the contents periodically, and examine for developing trends. Always look for social, economic, and political significance. Keep a separate category for anything dealing specifically with occupational therapy and with other health professions.

Ramsey and Robertson (1993) suggest the use of an "Issue Impact Tree" to help in the identification of trends. The following exercise is an adaptation of their work.

8. Select an issue that may be reflective of a trend, such as technology-based distance education, reductions in medical-based health care financing, affordable home-based technology, or another of your choice. Write the issue you've selected in the largest of the circles represented in Figure 3–1. Working alone or with a group, brainstorm on what you think may be major implications of this issue. Write these implications in the next larger circle immediately adjacent to the largest one.

Now think about second-level implications that may grow from the first level. Place these in the next group of circles. Either alone or as a group, come to consensus to determine which of the implications you believe are most likely to occur. A case example is shown in Figure 3–2.

Score them as follows:

1. Most likely to occur
2. Might occur
3. Least likely to occur

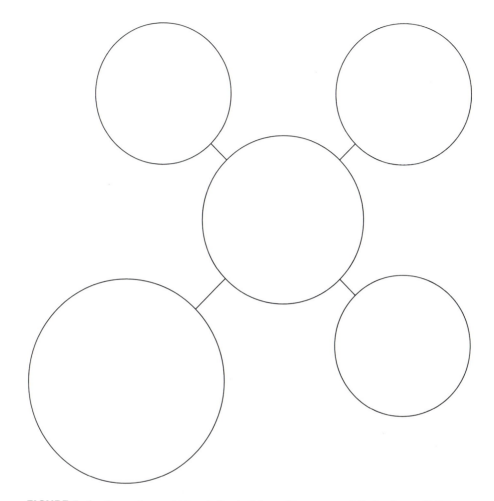

FIGURE 3–1   Issue Impact Tree (adapted from Ramsey and Robertson, 1993)

The parent-child community program case introduced earlier will help to demonstrate how an issue impact tree can be used to forecast possible futures for a possible program.

RESULTING IMPLICATIONS FOR FUTURE OCCUPATION-CENTERED PROGRAMMING

It is likely that the present and the next few years will welcome community- and school-based prevention programming and research targeting 1) violent behavior exhibited by children, 2) the nature of and time spent on computer games by children, and 3) the nature of parent-child communications and time spent in shared activities.

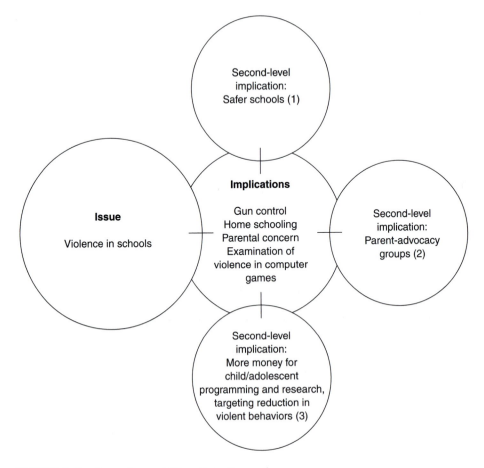

FIGURE 3–2 Issue Impact Tree, Case Example

The case example selected:

The nature of parent-child communications and time spent in shared activities around which to develop a community program

As we develop this case and others in future chapters, you will see how we continue to return to the information provided by trends analyses and the resulting futures forecasts.

SUMMARY

The planning of occupation-centered programs does not occur in a vacuum. An identification of trends based on past and present information will encourage the planner to anticipate the future and make forecasts regarding the potential successes of his or her proposed programming. Envisioning the future will prompt the planner to be prepared for changes in population, funding, and market demands.

It is intended that you use the results of the previous exercises to help you plan your future program(s). As a practitioner and program development specialist, it will be critical to your progress that you continue some ongoing analysis of trends. As a leader and as a manager, you may wish to place *futures forecasting* on a yearly retreat agenda; without it an organization cannot successfully complete five-year to ten-year planning. Skillful and sometimes intuitive futures forecasting can place you and your organization in the position of setting trends and designing futures rather than scrambling to keep up with those that are occurring. Begin now to establish habits that will place you in the forefront of futures forecasting.

REFERENCES

Bennis, W., & Slater, P. (1968). *The temporary society.* San Francisco: Jossey-Bass.

Celente, G. (1991). *Trend tracking.* New York: Warner Books.

Garretson, C. H. (1997). *Factors affecting Webmasters' sense of responsibility for information accuracy.* Unpublished thesis, Georgia Southern University.

Ramsey, D., & Robertson, S. (1993). *Breaking into new markets: Expanding roles in mental health.* Workshop resource book. Bethesda, MD: American Occupational Therapy Association.

Audio Transcripts

Evaluating the quality of information on the Internet. (1997). General Conference Session at the 12th Annual Computers in Libraries Conference, Arlington,Virginia. (Available from Alexandria, Virginia)

Tillman, H. (1996). *Advertising/marketing sources on the Internet.* Denver, CO: National Audio Video.

4

Program Development: What Skills Will I Need?

Learning Objectives

1. To develop a personally meaningful definition of occupational therapy
2. To practice the skills of effective/active listening
3. To practice the skills of effective verbal communication
4. To learn to recognize the distribution of personal time in balancing daily occupations
5. To explore the characteristics of an effective leader and manager
6. To assess personal knowledge and skills relative to community program design, development, and practice
7. To identify personal qualities, attributes, and behaviors in preparation for potential leadership roles in community programming

Key Terms

1. Program/Programming
2. Communication
3. Effective/Active Listening
4. Clinical Reasoning
5. Negotiation
6. Persuasion
7. Leader/Leadership
8. Manager

The focus of this chapter is learning how to identify the skills and information the planner will need to design and develop a *program.* M. J. Youngstrom defines **program** as "a specifically designed service that is aimed toward a specific goal and is designed to achieve clearly defined outcomes or results" (1999, p. 129). Specificity is important to this definition, for through specificity we are able to produce program results that are clear and measurable. A program designed by an occupational therapy practitioner may take several directions. For example, it may be therapeutic in its intent, that is, designed to provide therapy for those in need of *therapeutic intervention.* This intervention, the provision of occupational *therapy*, may include identification of specific needs (or screening), assessment, treatment, and evaluation for individuals of any age. Of course, programming of this nature may be developed to provide a new service not offered previously, or it may be developed to extend service in an existing occupational therapy department.

You will find the term **programming** commonly used in this text to denote the step-by-step orchestrated process of designing and developing a program (not to be confused with the actions to be performed by a computer). Although occupation-centered programs may be intended to solve problems, the order followed in planning programs for *people* is not always linear and, at times, may seem less than logical.

Occupation-centered programs may also be developed for individuals who are not candidates for *therapy* as defined by the need for treatment of disability or disease. Rather, because of life circumstances largely beyond their control, they are considered to be at risk for developing destructive life patterns that may diminish their opportunities for quality experiences. While programs for these populations may also involve screening and assessment, the intention is not to offer therapy. Screening and assessments are conducted to determine where the development of skills and the acquisition of knowledge and information will be required in order to reduce or diminish the potential for problems. Programs targeting the acquisition of skills, knowledge, and information neutralize risk. Whether our intentions are to provide therapy, to prevent problems by reducing risk, or to maintain health and wellness, the belief in *occupation* connects us.

Programs may also be designed to enhance and reinforce already present positive development. Because of occupational therapy practitioners' educational foundation and experience, programs can be carefully tailored to the specific needs of the individual. The understanding of occupation as an outcome of an intricate system comprised of the individual's values, interests, needs, and wants offers a unique perspective to programming not found in other professions. The appreciation of the intricacies of *occupation* coupled with a practical foundation in the analysis of tasks permits the occupational therapy practitioner to match the teaching of skills with the acquisition of abilities for positive occupation-centered outcomes. An occupation-centered perspective offers a particularly unique contribution to the development of programming for "at-risk" populations as well as programs targeting the maintenance of health. Programs designed by those with education and experience in occupation-centered perspectives, then, can be successfully adapted to any population in need of services.

The actual process of program development is a bit like solving a puzzle—one piece placed at a time, and the placement of each piece demanding our knowledge, skill and expertise. To help select the first piece of the puzzle, we might ask, "Just what do I need to know to begin the process of designing and developing a community program?" The answers are fairly simple. To begin, we need to know

- How to communicate clearly and effectively
- How to listen
- How to serve as a role model of occupational balance
- How to provide occupation-centered services
- How to provide leadership
- How to manage systems

And to complete the package, we need

- A solid occupational therapy professional education
- Strong professional and personal ethics
- Good common sense
- Energy and motivation to try something new

The Skill of Becoming an Effective Communicator

The first skill—or perhaps we should say the prerequisite skill—is to be an effective communicator. Most of us can communicate well enough to get the things we need and sometimes the things we want, but all of us can use some help in communicating effectively in many and varied situations. Effective **communication** is a skill to be learned, and we need to identify and practice the skills of finding and utilizing efficient and sufficient language to communicate ideas to anyone with optimal results. This is the key to marketing our program first to the agency or facility we may wish to have sponsor our program and then ultimately to the consumer.

EXERCISE 1
Learning to Identify Meaning and to Express Ideas

Much of what we will do as the designers and developers of programming will require that we be able to clearly express our ideas in an effective and meaningful way and that we *listen* with equal skills. The following exercise offers practice in synthesizing and expressing ideas and in finding the communicator's intended meaning. Try it with classmates or others. (The professional therapist may wish to skip these exercises; although a refresher can be useful, as we tend to take these skills for granted.)

1. Read the following paragraph:

> Every nation needs a past . . . some kind of core experience that will help people define who they are. Americans seek this with a desperation that

perhaps reflects their inherent poverty in this regard. Except for Native Americans, everyone came here from some other place . . . a place with rich traditions of its own. American artists and writers are continually looking for "roots" . . . for a way to build a cultural essence of some kind. They look to the small Midwestern town of 1910 or the New England village of 1750 or the Old West, but none of these symbols seem to stick, perhaps because all represent such a minute fragment of what it means to be American. (Bennis & Slater, 1998, p. 29)

2. Note below the main ideas you have gleaned from the paragraph, and share them with your partner, colleagues, or classmate(s):

_____

_____

_____

_____

_____

3. From the ideas you have identified, what do you find to be the *meaning* or *essence* of this paragraph? Note your views below, and share them with your partner, colleagues, or classmate(s); try using *occupation* and *community* in expressing the meaning:

_____

_____

_____

_____

_____

4. Discuss the steps of the exercise.

Was it easier for you to write down the components of the exercise than it was to express them verbally? Why, or why not?

The exercise asked you to identify the main ideas in the paragraph and then to assess the speaker's or writer's intended meaning. Is this how you usually assess spoken or written *meaning?* If not, how do you usually find the intended meaning in what someone says or writes? Note any ideas for discussion below:

_____

_____

_____

_____

Developing confidence through presentations of proposals helps students first discover and then build skills for effective marketing of occupation-centered community programs.

You may wish to choose other readings and continue these exercises with selected passages. After a few tries, you may be able to express your responses verbally first rather than write them. The intent of this exercise is twofold. First, it offers the opportunity to verbally express your thoughts and ideas to others, and secondly, it helps you to find the intended meaning in what you read and hear. Both are important to the successful process of program design and development.

Communicating to the Listener: Your Definition of Occupational Therapy

It is likely that on many occasions you will have to explain who you are and what you do as an occupational therapy practitioner. Perhaps first you will explain this to those who you hope will welcome your program in their facility, secondly to other professionals, and thirdly to consumers. Although many of the people with whom you come in contact will have an idea of what occupational therapy is (perhaps from the roots of the words themselves or from personal experience), it is unlikely that many will appreciate the diversity in practice exhibited by the profession. This may particularly be the case if you choose to develop community-based programming targeting prevention or maintenance.

If one of your student experiences provided the opportunity to explain occupational therapy to a group outside of the profession, you have a head start on this exercise. Experienced practitioners have likely developed their own definitions of occupational therapy; however, these definitions are usually tailored to a particular practice niche. If you, as the practitioner, are entertaining thoughts of designing and developing a program for a new niche, you may want to expand or change your definitions.

5. In your textbooks or the professional literature, find a definition or definitions of occupational therapy. Write the definition(s) below (use additional paper if you need more space):

_____

_____

_____

_____

_____

_____

6. Using a highlighter, note *key words* that you find *meaningful* in the definitions of occupational therapy. Write those words below:

_____

_____

_____

_____

7. Review the *key words* you selected. Use these words to write your own definition of occupational therapy—a definition by which *you,* as a practitioner, would like to be identified. Remember to keep your definition broad and not specific to only one kind of practice or to one kind of practitioner (for example, occupational therapist or occupational therapy assistant). Write your definition below:

_____

_____

_____

_____

_____

8. Write your definition of what occupational therapists or occupational therapy assistants *do* (what *you* wish to do). Again, keep your perspective broad, and avoid listing specific skills or roles. Begin to think of yourself as an *occupation-centered practitioner.* Write your definition below:

_____

_____

_____

_____

_____

_____

9. Using the definition you developed, translate it to use in the following scenario:

You wish to start a summer day camp for children who have been identified by parents and/or educators as emotionally-socially immature. It is not your expectation that any of the children will carry a diagnosis; but all may be seen to be "at risk." You have been asked by a mother who is interested in your program, "What does an occupational therapist do?"

Have a classmate, colleague, or friend role-play the question. Briefly write your response below. (You should also provide a verbal explanation. Remember to use the definition you developed in question 8 to structure your answer to the question.)

_____

_____

_____

_____

_____

10. Continue the exercise by applying the following scenario:

You have at least partially won the trust of the mother who now invites you to the Parent-Teacher Association (PTA) meeting to talk about occupational therapy. You can assume most of the audience will be interested in what occupational therapy can do for children, so you may wish to focus on this aspect. Consider how and why the above-mentioned children may be "at risk" and what kinds of assistance your camp might offer. This is likely your first opportunity to begin marketing your proposed camp program for "at-risk" children to a large audience, so you might also wish to include how mothers might recognize if their children would be good candidates for your camp.

This one may be a bit challenging, for there are several considerations that may be presently outside your experience. You may wish to first discuss it with classmates. Share your earlier definitions. When you are ready, briefly write below what you might say differently to this group and how your presentation style might be different. When you have written your responses, role-play your brief presentation to the group.

_____

_____

_____

_____

11. Try different groups with different interests, and critique each other in your responses. Maintain the essence of what occupational therapy is and what occupation-centered practitioners do.

You may want to follow your preliminary response with some specific purposes related to the different groups you are targeting, but resist the temptation to drift into splintered definitions appropriate to only very specific populations. Rather, think about your definitions in a broad way: *What does all of occupational therapy have in common? What do all occupational therapy practitioners strive to do regardless of their clientele?* Certainly you may wish to direct some of your responses to the specific concerns of your audience; however, if you find yourself explaining how to evaluate joint range or reciting the basic tenets of sensory integration, start again! Use the space below to make any notes you may need to structure your brief responses to new scenarios:

_____

_____

_____

_____

_____

Although critical, learning how to express our ideas and thoughts in a clear and succinct manner is only one aspect of communication. Often when we are new to practice, we become so concerned with trying to communicate our ideas (particularly to patients, clients, and caregivers) that we forget to or are unable to listen.

LEARNING TO LISTEN

In *Effective Coaching* (1999), Marshall J. Cook tells us that perhaps the best thing we can do for another person is to give that person our full, undivided attention. We all have attempted to talk with someone who was shuffling through papers, talking to someone else, or gazing somewhere over our head. If you are unable to drop everything to listen to someone who needs your attention, then it is best to be honest and ask that person to return when you are able to listen. It is a human tendency to engage in overlapping occupations, but the listening aspect of communication requires and deserves full attention, whether the speaker is a child, adult, client, coworker, or friend.

In his discussion of **effective listening,** Cook goes on to say that we must let the speaker finish before responding (1999, pp. 70–77). It is easy to interrupt when we *think* we know the intent of the communication. In therapy environments, where we often hear similar questions and concerns from our patients/clients, the tendency to believe we know the outcome of the communication may be particularly troublesome. Often we manipulate speakers when we interrupt or finish their sentences, particularly if they are not assertive enough to stop us. For many cultures, the therapist/professional represents a powerful authority position, and it would not be easy (and probably impossible) for the patient/client to redirect the communication.

Other characteristics of effective listening include hearing, reflecting, and re-phrasing. In the counseling professions, the term *active listening*—that is, listening for the emotional-feeling content as well as the information that is being provided by the speaker—might be used to collectively describe these characteristics. Active listening might include

- Hearing the words
- Reflecting on and rephrasing what was communicated
- *Hearing* the emotional-feeling content as well as the information

In summary, active listening describes the ability to hear and to *listen with total con-sciousness* not only to the words that are being spoken but also to the meaning and emotional content our speaker is expressing. Not only does this ability make us good friends and desirable companions, but also it is absolutely critical to our var-ied roles as therapists and as programmers/planners.

Whether speaking to an employee, a consumer, the owner of a building we would like to lease for our program, or a granting agency board, we must express our ideas clearly, *and* we must listen fully. It is not magical but rather a skill to be learned.

▰▰▰ EXERCISE 2 ▰▰▰▰▰▰▰▰▰▰

Active Listening

Practice the following exercise with a classmate, using "feeling" terms. These terms may seem awkward and artificial at first, but they are useful to initiate the development of the skill of active listening.

1. Your classmate or partner will express to you some event that happened during the course of the week; this should be an event that he or she found particularly meaningful (frustrating, happy, exciting, or perhaps disappointing).

You listen attentively. Face your speaker, and try to focus your eyes on the speaker's eyes as much as possible. You might wish to lean slightly forward, but be relaxed and natural. Through the course of this exercise, try to *tune in* to the feel-ings that are being expressed—not to just the words. The focus is away from what the speaker may be thinking and toward what the speaker is feeling. An example follows:

Your speaker tells you that she called her friend to go to a movie, and her friend said that she had to study. The speaker later saw her friend at the movie with a guy.

You could respond, "So, I guess you think she was avoiding you." This focuses on what your speaker might have been thinking, but a better, feeling response would be something like, "So, I guess you felt pretty left out."

You might be wrong in your interpretation, and your speaker might correct you. But if he or she does not, your communication will likely become unproductive. To avoid this, you can try rephrasing what the speaker has said, not only to focus on feelings but also to check the accuracy of your understanding of the content being expressed. When finished with this exercise, listen to your classmate's feedback of how effective you were in *reading* his or her feelings. Were you an effective and active listener?

2. Now complete the same exercise, but your classmate will receive your feedback.

Continue this exercise as long as you find it useful. Try it with family and friends. Remember to listen and respond to what you hear—at a *feeling* level.

It is worth noting the possibility of engaging in conversation with a speaker, particularly a client or patient, who is already so focused on *feelings* that you are unable to determine the accuracy of that person's *thinking* process. In such a circumstance, you will need to reverse from *feeling* responses to *thinking* ones in order to effectively and actively listen.

3. Before we move on, ask yourself the following question: "Am I an effective, honest, and open communicator?" If there are areas you would like to improve, note them below:

_____

_____

_____

_____

4. What might be some things you could begin doing right now to address the areas of communication you would like to improve in order to become a more effective communicator in your professional future? Note some ideas below:

_____

_____

_____

USING YOUR COMMUNICATION SKILLS TO NEGOTIATE

According to *Webster's Dictionary* (1975), to *negotiate* means "to confer or bargain, one with another, in order to reach an agreement." It is unlikely that you will move through your program design and development process without some **negotiation.** Negotiation does not necessarily mean compromise, and it is important to keep this in mind as we develop our goals and objectives for programming. Our identified need for services and our related goals will continue to remind us of our directive to provide quality programming in ethical ways. If some compromise must occur, it will not be within these dimensions. Shapiro and Jankowski, authors of *The Power of Nice,* put a bit of a spin on *Webster's* definition of negotiation by stating that "The best way to get what you want is to help the other side get what they want" (1998, p. 3). The multilevels of the needs assessment (to be discussed in chapter 6) will give us at least the surface characteristics of what is "wanted" for our targeted population by the community, the organization, or facility for whom we may provide service and then for those who will actually receive the services. Our ability to actively and effectively listen will allow us to identify the more subtle wants that may not necessarily be articulated by either group.

Jay Conger (1998) adds another characteristic of communication to the negotiation mix—the art of **persuasion.** He states that *effective persuasion* "is the ability to present a message in a way that leads others to support it" (p. 25). In our interests, to persuade someone is to first influence and then to convince them to support our ideas and plans for a community program.

Interestingly enough, as we expand our ideas regarding negotiation in the design and development of community programs, we are also talking about the skills that are relevant, even critical, to our clinical relationships with clients/patients. This refers to a therapist's abilities to negotiate the selection of treatment goals with the client/patient, or what in the past we may have referred to as "motivating" the recipient of services. We probably cannot truly *motivate* patients/clients for they must do that for themselves; rather, we negotiate and persuade.

Mattingly and Fleming (1994) provide another window of understanding for this intricate and delicate client/patient-therapist negotiation in what they describe as interactive reasoning, or collaborating with the person. They provide numerous examples of how therapists demonstrate skill in learning to interact with their clients/patients, that is, how they "collaborate." The therapist's ability to interpret what a person wants from therapy and the meaning that person attaches to the progress he or she wishes to make is perhaps the highest level of communication-based negotiation we could identify in our therapy process, and it is significant in our understanding of what Mattingly and Fleming describe as **clinical reasoning.**

LEADING AND MANAGING

All of the previously mentioned skills come together in helping us to identify ourselves as **leaders** and **managers.** We will first examine your present management skills and your potential to become a manager. The first task of good managers is to manage themselves and their own round of daily occupations.

Managing "Yourself" First

Do you currently represent yourself as a model for a healthy balance of occupations? Take a moment to reflect on your response and perhaps those of your classmates or colleagues. In particular, students are likely to say that they do not have

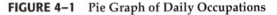

FIGURE 4–1 Pie Graph of Daily Occupations

enough time in the day or week and that they find themselves studying to the exclusion of leisure. Time, of course, is not infinite. It is likely that we do not manage time; rather, time manages us. But we are not victims. If we begin by making a daily, weekly, or monthly *map* of the way we spend our time, then we can learn to manage ourselves within the time we have available. These skills need to be learned as students. If we do not manage to balance our occupations today, it is not likely that we will in the future. It is *time* to begin!

Mapping Time for Our Physiological and Self-Care Needs

Physiology is perhaps the first and the most unrelenting marker when we anticipate carving out meaningful pieces of time for self-care. On a separate piece of paper, using the *pie* in Figure 4–1 to represent the time available to you in a day or a week and using colored markers or pencils to separate work/productive activity, play/leisure, and self-care, draw a slice in the pie to represent the percentage of time you require for sleep. For example, in a 24-hour day, do you require 6 hours, 8 hours, or more hours of sleep to feel your best? Be realistic and focus on balance. Too often students may abuse time by doing everything in excess (that is, studying for days, playing for days, or sleeping for days). Although it may contribute to the "charm" of youth, this is time-binging, and these habits are hard to break.

Now, on the same *pie*, draw a slice to represent the daily time you *require* to eat and the time you spend preparing food for yourself. Even though you may not be in the practice of eating to the exclusion of other tasks, note the time you require in order to feel good. This may be an appropriate place to acknowledge the art of overlapping occupations. For example, we eat, talk on the phone, watch television, communicate with others, and maybe get dressed all at the same time. Is this efficiency? Or is it waste? It probably does not matter; it exists for most of us and must be considered when we examine the ways in which we map our occupations.

Now, in order to attend to what remains of our physiological demands, note a slice for the time you require to go to the bathroom. Consider the time that is left. We have not attempted to define meaning in daily occupations, but this is implicit as we move on with this exercise. What occupations/activities have meaning for you, and what ones do not? It is likely that we feel more balanced when we have a distribution of meaning*ful* and meaning*less* activities in our day. After all, we can-not attend to a totally meaningful existence. We do not have the energy.

Mapping Time for Play/Leisure

What about play/leisure? Is it important to you to play everyday? Do you need that balance? It does not matter what activity you choose to represent play; that will depend on your values and interests and how you establish meaning in your life. Play may mean tossing a ball against a wall or rolling it to your cat; perhaps play means running three miles, engagement in sex, cooking, or another activity of choice. Although it commonly may be considered self-care, taking a bath or a shower uninterrupted is pure leisure for some, particularly for those with small children. If it is important in order for you to feel balanced, then draw in the time you spend doing it. If it is not important, if it does not hold meaning for you, or if you do not consider it true play/leisure, then leave it out of your map under this category. After all, one person's play may be another person's work.

Remember that even though you may not be in control of time, you are in control of how you decide to use it. In other words, you can set priorities. If you decide, for example, that you must obtain an "A" grade in every class even though you are not an "A" student (that is, you have to work so hard that you ignore balance in your life), then that is a priority you have established for yourself. Certainly this is not the result of a simple decision; there are layers of emotional dynamic at work. For instance, your parents may have strongly rewarded good grades, and perhaps you have confused your self-worth with that reward system. But our intention here is to help you develop your abilities to be a manager. Setting priorities is important to that process, so take some time and carefully consider your present priorities. Do they all represent meaning for you?

Mapping Time for Work

Again, it is important to recognize how much overlap plays a part in assigning meaning to occupations. For many people, their work is also their play; and even though to others they appear to work to the exclusion of play, in reality they may feel quite balanced.

Examine your typical day as a student or as a professional. If you are a student, do you spend the whole day in brain-wrenching scholarly endeavor? Maybe you cannot be where you wish to be (certainly classrooms or the workplace may be representative of restrictive environments); but how much time do you spend at work or school talking to friends, daydreaming, or sleeping? So let's realistically put time spent working, studying, and learning in your "pie." The time spent chatting, drinking coffee, and napping in the sun between classes or over lunch goes elsewhere on your time map.

Now take a look at what you have. Is there any activity in which you regularly engage that is missing? Is there anything you deem to be truly meaningful missing? Critically evaluate your map. You probably look more balanced in your daily/weekly occupations than you might have expected, and you probably have some empty space to use as you choose (play, self-care, and/or work). The human animal is fairly self-protective. We are skilled at balancing our occupations even when, at times, we believe ourselves to be balance-impoverished.

Remember this exercise, and complete it whenever you feel stressed regarding your balance of occupation(s). You may need to reexamine your priorities. Priorities change frequently when we are goal directed and as we move from one context to another. Are your priorities appropriate to what you wish to achieve? If so, you likely feel balanced, and you can maintain your health and well-being. If not, you may feel stressed, and it is time to make adjustments.

Now that you have completed the previous exercises, you should have a better sense of your *priorities* and how these priorities influence your personal *balance of occupations*. You have identified your *communication* strengths as well as those areas where you may need to do a little work on your communication skills. You now have a much better grasp of what it means to *manage yourself.*

THE CHARACTERISTICS OF A MANAGER

There are many resources available to you for the fundamentals of management (such as budgets, staffing, billing, and daily operations), and you will find them referenced in several chapters of this text. If you are aspiring to start a community program, then you either must be familiar with all of the expected operations of an occupational therapy department, or you must have access to the services of someone who does. If you are a student, then this book is intended as a supplement to an occupational therapy professional education management and supervision course or courses rather than as a replacement for such courses.

If you are a professional but have not had the opportunity to manage a department or program, then taking the time to closely observe the manager of your place of practice is strongly recommended. Also, if possible, spend time with a mentor who is successfully operating a program such as the one you are contemplating, with the goal of understanding the management of day-to-day operations. Arranging an additional internship or externship in management would be beneficial to students who are seriously considering developing and managing programs. Of course, the intent of a community program is to offer a service or services to a targeted population. The skills involved in delivering an occupation-centered service are implicit in your professional education and any advanced coursework, specialty practice, and/or credentials you may have earned beyond your professional courses and fieldwork.

Of course, management involves managing complex whole *systems* of both things and functions, but often those who are considered to be the best managers are known for their demonstrated abilities in the management of people. In his book *Winning 'Em Over,* Jay Conger (1998) talks about a revolution in management that is occurring in the business world today. This revolution is marked by a shift from a management model strongly anchored in the power of authority and hierarchy to one of persuasion and teamwork. Shapiro and Jankowski (1998) echo these thoughts in their book *The Power of Nice.* If such a shift is actually taking place in the world of business, then we might expect similar shifts in the business of health care. It seems likely that the upper tiers of health care management, the tiers that represent the transition to business and corporate influence, may be struggling with the shift from power-dominated authority to a friendlier model as well. Though these shifts are probably not entirely voluntary, Conger and others would suggest that Generation X is a strong part of the mix, forcing a more interactive management style.

The actual providers of health care—in our discussions, occupational therapy practitioners—have long extended their care-giving styles to blend with their management styles. In recent years, which have been marked by competitive and challenging times in health care, it would seem that many occupational therapy managers have felt apologetic for this more caring, people-centered management style and have aspired to be more authoritative and tougher (what they may have perceived to be more "business" oriented). It is interesting to note, at least according to Conger, that business may now be moving toward a more "people-friendly" model, a management model occupational therapy managers have long demonstrated and probably have developed from their therapeutic *ways of being.*

As mentioned earlier, in his discussions of the "new management," Conger elaborates on persuasion as a central concept for managers in developing relationships with their personnel/teams. He feels that the components of successful persuasion include "Building your credibility; finding the common ground; developing compelling positions and evidence; and connecting emotionally" (1998, pp. 43–46).

We might propose the question, "Who knows more about persuasion than the occupational therapy practitioner?" These concepts are also core to successful therapy, and the core skills we use as therapists are central to our abilities as managers and as leaders. The same is true of teamwork; occupational therapy practitioners have always seen themselves as participants in teams. For the students, working in groups (which is often perceived as never ending) represents the beginnings of the belief in teamwork as the most effective way "to get the job done." Therefore, the profession of occupational therapy has already acknowledged the importance of management by persuasion and teamwork. The goal now must be to solidify and refine these already-acquired professional skills and to avoid the authoritative, more linear model that is generally unresponsive to the needs of today's employee and appears to be rapidly moving toward obsolescence.

THE CHARACTERISTICS OF A LEADER

In his discussion of leadership, Townsend tells us that "leadership is unique to each person" and that in his estimation, "leadership is a matter of character" (Bennis and Townsend, 1995, p. 13). Both Townsend and Bennis delineate the qualities of a good leader to include controlled personal ambition, intelligence, and a clear and well-articulated communication style. Many current writers on leadership and management styles agree with these characteristics, particularly those centered around effective communication (Bennis & Goldsmith, 1997; Capodagli & Jackson, 1999; Conger, 1998; Cook, 1999; Shapiro & Jankowski, 1998). Writing about leadership from an occupational therapy perspective, Gilkeson (1997) describes the successful leader as someone who is unique. Yet she also notes that common traits that all leaders possess are "values, vision, communication skills, persistence, self-confidence, optimism, empathy, and observation" (pp. 3–4).

Drawing a distinction between leaders and managers, Bennis and Goldsmith (1997) note that "managing is about efficiency," and "leadership is about innovating and initiating" (p. 4). In their words, "leaders conquer the context" (p. 4), and the *context* of concern to occupational therapy practitioners—the environment of health care and health maintenance—is most certainly a flying carpet these days; to conquer it (even to remain upright on this uneven terrain), a leader must be agile, visible, and clever.

Can the leader and the manager exist in one person? Perhaps, but it is more likely that the most comprehensive leadership is produced by a team. This team must include a charismatic and visionary leader and managers who are effective and efficient in the understanding and control of multiple systems. The team members must be ethical, loyal to their cause, skilled, and above reproach. Bennis and Goldsmith note that the profound difference between a manager and a leader is that a "good manager does things right and a leader does the right things" (1997, p. 4).

In some circumstances, the development of a community program may pose a risk for the developer. The luxury of taking such a risk alongside a good manager may not be financially realistic. Therefore, the programmer often must acquire the skill sets of both a leader and a manager, at least in the beginning. Certainly the programmer is a leader; starting a new programming venture in the community would not occur to anyone else. But often the skills needed to *manage* the developing program have to be learned. Perhaps the *true* leader, and the *true* manager cannot ever really exist in one person; the personalities, the *ways of being* and the *ways of thinking,* are likely different. The wise leader, though, will certainly appreciate the intricacies of management. If not able to employ a management team early on, he or she will at least consult with one as development occurs.

Early in this chapter we discussed the importance of clear and efficient communication. The first task of the leader is to *sell* himself or herself and the proposed program, which requires the ability to engage others in the venture. Most likely the planner/leader first will need to obtain support for his or her potential program from those outside of occupational therapy. The nature of these early communications may be different from those that will follow. Soon after, though, the planner must engage the support of the team that will be carrying out the programming; the planner must gain the team members' trust and must encourage them to share in the excitement that comes with such an undertaking. The task of the *leader/manager* is first to recognize and then to supervise and manage the knowledge and skills of others in such a way as to form a successful and productive goal-directed team. Whether program personnel are aides, certified occupational therapy assistants, occupational therapists, other professionals, students, or volunteers, the planner's skills as a leader/manager will make the difference in the success of the program. A leader must clearly communicate his or her goals for a program and accompanying expectations for the performance of employees and others. It is also critical that a leader provide honest, direct, and open feedback regarding performance while not losing sight of the larger goals. A successful communicator will be able to provide honest and supportive feedback that will strengthen and empower the employee and the program.

EXERCISE 3
Reinventing Yourself as a Leader

Now that you are on your way to becoming a more effective communicator and you are developing an awareness of what skills are necessary to be an effective manager, you must begin the process of reinventing yourself as a leader. If you consider yourself to be a leader now, look at strengthening your capacities. Young, less experienced leaders are likely to have difficulty in delegating responsibility to a team. Not trusting anyone but yourself to do a job will lead to rapid burnout and, eventually, failure. Learning to delegate wisely is a skill that is initiated when the leader/manager first establishes a goal or goals for the program; from these foundational goals, he or she can then build a multiskilled team. The trust that is established around this team makes the process of delegating responsibilities much less hazardous. Comfort with the process comes with each successful experience.

The following exercise is adapted from Bennis and Goldsmith (1997).

1. What do you personally consider to be the qualities, attitudes, and behaviors of a leader? You may wish to think of those people who are considered to be leaders. List the characteristics below, and beside each one, note your skills and/or attributes in that particular area:

Qualities (for example, personal honesty)	Your Qualities
_____	_____
_____	_____
_____	_____

Attitudes
(for example, open/friendly)

Your Attitudes

_____

_____

_____

Behaviors
(for example, working hard)

Your Behaviors

_____

_____

_____

Carefully assess your strengths with regard to the above. Do you have leadership qualities that will assist you in the development of new occupation-centered programs? You may wish to discuss the results of your personal assessment with others. Most people have trouble identifying their own leadership qualities and tend to minimize their strengths in this area. Your friends, colleagues, and perhaps family may be able to help.

WHAT KNOWLEDGE AND SKILLS WILL I NEED?

We have discussed ways to develop our abilities to communicate clearly and effectively, how to identify daily and weekly time use in prioritizing for occupational balance, and how to recognize and develop the characteristics that make a good leader and manager, but there is one more thing we must do. We must recognize that what we must know (knowledge) and what we must do (skills) are the foundation upon which leadership and management develop; without them we have little about which to communicate. Although we have briefly touched on the importance of meeting the needs of our targeted community population, it is imperative that we avoid soliciting needs and wants that we cannot realistically hope to satisfy. Not only would this be unethical, but also it would be enormously stressful and foolish. Experienced professionals have a good idea of their knowledge base and their skills but often still need to do some *self-assessment* homework with regard to the information and skills necessary to successfully design and develop a community program. This certainly does not mean that if you identify a need in your target population but find yourself lacking in knowledge or skills that you must give up the idea for the program. What it does mean is that you must acquire the knowledge and the skills yourself or that you must engage the services of other professionals, paraprofessionals, or volunteers to help.

Students bring a variety of skills, expertise, and experience to the learning environment, and these skills need to be identified. For students, prior experience and resulting knowledge and skills are the foundation upon which occupational therapy principles, philosophy, and practice will be placed. Unique skills, expertise, and experience oftentimes produce the entrepreneur.

Occupational therapy practitioners as well as students may overestimate or underestimate their expertise and may often fail to anticipate the need for adequate resources. Thus, before you make your initial on-site appointment, complete the following checklist. This exercise will be helpful in achieving a good sense of what you can offer to any potential program, and as you develop your ideas for specific programming, it will help you to identify areas where you may need some assistance.

▰▰▰ EXERCISE 4 ▰▰▰▰▰▰▰

Self-Assessment of Knowledge and Skills Relevant to Designing and Developing Community Programs

1. Assessing What You Know: Your Present Knowledge Base

a. Your academic knowledge base. Consider what you have studied, including your professional occupational therapy education and other disciplines you might have studied previous to or following occupational therapy that you think might assist you in designing, developing, and working in occupation-centered community practice. Highlight your academic knowledge base below:

_____

_____

_____

_____

b. Your experiential knowledge base. Consider any previous or present experience that contributed to your present knowledge base that might assist you in designing, developing, and working in occupation-centered community practice. Such experience might include clinical practice, outcome/evaluation research, sales, managing, interacting with communities, or other areas. Highlight your knowledge gained through experience below:

_____

_____

_____

_____

2. Assessing Your Skills

Consider what you can do. Do you have expertise with particular modalities, tools, equipment, or assessments used in occupational therapy practice or other clinical practices? Consider any particular credentials you may have earned, certifications, or, for the COTA, service competencies. Do you have particular expertise with arts and crafts? A sport? Perhaps music? Do you have any other skills that may not be directly related to clinical practice but that might be useful when working in the community? Remember that we are also interested in prevention and maintenance of health. (*Note: Of course, we know that the above-mentioned skills are interelated with knowledge; but for the purposes of this exercise, we will separate them.*) Highlight any skills you may have below:

_____

_____

_____

_____

In later chapters, when you have selected your target population and have begun to discuss the service needs they may have and the kinds of programming that will help you meet those needs, you will want to revisit the above lists of knowledge and skills from your new perspective.

In conclusion, when you have selected your target population and know its needs, you will

1. Determine the knowledge and skills required to successfully meet the needs of the target population
2. Revisit the knowledge and skills of the planner and others that may be involved in developing the program

The difference between these two items will tell you where you must acquire additional knowledge/skills (if realistic and if time permits) or where you must find others to assist you (such as professionals, paraprofessionals, volunteers, or others).

SUMMARY

To return to our original question, we must ask ourselves, "What do I need to know to develop a community program?" Through the course of this chapter, we have identified the following areas of personal responsibility in preparing the foundation for program development:

1. The development of clear and effective communication styles
2. Knowing how to effectively and actively listen to others
3. Recognizing the responsibility to serve as a role model of occupational balance
4. Knowing how to provide occupation-centered services for our patients/clients/consumers
5. Knowing how to provide leadership
6. Knowing how to manage systems

The above characteristics, which are established on a firm base of professional ethics and personal integrity and sound occupation-centered practice knowledge and skills, will provide a foundation for the continued development of any additional expertise that may be needed to become an insightful and effective planner, leader, and manager. The resulting "package" will not be difficult to market!

REFERENCES

Bennis, W., & Goldsmith, J. (1997). *Learning to lead: A workbook on becoming a leader.* Reading, MA: Addison-Wesley.

Bennis, W., & Slater, P. (1998). *The temporary society.* San Francisco: Jossey-Bass.

Bennis, W., & Townsend, R. (1995). *Reinventing leadership: Strategies to empower the organization.* New York: William Morrow.

Capodagli, B., & Jackson, L. (1999). *The Disney way.* New York: McGraw-Hill.

Conger, J. (1998). *Winning 'em over: A new model for management in the age of persuasion.* New York: Simon and Schuster.

Cook, M. (1999). *Effective coaching.* New York: McGraw-Hill.

Gilkeson, G. (1997). *Occupational therapy leadership: Marketing yourself, your profession, and your organization.* Philadelphia: F. A. Davis.

International Webster new encyclopedic dictionary. (1975). Chicago: The Language Institute of America.

Mattingly, C., & Fleming, M. (1994). *Clinical reasoning: Forms of inquiry in a therapeutic practice.* Philadelphia: F. A. Davis.

Shapiro, R., & Jankowski, M. (1998). *The power of nice: How to negotiate so everyone wins—Especially you.* New York: John Wiley and Sons.

Youngstrom, M. J. (1999). Developing a new occupational therapy program. In K. Jacobs and M. Logigian (Eds.), *Functions of a manager in occupational therapy* (3rd ed., pp. 129–142). Thorofare, NJ: Slack.

CHAPTER 5

Getting Started: Developing "The Idea"

Learning Objectives

1. To explore ideas for occupation-centered programs
2. To discover a variety of avenues for developing programs
3. To learn how to locate a site for your program
4. To identify the purpose of your program and to begin to develop goals and outcomes

Key Terms

1. Program
2. Client/Member
3. Agency/Site
4. Community Profile
5. Target Population
6. Advocacy Groups

Case Example

A successful gardening program could begin something like this: "I love to work outdoors, and I think gardening is very therapeutic, so I'd like to start a gardening program for persons with psychiatric disability who reside in the community, or are homeless . . . . I'd like to staff it myself (an occupational therapist) but maybe would want to include a COTA (certified occupational therapy assistant) and the assistance of retired volunteer gardeners. All would help to raise vegetables, herbs, and flowers for local restaurants, and maybe some-day we would have a restaurant attached to the garden."

Is this a good idea? It appears to be. It is also occupation-centered in every way—for the **client/member,** the volunteers, and eventually the consumer of the product. Thus, we have the *seeds* of a community gardening program.

The community gardening program is the second of several case examples that we will weave through the chapters of this text to help illustrate the process of program design and development. The first case, the Parent-Child Education Program, was introduced in Chapter 3, and we will return to it later.

GETTING STARTED

But just how do we begin establishing an occupation-centered program? We might start by asking why programs are needed in the first place. In reply, we would suggest that a program is responsive to need. **Programs** are designed to clearly focus effort and activity in meeting the needs of an identified group. For us, as occupation-centered practitioners, these needs may be to develop knowledge and to provide information and skills in order to help our clients/patients/members/consumers first identify and then engage in meaningful occupations. These are our areas of expertise.

Ideas for programming are seldom spontaneous. Impetus for new programs come from a number of sources that may include: 1) other occupational therapists, such as the manager of your department (for example, when an outpatient clinic for pain management clients is needed; or a camp for children with learning disabilities); 2) patients and their families (for example, Parkinson's patients and spouses requesting an exercise program that they can enjoy together); or 3) other health care providers/professionals (for example, dentists/orthodontists who wish to help their patients manage temporal-mandibular-joint, or TMJ, pain). Greene and Cantalupa (1996) describe a process involving other professionals and services in their discussion of the development of the occupational therapy programming component of larger programs with psychosocial directives. In addition to the sources listed previously, the changing health care environment itself may be the impetus for ideas (for example, post-surgical hand therapy clinics or cardiac maintenance and wellness programs). Finally, the recognized need to bring together services for clients in a new or more efficient way that is more readily understood and accessed by the community may generate ideas for new programs (for example, child day care and therapeutic programming for children with disabilities coordinated with child day care for siblings). And, certainly, new programs may come as the result of a structured marketing plan originated by the insightful leader/planner.

Meeting parent-child partnership goals while learning about marine science is an example of combining occupations in the design of effective programming.

An example of sources for programming ideas can be seen in the parent-child program first introduced in Chapter 3, which came about as a result of networking with other professionals (teachers and education coordinators) who were familiar with other occupation-centered after-school programs originated by occupational therapy students. The expressed *need* was for some kind of programming that would strengthen parents' involvement in their children's educational pursuits, particularly in science. It was clear that the need was strongly occupation-centered and appropriate to our interests and abilities.

When we come up with ideas ourselves, most often they are based on something that we enjoy or something we think would be fun. The gardening program is a clear example of this kind of motivation. But the interest and accompanying skills motivating the development of a program could just as easily be horseback riding, keeping and caring for pets, arts and crafts, river rafting, scuba diving, or anything else for which we feel a profound affection. We also must harbor a belief in the activity's potential as therapy or as prevention.

As a psychologist, Jolkowski (1998) speaks of utilizing our interests in developing and marketing programs. He encourages the exploration of what he describes as *niche* markets. In his case, he extended his personal interest in music to develop group programming for musicians who were experiencing performance anxiety (1998, p. 5). Occupational therapy practitioners interested in music could develop similar programming but perhaps could target musicians with stress-related hand injuries or *those musicians who wished to prevent hand injuries.* Clearly, an understanding of *occupation* and the *meaning* invested in such an occupation as that practiced by the professional musician would place the occupation-centered practitioner firmly in the marketplace. In the same article, R. Phillips (also a psychologist) found his particular niche in the sport of golf, but the programming was similar in that it targeted performance anxiety (1998, p. 5). Again, for occupation-centered practitioners the niche might be expanded to help golfers avoid or treat golf-induced or golf-related injuries. Personal interest and skill in the *occupation* of golfing must certainly be advantageous in developing such a practice.

As mentioned earlier, a need might be expressed by someone in the community, a family member, or sometimes by a potential client or groups of clients. If we think we can fill that need, the beginnings of a new program may emerge. You could also generate an idea because you recognize what may become a lucrative endeavor, which may be one of the seminal ideas for a private practice; however, alone, it is not enough to design a program that will achieve results.

In summary, ideas for programs may come from the following:

1. Other occupational therapy practitioners
2. Patients/clients and/or their families
3. Other health care providers/professionals
4. The changing health care environment
5. The program developer's interests and skills coupled with a good marketing plan

Program Planning in a Classroom Environment: A Notation

If you are a student, your instructor will likely supply you with a list of community **sites** that have expressed a desire for programs. While these are often obtained by word of mouth, sometimes a letter is sent to community **agencies** explaining the goals and activities of your class and asking if they would like to work with occupational therapists and students. In this scenario, there is a mutual obligation. The agencies will contribute their time and ideas, and you will provide them with a program and a plan to make it happen. If possible, you can also contribute volunteer or independent study hours to get the program up and running, or the Student Occupational Therapy Association may wish to assume some leadership in continuing involvement (however, these opportunities vary from academic program to academic program).

If your program has a faculty clinical practice, perhaps faculty members can offer supervision. It is important that you do not promise the facility or agency something you are unwilling or unable to deliver and that early on you clarify any assumptions the agency may make regarding what you will do or time that you will contribute. You can and should, however, supply the agency or site with a carefully generated and thoughtful plan tailored to its specific needs.

This plan will include the services of an occupational therapist and perhaps one or more occupational therapy assistants and a strong case for why occupation is central to the plan; it is assumed that if the agency implements your ideas and professionals are hired, they will be occupational therapy personnel at some level.

A clear rationale for why occupation and why occupational therapy personnel are central to the plan must be included in all proposals.

Of course, if you are already a practicing occupational therapy professional, then the plan will include your services. If you are developing a plan as a certified occupational therapy assistant, then you should also include arrangements and costs for supervision. Your knowledge, interests, and expertise as occupation-centered practitioners are critical to the plan's success.

In all plans, it is important to keep occupation as the central organizing theme. The plans are designed by occupational therapy practitioners or by students who are aspiring to become practitioners. Each plan offers us the opportunity to describe the power of occupation and opens the door for potential involvement by occupational therapy practitioners. In our enthusiasm, we do not want to lose sight of this message or the potential danger of giving away our plans as student groups. Certainly the well-being of our consumer is of utmost importance to us, but we must be committed to protecting our professional futures as well. Even as students, if your plan is going to be implemented, you should try to stay involved with the program in some ongoing way.

Continuing these plans in the community is also an excellent way for the educational programs of the occupational therapy and the occupational therapy assistant student to become involved in a partnership. These partnerships go beyond academic exercise to "real life," and they are opportunities that students constantly request.

Sometimes in the classroom it is fun to generate ideas for programming without a community site or agency in mind. Although this may be useful as an exercise, the learning experience is enriched by the presence of an actual site/agency for involvement. Much of the significant learning occurs when the students begin the process of communicating and then negotiating with those who expressed the original need.

THE COMMUNITY GARDEN CASE EXAMPLE REVISITED

Let's return to the idea of a community garden for persons with psychiatric disability. What happens next? Even if gardening is not new to our experience, there is still some research to be done. Since community gardening is an idea that has come to fruition in many and varied ways, there are resources available to you. The occupational therapy-managed horticulture program at the Veteran's Administration Medical Center in Brentwood, Los Angeles, referred to as the "garden," is one of the longest running and successful ventures of its kind (Strege, Molina, & Jewell, 1991). Substantial information describing horticulture therapy and the therapeutic aspects of gardening is also available on the Internet. There are also many resources for gardening in general. Regardless of your selected modality, you can further your research at the library or on the Internet. The Internet has made the process of program development much more efficient than it was even a few years ago.

It is also important to note that although our community garden case example was greatly influenced by personal interest in gardening as therapy, it was also facilitated by the concerns of citizens who felt that persons with psychiatric disability (certainly, "idle" and homeless persons with psychiatric disability) present problems for the city. Perhaps this interpretation seems a bit brutal, but there are many and varied motives for the practice of good works, and the astute planner will stay abreast of them, cleverly mobilizing them toward positive outcomes for the clients.

In Chapter 18, we describe some of the characteristics of urban homeless, and we know that persons with psychiatric disability are a large part of this group. The development of programming for this population is challenging, even to the most experienced therapist. Clients are extremely varied in their interests, values, and skills, and it is not easy to find meaningful occupations for them.

The idea of a community garden in our example may be a possible solution. Our task, then, is not only to develop a garden in the community but also to *build a community* around a garden.

WHERE DO YOU LOCATE A GARDENING PROGRAM?

To expand on our case example, the location of the targeted population was an urban, downtown setting. The planning process was initiated by exploring the ways for people to garden in a large city, assuming that they have no property of their own. This exploration can be facilitated by contacting the botanical gardens, the city's Park and Recreation Department, or local nurseries. In some cities community gardens are sponsored by a University Cooperative Extension—Division of Agricultural Sciences. To find a site for your program, you also can

- Contact city or regional agencies for collaborative ventures.
- Contact the Chamber of Commerce, churches, or local businesses.
- Go to the telephone book, the library, and/or the Internet.
- Check notices at the local market.
- Ask people in the community.

Finally, another way to find a site is to simply walk around the neighborhood where you wish to provide your program. This is part of what we describe as developing the **community profile,** or getting to know as much as possible about the community/neighborhood where your program is expected to take place.

If most people reside in apartments or public housing, there is likely some empty lot set aside for a garden or an empty lot that could be developed in that way. Some of the urban garden sites are quite restrictive, and, of course the garden site in our example needed to be where the population to be served was located. It was not likely that the client/members would board a city bus and travel to the garden daily (although once the garden was established, perhaps they would). This ability to navigate the community, in fact, could have been one of the goals for the programming.

As we think about our program participants in this stage of the planning process, we must clarify the rather liberal use of terms we have used to describe them. During our planning process and before they actually become participants, we refer to them as our **target population,** or those we have *targeted* to receive our *services.* When the members of our target population become involved in our program, we may refer to them in several ways. In general, those participants who are not paying for services (that is, community gardeners) prefer to be referred to as *members,* and a club structure designating *membership* may be useful for many types of community programs. Although the term *outpatient* may be used, the more medical term *patient* is less used in community settings. *Client* or *consumer* are the common terms used to designate the participant of services for prevention, maintenance, and general wellness programs. Third-party payers may have a preferred terminology that you will certainly want to use if you are relying on them for reimbursement. Finally, when in doubt, ask the consumers how they prefer to be known. Often it may just be a term such as camper, gardener, or craftsman etc.

AFTER LOCATING THE SITE, WHAT COMES NEXT?
Planning in a Nutshell

If you are planning a gardening program such as the one described, some negotiation will likely occur as you select a site. Of course, early on you will have done your preliminary homework, and you will have drafted a plan for how you will proceed. Although not incorporated in this phase of planning, you may still be entertaining the future possibility of a small restaurant or maybe a vegetable/flower stand to begin. If you have not already located it, you have a good idea what kind of site/location you require (for example, slope, sun, shade, water, accessibility, and so on), how large it should be, and zoning requirements in case you intend to go ahead with plans for a restaurant. You have honed your communication/negotiation skills, you have determined how many client/members you can accommodate, and you have developed a preliminary list for what equipment/supplies will be needed to begin and an estimate of what they will cost. Certainly your supply and equipment list, staffing, and client/member selection will require additional work, but you have done enough to have a sound estimate of costs. Your credibility as a planner likely will be matched to the specificity of these early estimates, so be as accurate as you can be. An experienced planner definitely has an advantage over the beginner in this early stage of the process and will likely be more accurate in determining what will be necessary to begin; however, the novice can usually compensate with a bit more homework and preparation.

You might encounter the scenario, as in our case example, where urban leaders want something done but do not want to spend any money in order to do it. In addition, you might not know how much they will provide until you have presented your proposal. Thus, it would be advisable to identify some potential small, private granting organizations (such as garden clubs or family sponsors of local gardens and parks). These private granting organizations can be delegated to a secondary plan to be identified if you are not able to get the monies you need from your first organization.

Attracting the Volunteers

A significant challenge for a project such as the one we are describing is in attracting the potential client/members to the site to begin the work of gardening and to get the volunteer help that will be needed to develop the program. You have already contacted the local gardening clubs to solicit the assistance of volunteers who have a strong commitment to gardening (this, of course, was included in the draft plan to the city or other decision-making group). Perhaps you also have access to students. Although they might not be gardeners, enthusiasm is an equally strong attribute. Finally, we cannot overlook the fact that the presence of youth and free food have assisted in the marketing of a number of community programs.

While accessing volunteers to supervise the gardening seems simple enough, helping them feel comfortable with your client/member population may not be so easy. You now must market your idea and your targeted population to your volunteers, and you will need to know the needs of both groups. Finding a confidant on the garden club board may help, or perhaps you know someone who has an established relationship with your proposed volunteers. The intention is to utilize any networks you have established in order to help you get started.

First you need to explore any preconceptions your potential volunteers might have regarding persons with psychiatric disability and the homeless. You will need to know how to present factual information so that it will be heard in the most productive way. Reading from the *Diagnostic and Statistical Manual of Mental Disorders* or quoting statistics for how many persons with psychiatric disability who are homeless populate the city will not be convincing. An **advocacy group** can provide a strong incentive to your potential volunteers based on realistic information and an emotional investment. These are groups of persons who *advocate* for a particular group of people—generally people with disabilities and/or those with special needs. Advocates may be persons who are disabled themselves, relatives or friends of these persons, and professionals. You might wish to contact local advocacy organizations such as Parents of Young Adults with Schizophrenia or other advocacy groups with similar interests. Utilize community resources such as Directories of Social Services for your city or county to find the groups that might be best able to assist you.

You may have years of experience working with persons who have chronic psychiatric disability, or you may have little or no experience. But a critical skill in marketing to nonprofessionals is to understand their experience and their views and to not minimize either. The average person knows about mental illness/psychiatric disability from the media or from brief personal encounters with a delusional and hallucinating person living on the streets. Neither image presents all there is to know, but your marketing task is to skillfully distinguish between the realities and the myths. Further, you must provide an incentive that is meaningful to your volunteers. Assuming you accepted this challenge because it has meaning for you, then sharing your commitment to this venture with your volunteers should not be difficult. If you accepted the challenge with little real interest, then it is doubtful that you will be able to mobilize the help you need.

Attracting Your Clients/Members

Once you have your cadre of occupational therapy personnel and motivated volunteers, you can begin recruiting client/members from your targeted population (those persons with psychiatric disability who live in the community or are homeless). You may want to arrange for a van or a truck to literally drive around and encourage people to come with you. If you have homeless shelters or missions in the area (and you probably do), solicit their assistance in providing transportation for your clients/members. If homeless persons with chronic psychiatric disability are indeed a problem for the city, then the police or volunteer police organizations might help bring them to your garden. Another option is to solicit the assistance of churches or other volunteer groups working in the area.

Once your clients/members have arrived, it will be the enthusiasm and caring of your volunteers and the skills of your occupational therapy personnel that will keep them there. It is important that your first group of participants be involved in the actual building of the garden plots and in the initial development of the gardens, for this group will become your future supervisors, perhaps your board members, and your strongest advocates.

Although our case example was designed for an urban area, you can do the same thing in a suburban or rural area. In these locales you might not find a large population of homeless persons with psychiatric disability or adolescents who are delinquent youth offenders, but you can apply a similar concept with other groups

Bringing participants from several programs together to share the carving of the garden "harvest" can meet program goals in fun and creative ways.

who are in need of your services. Gardening on a smaller scale—even in pots—has been very successful in nursing-rehabilitation facilities, in residential facilities for persons who are developmentally delayed, and in numerous school-based facilities.

If we expand our ideas to residential housing for the well-elderly or adults who are developmentally disabled living in the community, then a shared community garden is an excellent way to keep these populations connected to their neighborhoods and to meaningful activity. In addition, grouping client/members of different ages and abilities together with volunteers of different ages and abilities is recommended in an effort to *create community*—something we should facilitate at every opportunity.

Whereas suburban and rural areas often have fewer restrictions on establishing gardens and on selling the produce than urban areas do, finding small granting agencies or donations in these areas may be more difficult than in the city. These are reasonable tradeoffs in many ways, and the opportunities to make the garden a "paying proposition" with the therapeutic rewards of sharing dividends may outweigh the opportunity for donations. However, do not automatically assume that grants and donations are not available in rural areas; start-up monies, in fact, may be there as well.

BEGINNING TO THINK ABOUT TENTATIVE GOALS FOR YOUR PROGRAM

Through our garden example you see how an idea takes shape and grows into a program step by step. Throughout the course of this evolution, it is wise to continue to return to our purpose—the need for our program—and to ask the following questions:

Why is a program needed?
Why this program?
How is it occupation-centered?
How will it have meaning for the client/member?
What do we expect will be the outcomes of the program?

When we begin to define our purpose and think about outcomes (or what we expect will happen), we are beginning to develop the goal or goals that we will use to guide programming. These are early, tentative goals to provide direction as we proceed in the planning process. These goals are not intended to be fully developed, and they are not yet accompanied by measurable objectives—that will come later. For now, they serve to define and structure our *purpose*.

In our community garden case example, the central idea or tentative goal based on what was perceived to be the need was to establish a *community* for homeless persons and others with chronic psychiatric disability in the city. Secondly, another tentative goal was to provide a variety of meaningful choices of occupation for those involved in the program. At this point in the process, these goals are very vague statements, and it might be difficult to write objectives that would be measurable or outcome based. They do, however, define our *purpose,* and they provide a good foundation for the more formal goals and objectives that will follow.

■ EXERCISE 1 ■
Trying Out Your Ideas

Now that you have an understanding of what is involved, try brainstorming some programming ideas of your own. Have some fun with this. At this point, the ideas do not need to be practical, and you do not need to know exactly how you will carry them out. If you are a student, your instructor has likely provided a list of potential sites that may have expressed needs, so start your brainstorming with these in mind. If you are a professional and have an idea, continue to develop it.

1. Write your ideas below:

_____

_____

_____

_____

_____

2. Who is your target population? What special needs does this population have that must be considered in your planning?

In our community garden case example, the population consists of homeless men and women with psychiatric disability, and there is the possibility of children accompanying their parents. In our parent-child case example introduced earlier, the population is comprised of inner-city fourth-grade and fifth-grade boys and girls and their parent (mother, father, or other home-care provider). When we think of "special needs" as occupational therapy students and practitioners, we often think of physically, emotionally, or cognitively disabling conditions. Certainly, these things must be considered in our community work; however, we must also consider the "special needs" prompted by socioeconomic circumstances. The clues to these considerations in our case examples are *homelessness* and *inner-city*. Both of these considerations will require our attention as we address the needs of our case example populations and as we develop their service profiles.

Describe your targeted population and its special needs below:

_____

_____

_____

_____

_____

Will the special needs of this population require specific programming? Adaptations? Other considerations?

_____

_____

_____

_____

_____

Persons who are homeless with psychiatric disabilities not only must deal with the repercussions of their particular illness, but they also must develop their own adaptive survival measures to remain safe and nourished. The adaptive strategies that permit survival on the street must be understood and appreciated by planners in order for community programs to be successful.

The first "special need" noted by the parent-child program planners was, in fact, their own. To be responsive to several of the participants, it was necessary for some of the planners to speak both Spanish and English; the need to translate the written materials into Spanish was also quickly apparent. There were also other concerns prompted by the inner-city public school environment and the multicultural considerations of the children and parents.

3. Have the case examples prompted your consideration of any other needs your targeted population may have that will influence your program planning? If so, note those needs below:

_____

_____

_____

_____

_____

4. If you have identified additional needs, what will they require of you and of your program?

_____

_____

_____

_____

_____

5. Stop and ask yourself the following questions, and note your responses in the space provided.

Why this program?

_____

_____

_____

How is it occupation-centered?

_____

_____

_____

How will it have meaning for the client/member/participant?

_____

_____

_____

What will be the purpose? What do we want the outcomes to be? Remember these are outcomes for the *program*—the collective outcome for all of the participants.

_____

_____

_____

_____

What might be a tentative goal or goals relative to the purpose for *all* participants in your program? What do you want to accomplish for all participants?

_____

_____

_____

_____

Note that with the community garden, we stated that the primary purpose, or tentative goal, was to establish *community* for all of the participants. And for the parent-child program, the primary purpose, or tentative goal, was to build parent-child *teams*.

6. What are your ideas for where the programming that you are proposing might be accomplished? Do you have a community site in mind?

_____

_____

_____

_____

_____

The process of locating a program site may be very different. In our gardening case example, the idea was developed before actually locating the specific population or the site. The program held certain advantages for the city, and in fact, when the plan was proposed, assistance was offered in finding a suitable garden site, without cost, adjacent to an established community garden.

The location of a site for the parent-child program took several turns before resolution. In the early planning stages, where you are now, it seemed obvious that the program should be held at the school. Previous to actually doing the needs assessment, it was believed that the program would be conducted immediately after school and that the children would be joined in one of the classrooms by their parents. This also seemed to be a convenient place and time for the occupational therapy coordinator and students who would be conducting the program. Most of the activities were appropriate to the tables, chairs, and desks of the classroom, so it seemed the perfect place. In fact, much of this early brainstorming was on-target; however, a detailed assessment of need helped the planners to design a program much more appropriate to the concerns of the participants and, therefore, much more successful.

7. Continue your brainstorming by noting some ideas for the following considerations. Remember that these are very early, tentative ideas; however, they will help structure the remainder of the process.

Who might carry out the day-to-day operations?

_____

_____

_____

_____

What equipment/supplies would you need to support the programming you are considering?

_____

_____

_____

8. Have you discovered areas where you will need to conduct more inquiries, do more research, or review previous learning in order to prepare a proposal? If so, in what areas? List them below, and note where you might go for more information.

Unanswered Questions   Possible Resources

_____   _____

_____   _____

_____   _____

_____   _____

_____   _____

9. Have these cursory exercises caused you to alter your initial idea or plan? If so, in what way? Note your response below:

_____

_____

_____

_____

_____

Present your idea or the idea of your working group in a brief proposal to classmates. If you are a professional, present your idea to colleagues or others who could provide constructive feedback. Have their suggestions caused you to alter your initial plan? If so, in what way? (Note: making alterations in your initial plan during the development process is almost always necessary, but it should not mean that you compromise your initial idea.) Note your response below:

_____

_____

_____

_____

_____

If classmates or others found your idea amusing, remember that all great leaders and planners were probably ridiculed at least once! Observers of a young midwestern artist in 1923 struggling to start a film-making business based on a "mouse" must have laughed long and hard; but undoubtedly their grandchildren visited Disneyland and certainly recognized Mickey Mouse (Capodagli and Jackson, 1999). And most told Debbi (Mrs.) Fields that she could never survive "just selling cookies." She now not only survives but also has over 650 domestic locations and 65 international locations in eleven countries (http://www.mrsfields.com/the_story/story-bottom.html).

If your idea is larger than your present abilities, save it for the future. This reveals an important point: Begin now to keep a journal or file of ideas for programs. Many great ideas were probably first recorded on cocktail napkins; the same can hold true for great ideas in occupation-centered programming! Your occupational therapy professors and instructors and your colleagues drop interesting ideas for practice and program development all of the time. Occupational therapy journals and publications frequently highlight entrepreneurial practices, as do the journals and newsletters of other helping professions. An idea does not have to be yours alone to be successful. Consider all of these ideas to be "pearls of programming wisdom," and write them down to stimulate your future program-planning ventures.

In a few years when your practical wisdom and experience match your present creativity, intellect, and enthusiasm, pull out the journal or file and see what interests you. If you are already a practitioner, you probably have lots of ideas; still take the time to organize them in a file, and when you feel the need for a change, page through the file and take a good look around you. You will most likely find opportunities just waiting to be discovered.

SUMMARY

Generating your ideas for programs is the first step in getting your foot in the door. This is followed by careful and detailed planning that might include asking lots of questions and pursuing the answers in the community, in the library, and on the Internet. Learning as much as you can about the needs of your proposed population and brainstorming ideas for why, where, and how the program may be conducted will prepare the way for the detailed work that is to follow.

REFERENCES

Capodagli, B., & Jackson, L. (1999). *The Disney Way.* New York: McGraw-Hill.

Greene, S., & Cantalupa, M. (1996). Program development. In M. Brinson & K. Kannenberg (Eds.), *Mental health service delivery guidelines.* Bethesda, MD: American Occupational Therapy Association.

Jolkowski, M. (1998, October). *Practice Strategies, A Business Guide for Behavioral Healthcare Providers.* Washington, DC: American Association for Marriage and Family Therapy.

Strege, M., Molina, M., & Jewell, J. (1991, August). Vets' gardeners reap a full harvest. *Advance for Occupational Therapists, 5*(31).

Internet Resources

Mrs. Fields Cookie Company:

http://www.mrsfields.com/the_story/story-bottom.html
email: marcelenew@mrsfields.com

Community Gardening:

The American Community Gardening Association provides links to university and college horticultural extension programs; community gardening specific to states and locales, and general community gardening information, including getting started, organizations to assist, and funding. You can contact this association at http://www.communitygarden.org/links/index.html.

Children's gardening and community gardening grants (including opportunities for free seed, tools, plants, garden products, and assistance), ideas, projects, products, books, and manuals:

http://www.hort.vt.edu/human/CGgrants.html
http://www.hort.vt.edu/human/commgrants.html
http://www.hort.vt.edu/human/CGmoreres.html
http://www.hort.vt.edu/human/CGbooks.html

Profiling the Community, Targeting the Population, and Assessing the Need for Services

Learning Objectives

1. To recognize the layers of inquiry necessary to determine what services are needed by a population
2. To learn how to profile a community for information to support the need for services
3. To develop a profile of your selected community
4. To understand the characteristics of the service profile as it is used to support the need for specific targeted population services
5. To develop a service profile for your selected population
6. To explore the options for the needs assessment
7. To conduct a needs assessment for your selected population

Key Terms

1. Assessment of Need/Needs Assessment
2. Community Profile
3. Service Profile
4. Population
5. Condition
6. Context

7. Interview
8. Focus Group
9. Survey

At this early stage of the planning process, we are asking a set of fairly straight-forward questions. These questions were first entertained by the potential planner during the "idea" stage: Are services needed? What kind of services are needed? Are *my* services needed? Walt Disney once said, "You don't build the product for yourself. You need to know what the people want and build it for them" (Capodagli & Jackson, 1999, p. 59). Although he was talking about the design and planning of the first *Disneyland* theme park, this statement by Walt Disney is appropriate to our discussions of need. His statement prompts us, as community program planners, to remember that if we are more responsive to our own personal needs than we are to those of our targeted population, we may have a hard lesson to learn. Sometimes we are so impressed with our idea and so committed to it that it causes us to ignore the results of the assessment of need; sadly, the resulting program does little to serve the population.

There are several *layers of inquiry* necessary to determine what programming services are needed by a population. These layers include knowing the community where you will provide services; knowing the targeted population that will receive services; knowing your own potential for providing services; and if you anticipate working with an agency/facility, knowing what that administration wants for its client/patients and knowing what the client/patients want for themselves. If any of these areas are neglected in the early stages of planning, it is likely that you will not be as successful as you could be.

In summary, layers of inquiry to determine what programming services you will provide are as follows:

1. Know the community where you will provide services.
2. Know the targeted population who will receive services.
3. Know your potential for providing services.
4. Know what services the agency/facility administration wants for the clients/patients.
5. Know what the clients/patients want for themselves.

KNOWING YOUR PERSONAL POTENTIAL FOR PROVIDING SERVICES

In Chapter 4 we discussed ways to ascertain your present foundation of personal and professional knowledge and skills. If you participated in the exercises provided, you have a good sense of what you can offer a potential program. It is important to remember, regardless of where you are in your occupational therapy program of study or in your career, that you *do* possess a considerable amount of both knowledge and skills. Many, if not all, students today have had previous work, family/home, and academic experience. Often these are the experiences that bring a unique perspective to your practice, particularly in the less proscriptive environment of the community. In the context of *community*, we are truly defining and creating a new practice—not only for the community and the population that resides within it or is transitioning through it but also for ourselves as practitioners. Whether or not the particular practice has occurred previously, *this community* coupled with the uniqueness of the programmer sculpts a totally new *practice* that cannot be duplicated in other settings.

PROFILING THE COMMUNITY

As discussed earlier in this text, *community* is a complex concept and one that the potential programmer must explore at many levels. By examining one level at a time, we will investigate the community broadly to create a description of what factors exist that may impact our developing plans. We are referring to this description or brief picture as the **community profile.** In creating this profile, the Aspen Reference Group suggests that the planner contribute equal attention to both the community demographics (that is, age, sex, ethnicity, education, and so on) and to the social demographics, or those community social and medical services that presently exist as well as those that are lacking (DiLima & Schust, 1997, pp. 73–74). The addition of social demographics will not only help the planner know if his or her services are needed, but it will also help the planner know what services are needed to complement those that may already exist. Forming complementary services to those that are presently being provided is often the most successful way to enter a community.

Youngstrom (1999) offers suggestions for identifying service needs that are appropriate for the experienced professional who may have expertise to offer and who is looking for a community where this expertise will be most needed (that is, establishing a private practice). Youngstrom recommends that the following questions be used to structure the early planning process, or what we are describing as the community and service profiles (1999, pp. 197–198):

1. What is the event of the given problem? or How often does it occur?
2. How many individuals does it affect?
3. How frequently does it occur?
4. Is it expected to increase? (that is, identification of trends)
5. How and to what degree is the problem being addressed currently within the community? Who is addressing it?
6. What are the factors that contribute to or sustain the problem?
7. Will your proposed program address one or more of the contributing factors?

Collecting demographics that include service dimensions for the community will help us to determine if our proposed programming presently is being offered; with further investigation we could know if additional services are warranted, perhaps with alternative methods of delivery. The sum of all of the observations and

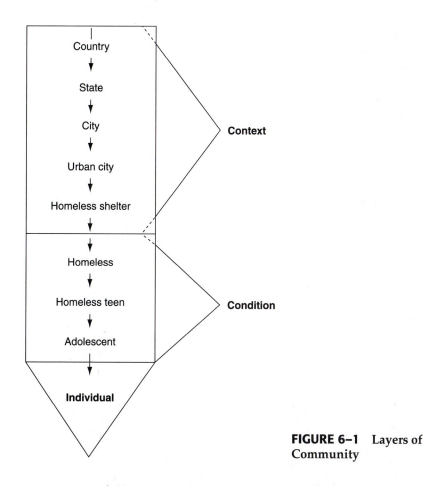

FIGURE 6–1   Layers of Community

research we conduct will result in a description, or profile, of the community or communities where our targeted **population** resides and engages in occupation (and the community, if different, where we will provide services).

In many instances the programmer may feel some familiarity with the larger community. Perhaps, for example, he or she has lived in the community such as suburban Denver, Colorado, for some time. But if programming is being considered in a downtown Denver sanctuary for runaway teenagers that may be frequenting Laramer Square, then the programmer must explore and understand the specific *community*—in our example, *downtown urban Denver*. The next level to be considered is the community of the homeless in urban Denver and the community of runaway homeless teens which is perhaps similar in some ways but likely very different in other ways. Of course, communities are made up of individuals. Each homeless teen in our example brings with him or her the remnants of the cultures and communities from which the teen may have recently sought exit. These multilayers of *community* always exist and must be explored and understood in order to define and develop the most effective programming possible (see Figure 6–1).

DEVELOPING THE PROFILE OF YOUR SELECTED COMMUNITY

Before you make your first visit to the site where you will develop your occupation-centered community program, locate it on a map. Mapping will provide you with a sense of where your selected community is located with respect to adjacent communities. The location of landmarks, public buildings, and public services will be useful information as you begin to develop specific objectives for the program. As you develop your program, you may find that you will rely heavily on public services; if this is the case, you will want to obtain more specific and detailed maps such as those of transportation networks and public services. Determining the boundaries of ethnic neighborhoods and accompanying services adjacent to your selected community may be useful information. While these boundaries sometimes are fluid, permitting easy passage of persons and things from one neighborhood or community to another, they also can be fixed by language, social custom, and culture. Either circumstance may affect your targeted population and the range of services your program will provide.

For most of our program designs and plans, we will seek the support of an agency/facility in order to assist us with our work. This does not preclude the possibility that programs can develop without such agency/facility support or sanction (that is, private practices). However, it is strongly recommended that student learning experiences be structured to include work with an agency/facility. Once you have mapped the location of your agency and the neighborhood/community, it is time to collect some demographical information. Census data is often the place to begin to establish a foundation for understanding the community.

When you have enough information to develop a brief profile of your identified community, it is time for a visit in order to match what you have learned with what you can observe. This is sometimes done enroute to your first on-site appointment, but you can also explore the area before you schedule the appointment to begin the process of determining the programming needs. Either way, this first visit will permit you to make some useful observations and to ask yourself some questions pertinent to your program design and development. As you begin to explore the community, you might ask yourself the following questions:

What is the standard mode of housing?
Are there playgrounds, parks, and recreation facilities?
Are there adults and children on the streets? If so, what are they doing?
Are police visible?
Are there as many churches and schools as there are liquor stores and
    convenience stores?
Is there graffiti, including gang signs?
Do these observations match the statistical information I have gathered?

When you arrive at the site for your first appointment with the administrator or another professional, you have already gleaned substantial information from your demographical research and these early observations. You will have established the foundation for any questions you will wish to ask in order to center your targeted population in the community. It is important to remember that sometimes the population to be served by a program may live in a completely different community or many different communities. This is an important question to ask, and the answer might prompt you to extend your community profile to other communities in addition to the one where services will be located.

Your observations might also prompt the need for community information beyond what you have collected previously. In addition to census bureau data, you might wish to examine national and local marketing and survey data; government documents, reports, and statistics; or data from other agencies. Your collected information may include ranges of income, the incidence of single-parent families, employment, education, religion, ethnicity, crime and police statistics, and other information of specific interest to you as you develop your ideas for programming. Many times the facility/agency can provide you with some of this information since it is often used to justify funding for programs and, in fact, might justify the funding for the one you are proposing. You might also want to consider community newspapers, newsletters, or posted materials describing local interests and events. Items posted on a town hall or grocery store bulletin board can tell you a great deal about the community.

Considering the information provided to structure the dimensions of a community profile; think about how you will develop the profile of the community or communities where your anticipated population resides as well as where the agency/facility is located. As suggested earlier, begin by locating the agency/facility on a map; in the following exercise, note any generic information the map might provide, such as landmarks, public facilities, and so on. Also determine what route you might wish to take when you make your first visit to the site. Locate a route that will provide you with optimal observational information to assist you as you develop your profile. Even if you are already familiar with the location, locate it on a map to visually center it with regard to surrounding communities.

EXERCISE 1
Initiating the Profile of Your Selected Community

1. Using a highlighter, draw what you presently perceive to be the boundaries of your selected community on a map. Note surrounding communities, locations of freeways, and other points of interest.

2. Record below any information you are able to glean from your map review, including landmarks and public facilities (libraries, parks, and so on). If you are already familiar with the location, use what you know to supplement the map review.

_____

_____

_____

_____

3. Develop a brief profile of the community you have selected using demographic information from the census bureau or other resources of your choice. This profile should provide you with a foundation from which you can extend your research as you continue to investigate the community. Record your responses in the space provided.

    a. Socioeconomic data:

_____

_____

_____

    b. Level of education:

_____

_____

_____

    c. Nature of family households (that is, single-parent, extended, and so on):

_____

_____

_____

    d. Ethnicity and religion:

_____

_____

_____

    e. Other data you may wish to collect:

_____

_____

_____

PROFILING OUR ANTICIPATED SERVICES

As students, when you are preparing to select an agency/facility for which you wish to design and plan a community program, you are informed of the population that agency serves. Experienced therapists most often wish to expand or extend programming within their area of experience and expertise (that is, public school therapists may wish to extend programming to after-school or day camps; acute care therapists may wish to develop outpatient services). In these examples the therapist may wish to solicit the assistance of an agency/facility with which he or she is already affiliated. In many instances, the therapist may seek referrals from other agencies as well. In expanding or extending services, conducting an investigation of the services already available, as mentioned earlier, would be important.

It is also important to remember that seeking support *from* an agency/facility is a different relationship than one where a program is developed *for* an agency/facility. The latter circumstance is suggested as a good first student experience. Of course, students may not have had sufficient experience to develop expertise with a particular population, as we might expect from a practicing therapist. However, selecting a population on the basis of interest and sometimes previous experience in a different context is an equally valid way to begin programming.

Although the potential population cannot be fully explored and understood outside of the context of the specific community, we can and should carefully research both before developing an interview format and instrument to facilitate the specific assessment of needs. As we have suggested with the early development of the community profile, it is best to begin with a map or maps. By gathering necessary demographic data we can also "map" our expected population by finding out all we can about it before going on site. With some preliminary information about the community and about the expected population, we will be prepared to ask the most useful and focused questions when we first meet the administrator or professional who will contribute to the needs assessment.

To return to our earlier case example, at the core of the potential program in downtown Denver and composing one level of community is the *adolescent.* Our first challenge will be to understand the developmental characteristics of adolescence. Only later, after reviewing what we know of adolescents, do we consider the needs imposed by the complex layers of community. In our example, homelessness may be the next characteristic to investigate. Homeless, runaway teens may or may not be the same homeless, runaway teen in New York City, Denver, Las Vegas, or Los Angeles. While knowing something about one community will likely tell us something about the others, it will not tell us everything. We may know statistically that, nationwide, runaway teens are likely to have attempted suicide, have been abused, and are addicted to drugs and/or alcohol (see Chapters 18 to 20). But those characteristics may or may not be present to the same degree in every community of runaway teens. To continue our understanding we must learn something about shelters, sanctuaries, and transitional centers. These settings may provide the context for programming and are, in themselves, yet another layer of community. This community is sometimes self-selected by the homeless teen; but often it is imposed by social services or the police. Therefore, the population of one shelter-community may represent programming needs differing from another based on whether it was chosen by the teen or ascribed by authorities.

As you can see from the previous example, before even going to a specific site, we have at least three or more areas to research if we anticipate program development to meet the needs of homeless teens. We must develop a profile of the population—in our example, *adolescence.* We must learn all we can about the **condition** of *homelessness* and particularly about homelessness during adolescence. We have also mentioned the conditions of substance abuse and abuse by others. Learning what we can about these conditions will further strengthen our profile. We must also investigate the **context** for services: *shelters, sanctuaries,* and *transitional centers.* The sum of this information will provide us with the profile of anticipated community-based services for this population, our **service profile.**

Population, condition, and context = service profile

We know that the population cannot be fully explored and understood outside the context of the specific community. But we also know that the above information will be adequate to assist us as we prepare more targeted questions to ask when we go on-site to first visit with those persons (administrators or other professionals and service providers) who will assist us as we continue to develop our program design. We have mentioned credibility as one of the prerequisites for developing a successful working relationship with the agency, or others who may assist us. A carefully researched and insightfully written community profile and anticipated service profile will go a long way to establish your credibility. If your anticipated population is one with disability then you must include the disability in your research of conditions. Remember that we are developing a service profile for the population which is simply a place to begin. Certainly not all adolescents, or all adolescents who are homeless, or all adolescents who are substance abusers exhibit the same individual profiles, nor do they have the same needs. However, they have many characteristics in common, and those are what we hope to identify with this early research. Later we will determine where the needs of our specific population may differ from the general population.

It may be useful to mention that the experienced therapist who is considering developing a new program but is not yet ready to target a specific site may wish to postpone the community profile, first observing and researching service populations similar to what is anticipated. The community selected for observation of the population may be different from the one where programming will eventually be developed, but there is useful information to be gained. By understanding the general needs, of the population—developmentally, clinically, and socially—you can then develop the community profile when the site has been selected. You will know the parameters of your profiles, and you will know how your knowledge base and skills are matched to what the anticipated need will be. You will also have a much more realistic idea of the resources that will be needed whether you gain the expertise to supply these or you glean them from the community.

EXERCISE 2
Developing the Service Profile

The following are examples of populations for whom occupation-centered community-based programs have been designed; use them to practice identifying the population, the condition(s), and the context to develop a service profile.

Population, Condition, and Context:

1. Junior high school adolescent girls between the ages of twelve and fifteen who are pregnant or raising an infant while attending school
2. Well-elderly men and women between the ages of 65 and 94 who are living in a low- to moderate-income inner-city transitional apartment complex
3. Young adults with low vision who are living at home and working in the community

1. Discuss the above examples with your instructor, other students, or colleagues. Organize the information provided for each of the above examples into the following categories:

The population:

a. _____

_____

b. _____

_____

c. _____

_____

The condition(s):

a. _____

_____

b. _____

_____

c. _____

_____

The context:

a. _____

_____

b. _____

_____

c. _____

_____

Developing the Service Profile for the Population *You* Have Selected

2. Review all of the information you have for the agency/facility you have selected and the population it serves. Provide a brief but comprehensive description below (as was done in the previous example):

_____

_____

_____

_____

Discuss your description, and with the help of your student group or colleagues, separate out and delineate the following categories as you did in the previous examples:

Population:

_____

_____

_____

Condition(s):

_____

_____

_____

Context:

_____

_____

_____

When you have completed the above exercise, you have the anticipated service profile for the population you have selected. With this profile, you are now ready to research your textbooks, library, and Internet resources to learn as much as you can about 1) the population, 2) the conditions expressed and experienced by this population, and 3) the context in which services will likely be conducted. You will have generated enough information with this recent research and the preliminary community profile to begin a program-development file for this specific program. You can index the file in the same way the chapters of this text are organized, or you can develop your own system. By the end of the process, you will have collected a substantial amount of information and resources from which you will develop your formal program proposal.

When you have completed the research to further develop the anticipated service profile, you are ready to develop the formal needs assessment. The results of the needs assessment will help us identify areas where we may wish to do further research to enhance the accuracy of what will become our specific service profile and to complete the data collection for the community profile.

THE NEEDS ASSESSMENT: PHASE I

The earlier preliminary work we have accomplished to develop our community profile and the profile or our anticipated services sets the foundation for what we are beginning to define as the needs of this particular population in this particular community. But up until now we havebeen working primarily demographic quantitative data collected by others and with some qualitative generalizations formed through our observations. Perhaps we also have had brief conversations during an early, informal community visit. For example, from our preliminary research into the demographics of the community we might know that there is a certain number of adolescent girls with infants living in their single mother's households, and we might know that these girls did not finish high school. We might also know that pregnancy prevention, parenting classes, or other such services for these girls is nonexistent (or exists but appears to be ineffective). Perhaps we also have talked informally with a school counselor, a minister, or a teacher who confirms some of this data.

But at this point in our inquiries, we have not formally asked other professionals in the community what kinds of services are needed for these girls and their families, and we have not asked the girls or their families what kinds of services they need (such as for education, skill building, prevention, remediation, and so on).

In short, we still must formally or specifically assess or define the needs of our community population. In other words, we now must conduct the formal **needs assessment.** Generally the formal process of assessing the need for services is done in two phases. Phase I assesses the needs of the targeted population from those who may be involved with them at some level; Phase II assesses the perceived needs from those of the target population themselves. Those assessed in Phase I might include other health care professionals, teachers, counselors, police, parents, spouses, and caregivers. If we are working with an agency, the first phase of the needs assessment is initiated with the professional(s) at the site (the facility, institution, or agency). For the above example, this may be the principal or the counselor at the school. Or if we know that there is a community agency already providing services to meet the needs of this population, we may go directly to the agency. We have indicated that it is advisable to be as familiar as possible with the demographics of the community and with the proposed population before going on-site. From this information, you will develop the structure of this first **interview** with the agency representative(s).

If you are a student, this visit begins with your self-introduction (or the introduction of your group). This interview also includes the purpose of your visit and sometimes includes an explanation of the parameters of your assignment and explanations of occupation-centered practice. Much of this will depend on how your instructor elects to structure the experience. Although this chapter focuses on *need* as the starting place for program development, it is worth mention that our assessment of need often becomes complicated by *want*. It is important to clearly distinguish between the two. We certainly do wish to help the agency/facility achieve its needs; however, at the level of the clients/patients, we not only wish to address their needs but their wants as well. It is through our ability to meet needs and wants that we are able to offer programs that our target population find meaningful. If programing is not meaningful to our client/patient, there cannot be successful goal development or positive outcomes.

Our first interview is semistructured; it often begins appropriately conversational and consists of a discussion centered around the following core set of questions (the interview questionnaire) we have developed:

1. What is the purpose (that is, the mission and philosophy) of your organization?
2. What group of individuals (that is, your targeted population and others served by this organization) do you serve?
3. What are some of the characteristics (that is, their ages, abilities, and so on) of this population?
4. What kinds of programming (that is, treatment, prevention, group, individuals, and so on) do you presently offer?
5. Are there unmet programming needs (from the perspective of the interviewee) that you, as an occupation-centered practitioner, might be able to consider?

We describe this interview format as conversational because we will find that the interviewee's responses to our core questions will often prompt other questions. This is also your opportunity to introduce information you have collected from your earlier work developing the foundational community and service profiles. The interviewee can validate and perhaps dispute your information and may direct you elsewhere for more research. Although you or members of your group will ask the questions, it is very appropriate to note the responses under each question and for all members of the group to do this. In these interviews it is expected that you take notes, and if all members present do so, you are not likely to miss important information.

When you have completed this interview, you can use the answers to your interview questionnaire to check the accuracy and scope of your preliminary community and service profiles. Based on the information you have received, you might find that you do not need all of the information you have collected to form a comprehensive picture of the population identified by the agency. To this end, you might want to synthesize from the earlier work information specific to the group where needs have been identified by the representatives of the agency/facility. Even if it is not presently needed, retain all of the demographic and observational information you have collected for future options such as the extension of services or alterations in the way services are provided.

THE NEEDS ASSESSMENT: PHASE II

There are several methods used to assess the need for services; we already mentioned one of these—the *interview*—in our discussion of Phase I. When this method is used in conducting formal research to obtain quantitative data, the interview instrument (the interview questionnaire) establishes a prescribed, structured set of questions that is given to each participant. There are no open-ended questions. The interview format we have described for use with the agency/facility or other community service providers is not entirely true to the above definition. We are using a structured set of questions we want interviewees to answer, but we are also hoping to generate more questions. We can appropriately call this approach a semistructured interview, which is more characteristic of qualitative research methods where in-depth interviews are conducted via probing and open-ended questions. This would seem to fit our more conversational open-ended exchange. Our interest in having a core set of questions answered and perhaps generating more questions makes this method very appropriate for Phase I of our needs assessment.

If we decide to again use an interview questionnaire when we prepare our second set of questions targeting the specific needs of the population for whom we wish to develop programming, it is likely that it will not be as open ended as the first one prepared for the agency or other care providers. We use the results of the first interview to prepare the second interview questionnaire, which is more focused and contains fewer, if any, open-ended questions.

Also very appropriate to assessing the need for community-based programs is a **focus group.** A focus group may be used in Phase I, Phase II, or both. Although a focus group typically is a fairly small group (usually six to ten members), the group can consist of up to approximately thirty members when there are several planners conducting the group. With several planners, one or more may take notes, or one of the group members might be asked to record on a flip chart. If the group agrees, audiotaping is a good way to capture all of the discussion. Members do not usually know each other but probably share some common characteristics that relate to the focus of the group. For successful outcomes, Dumka and Michaels (1998) recommend careful consideration to seemingly simple things such as a convenient and comfortable location and a convenient time. The group *focuses* on a set of questions provided by the facilitator (planner). Like an open-ended interview, the intent is not only to get questions answered but also to generate questions. When used as a Phase I assessment, the planner guides a group of interested community members (such as professionals and service providers) through increasingly focused issues related to the core set of questions or concerns and utilizes the same process for a Phase II assessment with potential clients/patients/members. When used as a Phase II assessment, the questions prepared for the focus group will likely have been generated from previous Phase I interviews; in some cases, the process of formalized needs assessment may begin with this group. Generally the focus group generates diverse ideas and allows members to influence each other by listening and responding to the ideas presented in the discussion. A successful focus group experience can result in a developing network of support for the program.

DiLima and Schust (1997) recommend the use of a focus group when we wish to find answers to the complicated issues of health beliefs and behaviors, barriers to health care, and cultural influences on care. These issues often make the difference in the success or failure of a community program. Using members of such a focus group for a continuing Advisory Council or developing new focus groups during programming can assist in finding answers to programming questions in an efficient and effective manner.

In some cases, when the use of interviews or focus groups is not practical (for example, the population may be quite large or is not readily accessible, or respondent anonymity is desired), a **survey** may be the preferred instrument. A survey is most often conducted via a questionnaire that is distributed on-site or by mail. Its intent, of course, is to collect information from a sample of the population. In our case, we wish to collect information with regard to the community programming services people may need and want. As in the other methods described, our sample, or those we wish to survey, will be selected from our initial target population.

Our survey questions are developed around the initial identification of need provided by the facility, but they are now developed toward the specific sampling of our proposed population. For those wishing to know more about the sampling method, Fink and Kosecoff (1985) and Fowler (1993) offer an in-depth exploration of survey design and development.

Thus, methods that can be utilized in assessing the need for community-centered services include:

1. Structured or semistructured interviews
2. Focus groups
3. Surveys

All of the aforementioned methods are appropriate for the student programmer as well as the experienced therapist. Depending on the characteristics of the population and the nature of service provision, there are additional mechanisms for obtaining data related to needs.

For example, never neglect information that has already been collected, *assuming permission to review can be obtained.* We have already discussed ways to access demographic data but there are other existing data banks that may provide programmers with useful information. Medical charts, institutional survey results, quality-assurance studies, end-of-year reports, and other such institutional information are all examples of existing data banks that may be useful to support the need for occupation-centered services. Local and regional regulatory agencies collect and maintain information on items such as indicators of health status, which may also be useful to preliminary programming work. Collection of data may vary from one region to another, but reviewing what is available in your area is well worth the time.

Remember that the questions designed to structure the needs assessment are prepared within the parameters of the therapist's expertise or that of previously considered resources (that is, other persons, instructional aids, or further training within a realistic time frame). In many cases one round of Phase II assessment following the first interview with the agency/facility or others may be all that is necessary; however, Phase II most often is a process involving several formats, each one more specific and more targeted. For example, following the review of survey results, the planner may wish to conduct focus groups or interviews. It is not uncommon that need may continue to be assessed while the programming is being conducted. For example, ongoing information regarding needs and wants may be gleaned from the care provider, patient, parent, child, social service worker, house manager, vocational counselor, and, perhaps others who are in contact with the population for whom you are providing services. This continuing assessment of need may be included in program evaluation if the programmer asks the clients/patients/members and perhaps others questions regarding satisfaction with services and what additional services they might need.

You will use the results of the needs assessment to guide the establishment of goals and objectives for programming. It is important to remember that the needs assessment *guides* the services that will be provided but does not establish them. The establishment of programming will require substantial negotiation between everyone involved in the process. For example, the needs identified in Phase I and those identified in Phase II may be in disagreement, or the needs as they are identified may be outside the purview of the programmer. It is the task of the programmer to ensure that once negotiations end, he or she has crafted a program that represents the needs of all of those concerned.

In summary, the following are steps to identifying the needs of your targeted population:

1. Develop the community profile
2. Develop the service profile
3. Conduct the first phase of the needs assessment (interview the agency/facility director or others involved with the target population)
4. Conduct the second phase of the needs assessment (select a methodology and obtain the needs as identified by your target population)

EXERCISE 3

Developing the Needs Assessment
Phase I of the Needs Assessment

Develop the specific questions you will ask in your initial interview according to the parameters recommended earlier: What is the purpose of your organization (mission and philosophy)? Who do you serve? What are the characteristics of your service population? What services do you presently offer? Are there any unmet needs?

1. Based on what you have learned while developing your community and service profiles, write below the questions you will ask when you have your first

interview with the representative(s) of the facility/agency where you expect to develop your program. Your questions will provide a structure so that you do not forget anything you wish to know, but they may be altered as you move through the interview.

Drawing from our previous case example, the work accomplished in developing the community and service profiles for the homeless adolescents in Denver might prompt the following question to the director of a sanctuary:

I see from your mission statement (hanging on the wall when you entered the building) that you provide free meals, a shower, and a bed in a safe environment for adolescents who are homeless. Are there other services you provide as well?

The answer will satisfy several of your questions and will likely prompt the director to think about other things he or she does or wishes to do at the sanctuary.

Draft the questions you will ask below:

_____

_____

_____

_____

_____

2. Are there others you would like to interview as part of your Phase I assessment? Note below who they might be and what questions you would like to ask them:

_____

_____

_____

_____

_____

_____

3. Following your first interview, are there persons you would like to add to the above list? Any you wish to delete? Will you need to alter your questions? If so, note the changes below:

_____

_____

_____

_____

_____

_____

_____

4. Following your first interview, review the answers to the questions you listed previously. Are there any areas you will need to research further before developing your Phase II assessment? If so, note them below:

_____

_____

_____

_____

5. What did the director identify as an unmet need or needs?

The mission of the sanctuary for homeless adolescents identifies the purpose of the sanctuary to be the satisfaction of what Maslow (1970) would describe as basic biological needs—physiological needs and safety. In keeping with this purpose and the characteristics of the population (adolescents), the director might identify an unmet need of programming for "safe sex."

Note below any unmet needs that were identified during your interview:

_____

_____

_____

_____

6. Review all of the information you have to date, including the results of any additional research or interviews you may have conducted. Discuss the unmet needs that have been identified during your Phase I assessment process. Ask the following questions.

a. Are the identified unmet need(s) appropriate for occupation-centered programming? Why or why not? If you said no, you might need to return to your definitions of *occupation*; they may be too limiting. Note your responses below:

_____

_____

_____

_____

"Safe sex" was identified above as an unmet need for our community of adolescents. Is sexuality occupation, and is it, therefore, appropriate to our interests as occupation-centered programmers? To help answer this question, we might turn to occupational science. The activities and behaviors associated with sexual expression lend themselves to the three major research orientations of occupational science as described by Clark, Wood, and Larson (1998). These activities and behaviors exhibit directly observable aspects of occupation (form); collectively they serve adaptation (function), and they provide significance within the context of the adolescent's life and in the culture (meaning).

If we use the parameters of form, function, and meaning to understand the occupational patterns of developing sexuality in our population, and if we further use them to consider the multiple expressions of sexuality as adaptive responses to the potentially dangerous context of homelessness, we have the scaffold on which to build a significantly meaningful program. If we add to this developing theoretical construct what we know of the adolescent's developmental "window" for cognition, emotion, and morality, we further strengthen the potential for a successful program (Austin, 1995; Cronk, 1992; Garsee and Schuster, 1992; Schuster, Cronk, and Reno, 1992). For the creative occupation-centered programmer, meeting the need for "safe sex" is more than displaying a basket of condoms and a few pamphlets. This seemingly simple need might open a door to multiple programming objectives.

▰▰▰ EXERCISE 4 ▰▰▰
Phase II of the Needs Assessment

1. Review the recommended methods for assessing the needs expressed by your targeted population. Match these methods to what you know about the population. Discuss the pros and cons of structured or semistructured interviews, focus groups, or surveys. You might wish to review the references at the end of this chapter or other sources for additional information.

Select the method you wish to use, and begin to develop the instrument. Remember that you begin with the needs that were identified in Phase I (assuming that these were acceptable to you and that you have the knowledge and skills to provide programming to meet them). Also remember that during all phases of assessment, you can negotiate.

In our "safe sex" example, a focus group might be successful with our population of adolescents, particularly if it could be organized at the time of a meal served by the sanctuary. Group process might diffuse some of the suspiciousness that individual interviews would likely prompt. A survey could be tried to supplement the focus group, but it is not likely that this population would fill out even a brief survey unless a substantial reward were offered for doing so. Occasionally rewards (such as food, movie tickets, or concert tickets) are given to solicit cooperation in the types of programs we are suggesting, but if true need is defined, then this should not be necessary.

The first question or questions for our focus group would be designed to determine if the group supported the Phase I identified need for "safe sex." As the answers to this question or questions emerged, we would then develop further questions to identify what sexual behaviors are being practiced and what this population means by "safe sex." If new needs are introduced in the discussion and we feel we could design programming to meet those needs as well, we would take note of them and bring them back to those first interviewed in Phase I to see if there is consensus. This process is what we described as *negotiation*. In many ways we are the arbitrator/negotiator between the agency and our targeted population. We must meet the needs of both in order to receive the cooperation and support that we will need to offer the program.

    a. Note below the method you will use to conduct your phase II needs assessment:

_____

_____

_____

    b. Draft the questions you would like answered to support the identified Phase I needs. The nature of your questions will likely be different depending on whether you wish to use an interview questionnaire, a focus group, or a survey. You might also wish to offer some programming options based on Phase I needs, particularly if you use a survey instrument. Chapter 18 offers an example of a Phase II survey that defines what kinds of programming the respondent can expect.

_____

_____

_____

_____

    When you have your draft of questions, develop your final instrument.

c. When you have field tested your instrument, discuss the responses with your instructor, your group, or colleagues. Do you have the answers you need to develop one or two goals for your program and related objectives? Do you need to draft another instrument or try a different methodology? It is often the case that you will need to assess your population again for more focused questions. If you have what you need to begin the design of the program, you can always return later with more rounds of focused questions (such as where and when would you like the programming to be conducted).

SUMMARY

In this chapter we discussed the multiple layers of inquiry that must be conducted in order to design and develop a community-based occupation-centered program that meets the needs of our targeted population. Our first layer of inquiry resulted in the development of a community profile. We explored the demographics of our community and matched this information to our on-site observations. To our community profile we added the profile of our targeted service population. This service profile represented the characteristics of our targeted population through our understanding of conditions and context.

The next layer of inquiry was represented by the Phase I assessment of need. This needs assessment was conducted through a semistructured interview with a representative of the agency/facility where we would access our targeted population. Through this interview and perhaps others, we would determine what services the agency/facility already provided and what the agency/facility considered to be needs still unmet for our targeted population. We then would evaluate the expressed need for appropriateness with occupation-centered programming, and we would evaluate our skills and expertise to determine if we could realistically meet the need as expressed. We would also determine the accuracy of our earlier work and what areas we might need to further research.

Using the Phase I results, we then determine the methodology we wish to use to assess the needs as expressed by the targeted population (Phase II). An instrument format appropriate to the methodology is selected, and questions are developed to determine if the targeted population supports the needs expressed by the Phase I respondents. Depending on the responses of the targeted population, we may then return to those we questioned in Phase I and begin the process of negotiation between the two groups. We may find it necessary to return to the targeted population with more specific questions with regard to how the program will be implemented, and we likely will continue our processes of assessing unmet need throughout the program via our program-evaluation procedures. When we are comfortable that we have identified the needs for which we will develop programming, we are ready to draft our goals and objectives.

REFERENCES

Austin, E. W. (1995). Reaching young audiences: Developmental considerations in designing health messages. In R. Parrott & E. Maibach (Eds.), *Designing health messages: Approaches from communication theory and public health practice* (pp. 114–143). Thousand Oaks, CA: Sage.

Capodagli, B., & Jackson, L. (1999). *The Disney way.* New York: McGraw-Hill.

Clark, F., Wood, W., & Larson, E. (1998). Occupational science: Occupational therapy's legacy for the 21st century. In M. Neistadt and E. Crepeau (Eds.), *Willard and Spackman's occupational therapy* (pp. 13–21). Philadelphia: Lippincott-Raven.

Cronk, R. (1992). Cognitive development during adolescence. In C. Schuster and S. Ashburn (Eds.), *The process of human development: A holistic life-span approach* (pp. 513–531). Philadelphia: Lippincott.

Dignan, M., & Carr, P. (1992). *Program planning for health education and promotion.* Philadelphia: Lea and Febiger.

DiLima, S., & Schust, C. (Eds.). (1997). *Community health education and promotion, A guide to program design and evaluation.* Gaithersburg, MD: The Aspen Reference Group.

Dumka, L., & Michaels, M. (1998). Marketing prevention services in a community context. Workshop conducted at the American Association for Marriage and Family Therapy, Annual Conference. Dallas, TX.

Fink, A., & Kosecoff, J. (1985). *How to conduct surveys: A step-by-step guide.* Newbury Park, CA: Sage.

Fowler, F. (1993). *Survey research methods.* Newbury Park, CA: Sage.

Garsee, J., & Schuster, C. (1992). Moral development. In C. Schuster and S. Ashburn (Eds.), *The process of human development: A holistic life-span approach* (pp. 330–350). Philadelphia: Lippincott.

Krueger, R. A. (1988). *Focus groups: A practical guide for applied research.* Newbury Park, CA: Sage.

Maslow, A. (1970). *Motivation and personality* (2nd ed.). New York: Harper and Row.

Morgan, D. (1993). *Successful focus groups: Advancing the state of the art.* Newbury Park, CA: Sage.

Rissel, R., & Bracht, N. (1999). Assessing community needs, resources, and readiness: Building on strengths. In N. Bracht (Ed.), *Health promotion at the community level 2: New advances* (pp. 59–71). Thousand Oaks, CA: Sage.

Schuster, C., Cronk, R., & Reno, W. (1992). Psychosocial development during adolescence. In C. Schuster and S. Ashburn (Eds.), *The process of human development: A holistic life-span approach* (pp. 532–543). Philadelphia: Lippincott.

Youngstrom, M. J. (1999). Developing a new occupational therapy program. In K. Jacobs and M. Logigian (Eds.), *Functions of a manager in occupational therapy* (3rd ed., pp. 129–142). Thorofare, NJ: Slack.

Related Web Sites

Developmental Research and Programs, Inc. (will send free copy of their *Communities That Care Youth Survey* instrument):
www.drp.org

KIDS COUNT Data Online (summaries of state and national data regarding educational, social, economic, and physical well-being of children):
http://www.aecf.org/

7

Writing Goals and Objectives: Developing the Program

Learning Objectives

1. To review steps to accomplish in preparation for writing program goals and objectives
2. To learn to recognize and develop empowering goals for occupation-centered community-based programs
3. To learn to develop measurable objectives to support a program goal
4. To appreciate the complexity in developing a program goal and accompanying objectives to meet multilevel missions and Phase I and Phase II needs
5. To understand the relationship between the program goal, related objectives, and the design of programming
6. To understand the relationship between theoretical frames used to guide practice and the program goal and accompanying objectives
7. To explore the relationships between your program goal, the accompanying objectives, and your selected theoretical frame of reference for practice
8. To appreciate the process of clinical reasoning as it may be used to describe the complex course of helping your patients/clients/members reach their goals

Key Terms

1. Goals
2. Objectives
3. Measurable Outcome

4. Mission
5. Theory
6. Theoretical Frame of Reference
7. Clinical Reasoning

Using imagination and creativity, occupational therapy practitioners and occupational therapy students develop inventive and creative ways to engage their patient/clients in meaningful occupation. Because they have many ideas and know how to access resources, the development of programs is seldom a problem. But developing realistic, needs-based, measurable goals and objectives for community-based programming at times is challenging.

Let's consider what we have accomplished. First we explored our knowledge, skills, and experience in preparation for program development. We then considered the general population with whom we would like to work, and we developed some ideas for occupation-centered programs that might be appropriate for this population. This was followed by practice in matching these ideas to tentative goals and program outcomes. Next we selected our facility/site and specific population, and we developed our community profile and our service profile. A visit to our facility (or programming site) helped us to obtain the facility's mission and goals, to learn something more about the population, and to gain some sense of the unmet need for services. Through these efforts, we accomplished Phase I of the needs assessment. We then went to the targeted population and conducted Phase II of the needs assessment. Based on the results of all of these processes, we can now initiate a firm plan for developing an occupation-centered community program. The next step is to write a goal or goals and objectives for the specific community program we are developing.

To summarize, the steps to accomplish in preparation for writing goals and objectives for programming are as follows:

1. Investigate what you can bring to programming—your knowledge, skills, and experience.
2. Explore ideas for occupation-centered programs.
3. Select your population and identify what you believe will be the purpose of the program (considering tentative goals and outcomes).
4. Develop the profiles of the community and the service population where you wish to conduct your program.
5. Conduct Phase I and Phase II of the needs assessment.
6. Compare the results of your needs assessment with what you have accomplished thus far:
   a. Do you need more information? For the community? For the service population?
   b. Will your skills and knowledge base permit you to meet the expressed need?
   c. Do your earlier ideas regarding the tentative purpose and outcomes of the program still fit?

LEARNING TO WRITE GOALS FOR OCCUPATION-CENTERED COMMUNITY PROGRAMS

Occupational therapy practitioners and students have spent a considerable amount of time drafting goals. Practitioners familiar with Medicare and other insurers have learned that the key to reimbursement for services is a patient goal that is functional, measurable, and objective. In the language of patient care, the term goal is used to describe what happens following evaluation by the therapist. A **goal** is what you aim to have happen, or your target. In general, a treatment plan developed by a practitioner will establish long-term goals (what will be accomplished at the end of the treatment process) and short-term goals (what will happen along the way to the accomplishment of the long-term goal).

For example, a *long-term goal* for a head-injured patient might be

1. Patient will be able to shop independently for necessary grocery items;

and the accompanying *short-term goal* would be

(1.a.) The patient will be able to generate a shopping list with minimal assistance.

You might have considerable experience writing goals using the above structure; even if you do not, you likely have used "goals" to structure your personal growth and progress. Over time many of us have had the goal to lose or to gain *something*. For example, we might aspire to lose weight or to gain friends. Goals are what we often vow to do in the passion of some fairly intense emotion. If these are left as general goals, then nothing much happens. But if we attach a short-term goal—an **objective**—results are likely to follow.

Consider the following example:

Goal: I will lose ten pounds.

Objective: I will not eat desserts for three weeks.

Or, to be more realistic, a better objective would be:

I will eat desserts only on Wednesday and Sunday for two weeks.

These objectives, of course, would be meaningless for someone who never eats dessert anyway, so we must know something of the circumstances before setting goals and objectives. Using the above example, perhaps the goal was generated by a friend or family member who suggested that you might lose some weight. This would be analogous to what we have described as our *Phase I needs assessment*, which included perception of need from someone other than the targeted population (in our example, the one who will have to do the work to lose the weight). We then ask the person who will have to lose the weight, "Do you feel you need to lose weight?" or "Are you overweight?" or "Do you want to lose weight?" These questions constitute the *Phase II needs assessment*. Of course, the methods differ when we are assessing need from our community, but the intent remains quite similar.

In our developing language to describe the processes of occupation-centered program development for the community, our use of the term *goal* will be reflective of the needs of the community of clients/patients/members, and the use of the term *objective* may take into account the profiles of individual participants. When our goals and objectives are tightly connected and our objectives are *measurable*, we can determine the effectiveness of the *program*. Of course, it is our interest that the goals of the program benefit all of the clients/patients/members; however, unlike individual goal setting, if not all participants meet their personal objectives, this does not mean that the program is a failure. This distinction between goals developed for ourselves or for individual patients and the goals we will develop for occupation-centered community programs and, most particularly, our expectations for outcome will take some practice. This is quite a different orientation from what we may have become accustomed to. When writing goals for a community as opposed to an individual, we must consider the needs of the *community*, and we must write goals for the *community* (of individuals). By assessing the need from both those who are observing what they believe to be the need(s) of the service population and those who are directly receiving services, we have a good idea of goals that will be meaningful for everyone involved.

Our shared knowledge base and our understanding of occupation permit us to translate the expressed "needs" into goals that are meaningful for occupation-centered intervention. In our community gardening example, the city officials who responded to the Phase I needs assessment expressed the need to find a place other than the street and the city parks for the homeless population, including those who were homeless with psychiatric disability. And something was needed to keep

The making of "Whale Tail Party Hats" symbolizes the celebration of parent-child empowerment, awareness of our connection to the larger environment, and accomplishment of a fun and creative task.

them busy. In the parent-child program example, the children's teachers wanted parents to become involved in their children's education, and the administrators of the Sea Grant Program specifically wanted to encourage the children's interest in science and science-based careers.

In discussions of the above Phase I needs, an attempt was made to synthesize and distill the expressed needs into what was considered to be motivating and inspirational language. It was believed that the needs expressed by the city officials could be satisfied and that the population would benefit from the creation of an occupation-centered community. In the second example the response to teachers and administrators was to create a parent-child program around the development of *teams* and *team-building* to focus on the academic progress of the child and, again, to go beyond to benefit the parent-child relationship in many other ways. Before conducting Phase II needs assessments, the concept of community was researched and translated into occupation-centered language. What is meant by *teams* and *team-building* and what this might have to do with parenting was also explored.

The broad goal of the gardening program, then, might be *to build community* and the broad goal of the parent-child program might be *to build teams.* The broad goal of our homeless adolescent program might be *to encourage self-efficacy.* You will recall that the Phase I need for the population of adolescents who are homeless was simply for "safe sex." Based on our community profile and our service profile, we believed that we could meet the expressed need to explore safe sex with this population, but our discussions prompted us to consider what *safety* might mean to these adolescents in the practice of their daily occupations. The issue seemed much larger than the Phase I expressed need; the issue seemed to be about self-efficacy. Thus, our broad goal for this program was *to encourage self-efficacy.*

In all of these examples, we are careful not to negate the Phase I need. In the discussions of that need, we develop a language for the Phase II assessment that offers more definition and perhaps not only explores the need(s) already identified but also might offer a few additional options. Our Phase II focus group might include not only questions for discussion around what the adolescents themselves identify as sexual concerns (such as safety) but also other daily/weekly occupations where safety might be an issue (such as drugs, solicitation for prostitution, and so on). The questioning could include consideration of the factors involved in self-protection (for example, issues of confidence, information, and skills that impact self-esteem and self-efficacy). We then can develop objectives for occupation-centered programming that are closely aligned with both Phase I and Phase II needs, and in this way we continue to invite the support and cooperation of both groups. With this support, the program becomes a part of the community.

The above goals and others like them are empowering; they virtually invite investment and interaction of the participants. They not only excite us but those who may wish to fund our programs as well. However, as they stand now, they tell us very little. Trying to evaluate the goals of *building community,* or *teams,* or encouraging *efficacy* in such a way that you can measure your effectiveness is not possible. Goals are not measurable as they are expressed; thus, we then couple these lofty, idealistic statements with clear, sound objectives that *are* measurable.

WRITING MEASURABLE OBJECTIVES TO ACCOMPANY PROGRAMMING GOALS

From our research and our dialogues, we develop one or perhaps two goals for occupation-centered community-based programs. Our goals are sufficiently global and comprehensive so that we will not need many to address the expressed needs for programming. Settling on appropriate goals takes some work, and in the process we must offer definitions and *tease* out meaning. When considering the previous examples, what does *community* mean? What about *team-building* or *self-efficacy?* As we grapple with the many ways we can translate the expressed needs into goals, we generate terms and phrases that will become our **objectives.**

DiLima and Schust provide us with a list of characteristics for community programming objectives. They recommend that objectives must be performance, behavior, or action oriented. They must be clear and must state the level, condition, or standard of performance that is expected. They must be results oriented and must have stated outcomes that are directly observable. They must have a specific time for completion, and, perhaps most importantly, they must be measurable (1997, p. 209).

To summarize, the objectives for community programs

1. must be performance, behavior, or action oriented.
2. must be expressed in clear language.
3. must state the level, condition, or standard of performance that is expected.
4. must be results oriented.
5. must have stated outcomes that are directly observable.
6. must be oriented to time.
7. must be measurable.

When we write objectives, we select from an assortment of verbs. Some examples include to learn, explore, promote, discuss, evaluate, identify, understand, determine, illustrate, recite, write, construct, define, demonstrate, challenge, accept, or support. Certainly there are many more from which to choose. With whatever we select, however, we must be able to determine when it has occurred; we must be able to **measure the outcome(s).** Our choice of *verbs* indicate the *action* that will be performed. We will then follow the verb with a *noun* that will identify the expected *outcome.* We then finish with *what level or condition* we expect and *when* we expect it to occur. Note the following example:

> The members will **demonstrate** their **commitment to the community** by **working in the community garden six hours each week** for the **twelve weeks of the program.**

You may have only one goal, but several objectives may be required for the participants of your program to be able to satisfy the goal. Your objectives offer the structure for your program. Keep them as simple and uncomplicated as possible, for you will have only a certain amount of time to accomplish them and everyone involved in the program—therapist, client, volunteer, and student—must be able to observe and recognize when the objectives have been accomplished.

For example, your goal for a day camp may be to encourage movement and socialization through play. You may enroll six children (or perhaps as many as twelve) for four five-hour days each week (or perhaps four two-hour days each week) for a period of two weeks; then you will have another group of children. Regardless of the number of children you decide to accommodate or the specific daily schedule, the objectives to meet the goal of encouraging movement and socialization through play must be accomplished in two weeks. Consider the following example of a measurable objective to meet this goal in the time specified:

> The children (or each child) will participate in one group game each day that will require movement through a flexible crawl tube.

Anyone working in the program described can observe and note when the objective has been satisfied; however, it would be virtually impossible for observers to *consistently* note the "encouragement of movement and socialization through play." There are four terms—*encourage, movement, socialization,* and *play*—all open to broad, subjective interpretation; none is measurable without a specific objective. You might wish to practice defining these four terms for yourself; in the process, you will have begun to generate objectives for such a program.

THE INFLUENCE OF "MISSION" ON GOALS, OBJECTIVES, AND PROGRAM DESIGN

We cannot draft goals and objectives for programming without first having sufficient knowledge of the umbrella organization (that is, that organization that sponsors or supports the selected facility/agency) and the **mission** and purpose of that organization. Our Denver sanctuary, for example, might be sponsored by Catholic Charities; a similar program might be provided under the auspices of the Red Cross. The after-school, delinquency-prevention program we will be describing in Chapter 16 is provided under the multi-umbrellas of the Community Development Commission of the City Housing Authority, the University Extension Urban 4-H Club, and the City Parks and Recreation Department.

As we noted earlier, the mission of the sanctuary example was to provide free meals, shower, and bed in a safe environment. The need expressed by agency/ facility administrators or other professionals working in that environment will reflect the mission and the purpose of the sponsoring organization, and that must be our first consideration in the design for programming. It may be an obvious oversimplification, but we would not expect to design a for-profit program to provide services for the homeless adolescent population frequenting the sanctuary. We also would not develop a "wellness" focus for a community-based program to serve the needs of a hospital whose mission is to serve the acutely ill; *however,* it might be appropriate if the hospital's mission also includes concern and protection for the health and welfare of the community it serves.

Meeting occupation-centered program goals can be great fun for the planner and the participant!

When you review the programming narratives described in Part III, you will see that all of the examples work from an early identification of the mission of the institution, agency, or organization. This is of significance when you are developing programming to support a particular community mission. Of course, if you are developing a free-standing program, then you will establish a mission of your own from which your programs will develop.

The following case example will demonstrate how the multiple missions of several umbrella organizations and their combined needs can be translated and melded to form an occupation-centered program:

1. The Community Development Commission/Housing Authority expressed an original need to occupy the children who resided in housing authority projects during after-school hours until their parents returned home from work. Although not explicitly expressed, this need may have been prompted by recurring problems associated with graffiti, property damage, and gang violence.

2. Most of the children living in housing authority buildings attended a nearby public school. The teachers of the school supported the need for such a program and responded to this need with a structured way to encourage the children's after-school interest in education that would be engaging and fun. A science teacher at the school had heard a recent talk by primatologist Jane Goodall and wanted to sponsor a "Roots and Shoots" program for students.

3. The City Parks and Recreation Department sponsored the activities of a facility adjacent to the projects. They were interested in having the neighborhood children frequent their facility, particularly to encourage attendance at their weekend programming, but were understaffed in the afternoons when the housing authority needed programming. With the support of the school and the University Cooperative Extension, they had initiated an urban 4-H Club chapter earlier in the year, and most of the chapter's activities were conducted on Saturday.

Granted, this is an extremely complex example, but it is likely that you will have a number of missions to consider when you identify an opportunity to design a program. In the above example, the missions did not appear to be competing with each other; they seemed, in fact, to be mutually supportive, and the Phase I needs assessment solidified these observations. There are recurring *themes of community* throughout these missions. The missions of the school and the Community Development Commission of the City Housing Authority were directed toward the education, protection, and development of children. The school's specific mission was to provide education to children in grades two through five. The Housing Authority not only provided housing to low-income families, but it also financially supported programming for the children in the community through the Community Development Commission. The city Parks and Recreation Department encouraged the health and fitness of children and adults through selected activity.

Two additional organizations were embedded in this mix. Through the sponsorship of the University Cooperative Extension, the 4-H Club's mission is "to enable youth to make wise choices and positive contributions to society throughout their lives." The club's mission is articulated through its motto: to "pledge my HEAD to clearer thinking, my HEART to greater loyalty, my HANDS to larger service and my HEALTH to better living" (4-H Clubs of America: http://www.4h-usa.org/). The science teacher brought another mission to the forefront through his interest in sponsoring programming developed around Jane Goodall's *Roots and Shoots* projects for children around the world. Encompassed in the mission, the three major directives for this organization include a demonstration of care and concern for the community, the environment, and for animals (Goodall, 1978). This programming will be described in more detail in Chapter 17.

The combination of these missions provided an excellent opportunity to combine the interests and support of several organizations in the development of after-school occupation-centered programming for inner-city children. Skillful program design would be responsive to the sociocultural development of the children through a structure of *clubs* rather than *gangs*. Goals and objectives would support *community building, education,* and perhaps a *futures orientation.* As occupation-centered practitioners, there are very few missions we encounter with which we are unable to relate. The previous example provides multiple opportunities for engagement in community-building while providing personal growth for each child involved in the program. The following is an example of a suggested goal for a program that will meet the Phase I needs and the combined missions.

Combined Missions: *To Build* Community

Proposed goal: *To demonstrate* care and concern for the community through club projects that encourage *thinking, caring* and *helping.*

A suggested objective to help us meet this goal might be:

The children will cooperate to plan and carry out one neighborhood activity in the celebration of Earth Day.

"Roots and Shoots" club members learn that cleaning up their neighborhood supports their club's goal to empower children to create change for positive global futures.

In this example, we have used *caring* and *concern* as indicators of investment in shared community, and *to cooperate* has been defined as one measure of what we mean by *community.* Can you think of other ways to define *community?* Consider the above example. As it is expressed, does the goal capture all of the interests of those involved in providing mission statements? Does it capture all of the needs expressed in our brief description of Phase I assessment results? Does it generate excitement, interest, and spirit?

EXERCISE 1

Writing *Goals* and *Objectives* to Meet Multilevel Missions and Phase I Needs

1. Write below a goal for the combined missions example:

_____

_____

_____

_____

_____

Discuss your goal with classmates or colleagues. You might wish to reread the example, highlighting those portions that describe the collective missions and the needs.

2. Review the objective provided in the example. As the objective is written, you might suggest that it cannot be measured. How will you measure *to cooperate?* What might be a more measurable way to indicate cooperation? Rewrite the objective so that it is more measurable:

_____

_____

_____

_____

3. Now write a measurable objective (or more than one) for the *goal* you wrote in step 1 of this exercise:

_____

_____

_____

_____

_____

EXERCISE 2

Writing *Goals* and *Objectives* for Your Program

Review all of the information you have collected as you have moved through the exercises to prepare you for this step. Consider the data gathered to develop your community and service profiles. If you have a sponsoring organization, review its mission and purpose. Reexamine the results of both the Phase I and Phase II assessments of need. Discuss how you will respond to the need(s). What do you want to accomplish for your targeted population? Will you provide *prevention* by offering programming to reduce the risks of illness, disability, or criminality? Will you provide *remediation* for the effects of illness and disability? Will you provide *promotion and maintenance* of health and wellness? Or will you provide a combination of these things? You will want to revisit your early tentative ideas for goals developed in Chapter 5, and you might wish to return to some of the examples offered in this chapter. Write below your ideas for a program *goal*.

1. Ideas for a program *goal:*

_____

_____

_____

_____

_____

Review some of the *cognitive/emotional routes* you have traveled to come up with the goal you wrote in the previous step. What does the goal mean to you? How will you define it for your community?

2. Develop several objectives that will permit your population to achieve the goal you have established. Write these objectives below:

_____

_____

_____

_____

_____

Review your objectives according to the criteria listed on page 105. Are your objectives written clearly? Are they measurable? Do you include the action that will occur, the outcome, the condition, and the time? Does each objective directly relate to the program goal? If an objective does not contribute to the satisfaction of the goal, then it must be rewritten or deleted. If more practice is needed, continue to work on these exercises until you have achieved the tight linking and clarity you will need to further develop the program. The quality of your goal statement and the accompanying objectives will establish the success of your program.

Now you must outline what sort of programming you will provide, on what kind of schedule, and for how long. Your goal and the accompanying objectives will provide the structure for this process. Your goal describes what you feel is most important to accomplish. Your objectives define, refine, and delimit the qualities that characterize your goal. The objectives describe not only what your population will do but also how and when they will do it. Now your task is to develop the programming that will *enable* your population to meet the objectives that will satisfy the goal. It is a detailed and methodical process, and the links between actions and outcomes are equally as intricate.

WHAT PROGRAMMING WILL YOU PROVIDE?

As you have accomplished the planning tasks in preparation for the work in this chapter, you have been "flirting" with the program you will ultimately provide. Many planners begin with the idea for a program and then seek to position and justify it through the steps of program development. As indicated earlier, this is likely the way that most experienced practitioners begin; the excitement generated by the idea springboards the work necessary to bring it to fruition.

We have all of our traditional options and more for how to practice in the community. Earlier we discussed several roles—including prevention, restoration, maintenance, and promotion—we might choose to develop a structure for our programs. Certainly these roles are not mutually exclusive; one program might, in fact, provide a goal and objectives to meet several of these directives. Regardless of the directive we select, there are some assumptions surrounding community-based practices. Practice in the community suggests that we become a part of our practice site—the community. Whether we reside there or not, we understand it and share in its problems and victories. There is an implicit expectation that we are responsive to the needs of the community, just as we are responsive to the needs of our client/patient/member. We understand that our client/patient/member is not only a member of the larger community but many other communities as well, and it is our task to encourage and enrich this person's contributions to all of these *communities*. We are aware of and responsive to what we might describe as *the greater good*. Although community-based programs need not always be charitable in structure, there is an expectation of charity in spirit. Occupation-centered community-based practitioners share in common a pervasive altruism.

In summary, the shared assumptions for community-based practitioners, then, include the following:

1. We become *part* of our practice community.
2. We are responsive to the needs of our community.
3. We encourage and enrich the contributions to their many communities by our clients/patients/members.
4. We share with other occupation-centered community-based practitioners a pervasive altruism and a belief in the *greater good*.

These assumptions are directed toward strengthening community—and in the process, strengthening its members. Alongside those who receive our services, *we* are its members. The assumptions listed in the previous paragraph could be described in the same way we have discussed goals; they are empowering, and they help us feel connected to a greater purpose. But just as we have acknowledged with regard to goals, these assumptions do not structure what we *will* do; they only make us *want* to do! Where do we go from here?

THEORETICALLY FRAMING YOUR COMMUNITY-BASED PROGRAM

Practitioners develop organized ways of thinking about what they see, what they do, and how these things are interrelated. Reed (1998) describes this as **theory.** She suggests that occupational therapy theory is concerned with occupational endeavor translated through four major concepts: the person, the environment, health, and occupation (1998, p. 521). From our discussions of occupation-centered community-based practice, it would seem that we are certainly relying on occupational therapy theory to not only frame our discussions of this phenomena but also to guide our program design and development. In trying to understand and articulate the placement of occupation-centered intervention in the community, the author draws heavily on the theoretical orientation of occupational science (Clark, 1993; Clark et al., 1991; Clark, Wood, & Larson, 1998; Yerxa et al., 1990). In addressing the questions stimulated by the interweaving of *community, occupation,* and *intervention,* we are searching for meaningful ways to integrate these concepts into a practice discipline appropriate for today and the future.

In addition, as practitioners each of us brings to the community one or more **theoretical frames of reference** that offer structure for the way we provide comprehensive services to our patients/clients. In Mosey's definition, she suggests that frames of reference "provide a systematic description of and prescription for a practitioner's interaction with his domain of concern" (1981, p. 5). But how do we select a frame of reference that is the right one and the most comfortable one for us to employ in our practices? Selection of a frame of reference (or more than one) for practice is first based on one's belief system; that is, it is based on what we believe about the world and what we believe about the people who occupy it. If we believe people define their own purposes in life and act on the world with intention, then we would seek a frame of reference that offered respect for that belief and not one that might be antagonistic to it.

Occupational therapy practitioners commonly use the term *occupation* to describe how people act on or react to the world. The language of occupation is widely used today; however, there is still considerable variability in how this language is translated through the various theoretical frames of reference. Perhaps this is how it should be; occupation unites us, but our choices of frames of reference set us apart. This eclecticism will permit us to meet the wide variability of community-based need in many creative ways while remaining true to our foundations.

Although first based on our philosophical orientations, the next step in the selection of a frame of reference for practice may be quite pragmatic. Although not necessarily intended for this purpose, *Uniform Terminology for Occupational Therapy, 3rd edition* provides us with useful and practical guidelines in selecting frames of reference appropriate to our service population (American Occupational Therapy Association, 1994; Moyers, 1999). The contextual, temporal, and environmental characteristics of the population may prompt the choice of a frame of reference that will provide the most useful way to view the patient/client/member (for example, based on chronological and developmental age; life cycle; disability status; or physical, social and cultural considerations). In addition, problems in function demonstrated in one or more of the performance areas may suggest component deficits (such as sensorimotor, psychosocial, and/or cognitive deficits), thus helping us to further define appropriate choices of frames of reference. Consider the following example:

Our service population consists of children between the chronological ages of five to seven who have developmental ages of two to four. The children are experiencing problems that can include toilet hygiene, dressing, feeding and eating, functional mobility, socialization, and functional communication. Their immediate community consists of family and other children in the service environment. Given this information, we might consider investigating two frames of reference—sensory integration and neurodevelopmental theory—that draw from *developmental* models to structure and guide our practice with these children. We might also wish to combine these with some aspects of a behavioral frame of reference drawn from learning theory or others that might be appropriate to meet the remediation, maintenance, and prevention needs of this service population.

This example might also describe the ways we could structure our day camp program mentioned earlier. The goal for that program was to encourage movement and socialization through play. We could broaden the objectives for that program not only to address functional mobility and socialization but functional communication, feeding, dressing, and toileting as well. We could attend to all of these "problem areas" through the medium of play guided by the theoretical frame of sensory integration, or we could combine sensory integration and neurodevelopmental theory and perhaps add others.

Whether your occupation-centered intervention is intended to help your population reduce risk and thus prevent illness, disability, or criminality; to intervene and remediate during the illness or disability process; or to maintain and encourage wellness and normal development, selecting one or more theoretical frames of reference will provide the programming parameters for successful outcomes. If you would like to further research theoretical orientations and theoretical frames of reference used in occupational therapy intervention, review the recommended readings at the close of this chapter.

Before we continue, we must mention one more factor that contributes to the process of moving your patient/client/member from *need* to *goal*. This factor is **clinical reasoning,** or what Schell refers to as "the basis of practice" (1998, p. 90). In many ways, clinical reasoning defines an occupational therapy practitioner's "way of being." Clinical *reasoning* describes the multifaceted process that encompasses all of the ways we utilize the information we have collected about a patient or client and the community—that is, through our theoretical orientations, our practice knowledge, and our experience. It also captures what has been described as more covert practice enmeshed in the "stories" that we and our patient/client utilize to develop and meet our goals (Fleming, 1994).

▬▬ EXERCISE 3 ▬▬

Selecting Theoretical Frames of Reference to Guide Your Developing Program

1. Review the goal and the related objectives developed in Exercise 2. Discuss with your group and/or colleagues some potential frames of reference that will support the concepts of occupation for the program you are developing.

Perhaps you are already using one or more frames of reference in practice. Are they appropriate to structure the program you are proposing to meet the objectives and to satisfy your goal?

Note below one or more frames of reference that are compatible with and supportive of your program goal and the accompanying objectives:

_____

_____

_____

_____

_____

2. Are you comfortable with your selection(s)? Is there agreement between these frames and your philosophical orientation? Your beliefs about people? Your beliefs about occupation? Is there sufficient breadth to provide the structure for any assessment you might wish to do? Is there a good fit with your purpose of remediation, maintenance, or promotion and/or prevention? Make any notes with regard to these questions below:

_____

_____

_____

_____

The model of human occupation was selected to guide several of the programs described in this text. Because the model addresses the motivation for engagement in occupation, how one elects to pattern engagement in occupation, the relationship between skills and performance, and the influence of context/environment on occupation, it is sufficiently broad to meet the needs of a wide range of program participants. It is also appropriate to structure programs targeting prevention and wellness as well as those targeting intervention (Kielhofner, 1995; Kielhofner and Barrett, 1998).

The adolescent sanctuary program mentioned earlier in this chapter had as its goal "the development of self-efficacy." Objectives were developed to address the components of self-efficacy to include confidence, information, and skills. A review of the model of human occupation provides us with language (such as volition, personal causation, values, interests, habits, and roles) to structure our program. In addition, the attention to the influence of environment on our population—within the context of urban homelessness—must be understood in the design of effective programming. This includes attention to what Dunn and her colleagues describe as ecology, or "the interaction between a person and the context" with resultant effects on behavior and task performance (1998, p. 531). In Chapter 6 we noted the multiple expressions of sexuality as adaptive responses to the potentially dangerous context of homelessness; therefore, the theoretical construct of "adaptation" is significant to understanding our population's response to the community and to our programming; therefore, we might also find it useful to include Schkade's and Schultz's work on occupational adaptation (1998).

Clearly stated objectives guided by the selected theoretical frame(s) of reference provide the framework for the design and development of programming that will *enable* our service population to satisfy needs and to meet the goal of services. The following equation summarizes this relationship:

$$\text{Objective(s) + Frame(s) of Reference = Programming = GOAL}$$

Objective: Adolescents participating in the program will be provided with developmentally appropriate information and skills, which they can use to make informed choices about practiced sexual behaviors.

Frames of Reference: These might include the model of human occupation influenced by the theoretical underpinnings of *the ecology of human performance* and *occupational adaptation.*

Programming: Modules might be developed to include the acquisition of information and the development of skills structured around the subsystems of volition, habituation, and mind/body performance.

GOAL: To advocate for oneself by effecting positive change in one's relationship with the environment (efficacy).

Finally, to complete our equation, we must add clinical reasoning:

$$\text{Objective(s) + } \begin{array}{c}\text{Frame(s) of}\\ \text{Reference}\end{array} \text{ + } \begin{array}{c}\text{Clinical}\\ \text{Reasoning}\end{array} \text{ = Programming = GOAL}$$

EXERCISE 4

Designing Programming

1. Following your goal, your objectives, and the tenets of your frame or frames of reference, what are your ideas for programming? (Refer to your textbooks, resources at the close of this chapter, and to Part III of this text for examples of programs if you need some help.) Note your ideas below:

_____

_____

_____

_____

_____

Will your programming enable your service population to meet the established goal?

The mechanics of what materials we will select or develop to provide programming and exactly how we will structure it (that is, weekly, daily, or monthly) will evolve as we continue to develop the program. For the beginner, developing programming in a step-by-step process is the best way to learn. For the experienced therapist, the process is less linear and problems are more easily anticipated and controlled during the planning process. But even experienced practitioners are often surprised and challenged by community practice environments and populations. Often it might appear to be more akin to chaos than order. There is always an element of trial and error even in the best of planning.

SUMMARY

The results of our earlier work in profiling our community and our service population and in gathering the results of the two phases of the assessment of needs has resulted in a goal for our program, which includes what we wish to accomplish for and with our service population.

Goals provide us and our population with an attractive and empowering incentive that keeps us engaged in the process of moving forward. However, without objectives to help us define and then measure these goals, they are useless in helping us to design programs for the community. It is from these objectives that our day-to-day programming evolves.

In community practice, we approach the individual's need through the combined need of the population; however, we maintain our responsibility to the individual by adopting a way of thinking, or a theoretical frame of reference, to guide our understanding and our choices of intervention. Our selected frame(s) of reference can be compared to a pair of eyeglasses. When we put them on, we see the individual as an occupational being; but *how* we utilize occupation will be influenced by the theoretical orientation to practice that we have selected. The frame(s) of reference we select provide us with ways to consider and to utilize occupation-centered thinking.

How the program will actually look (the day-to-day activities) is a result of the goal, the objectives, and the theoretical frames of reference. It is a result of the goal we have established for program outcomes, the objectives that will structure these outcomes, and the theoretical frame or frames of reference we will utilize to provide the direction for how to achieve the desired outcomes.

When you feel comfortable with your goal, objectives, and frame or frames of reference and when you have some ideas for programming that will move your population toward the expected outcomes, then you are ready to go on to the next step of establishing specific programming to include planning for staffing, space, equipment, and supplies. Who will do it? Where will it be done? And what is needed to do it?

REFERENCES

American Occupational Therapy Association. (1994). Uniform terminology for occupational therapy, 3rd edition. *American Journal of Occupational Therapy, 48,* 1,047–1,054.

Clark, F. (1993). Occupation embedded in a real life: Interweaving occupational science and occupational therapy. *American Journal of Occupational Therapy, 47,* 1,067–1,078.

Clark, F., Parham, D., Carlson, M., Frank, G., Jackson, J., Pierce, D., Wolfe, R. J, & Zemke, R. (1991). Occupational science: Academic innovation in the service of occupational therapy's future. *American Journal of Occupational Therapy, 45,* 300–310.

Clark, F., Wood, W., & Larson, E. (1998). Occupational science: Occupational therapy's legacy for the 21st century. In M. Neistadt & E. Crepeau (Eds.), *Willard and Spackman's occupational therapy* (pp. 13–21). Philadelphia: Lippincott.

DiLima, S. N., & Schust, C. (1997). In *Community health education and promotion: A guide to program design and evaluation* (p. 209). Gaithersburg, MD: The Aspen Reference Group.

Dunn, W., McClain, L. H., Brown, C., & Youngstrom, M. J. (1998). The ecology of human performance. In M. Neistadt & E. Crepeau (Eds.), *Willard and Spackman's occupational therapy* (pp. 531–534). Philadelphia: Lippincott.

Fleming, M. H. (1994). Conditional reasoning: Creating meaningful experiences. In C. Mattingly & M. H. Fleming (Eds.), *Clinical reasoning: Forms of inquiry in a therapeutic practice* (pp. 197–235). Philadelphia: F. A. Davis.

The Jane Goodall *Institute for Wildlife Research, Education and Conservation* (1978). *Roots and shoots fact sheet.* Ridgefield, CT.

Kielhofner, G. (1995). *A model of human occupation: Theory and application* (2nd ed.). Baltimore: Williams and Wilkins.

Kielhofner, G., & Barrett, L. (1998). The model of human occupation. In M. Neistadt & E. Crepeau (Eds.), *Willard and Spackman's occupational therapy* (pp. 527–529). Philadelphia: Lippincott.

Mosey, A. C. (1981). *Three frames of reference for mental health.* New York: Raven.

Moyers, P. (1999, May/June). The guide to occupational therapy practice. *American Journal of Occupational Therapy, 53*(3), 247–322.

Reed, K. (1998). Theory and frame of reference. In M. Neistadt & E. Crepeau (Eds.), *Willard and Spackman's occupational therapy* (pp. 521–524). Philadelphia: Lippincott.

Schell, B. (1998). Clinical reasoning: The basis of practice. In M. Neistadt & E. Crepeau (Eds.), *Willard and Spackman's occupational therapy* (pp. 90–100). Philadelphia: Lippincott.

Schkade, J. K., & Schultz, S. (1998). Occupational adaptation: An integrative frame of reference. In M. Neistadt & E. Crepeau (Eds.), *Willard and Spackman's occupational therapy* (pp. 529–531). Philadelphia: Lippincott.

Yerxa, E., Clark, F., Frank, G., Jackson, J., Parham, D., Pierece, D., Stein, C., & Zemke, R. (1990). An introduction to occupational science: A foundation for occupational therapy in the 21st century. *Occupational Therapy in Health Care, 6,* 1–17.

Related Internet Sites

1. 4-H Clubs of America:
   http://www.4h-usa.org/

2. Jane Goodall:
   email: JANEGOODALL@wcsu.ctstateu.edu
3. Vast Spaces and Stone Walls: Overcoming Barriers to Postsecondary Education for Rural Students with Disabilities:
   http://www.tc.umn.edu/nlhome/g258/vitlink/heathl.html
4. Yahoo Online Index of Disability Web Sites:
   http://www.yahoo.com/yahoo/Society_and_Culture/Disabilities/
5. Jim Lubin's Disability Resource List:
   http//www.eskimo.com/~jlubin/disabled.html
6. Updated Versions of Disability Resources:
   http://otpt.ups.edu/Rehabilitation/Resources.html

Additional Recommended Reading

Allen, C. K., Earhart, C. A., & Blue, T. (1992). *Occupational therapy treatment goals for the physically and cognitively disabled.* Rockville, MD: American Occupational Therapy Association.

Ayres, A. J. (1979). *Sensory integration and the child.* Los Angeles: Western Psychological Associates.

Bly, L. (1991). A historical and current view of the basis of NDT. *Pediatric Physical Therapy, 3,* 131–135.

Coster, W., Tickle-Degnen, L., & Armenta, L. (1995). Therapist-child interaction during sensory integration treatment: Development and testing of a research tool. *Occupational Therapy Journal of Research, 15*(1), 17–35.

Dunn, W., Brown, C., McClain, L., & Westman, K. (1994). The ecology of human performance: A contextual perspective on human occupation. In C. B. Royeen (Ed.), *AOTA self-study series: The practice of the future: Putting occupation back into therapy.* Rockville, MD: American Occupational Therapy Association.

Dunst, C. J., Trivette, C. M., & Deal, A. G. (1988). *Enabling and empowering families: Principles and guidelines for practice.* Cambridge, MA: Brookline Books.

Fisher, A. G., & Murray, E. A. (1991). Introduction to sensory integration theory. In A. G. Fisher, E. A. Murray, & A. C. Bundy (Eds.), *Sensory integration theory and practice* (pp. 3–26). Philadelphia: F. A. Davis.

Hagedorn, R. (1992). *Occupational therapy: Foundations for practice. Models, frames of references, and core skills.* New York: Churchill Livingstone.

Kielhofner, G. (1992). *Conceptual foundations of occupational therapy.* Philadelphia: F. A. Davis.

Kimball, J. C. (1993). Sensory integrative frame of reference. Inc. P. Kramer & J. Hinojosa (Eds.), *Frames of reference for pediatric occupational therapy* (pp. 87–175). Baltimore: Williams and Wilkins.

Mandel, D., Jackson, J., Zemke, R., Nelson, L., & Clark, F. (1999). *Lifestyle redesign: Implementing the well elderly study.* Rockville, MD: American Occupational Therapy Association.

Nelson, D. (1988). Occupation: Form and performance. *American Journal of Occupational Therapy, 42,* 633–641.

Parham, D. L., & Fazio, L. (Eds.). (1997). *Play in occupational therapy for children.* St. Louis, MO: Mosby.

Parham, D. L., & Mailloux, Z. (1995). Sensory integration. In J. Case-Smith, A. S. Allen, & P. N. Pratt (Eds.), *Occupational therapy for children* (pp. 307–356). St. Louis, MO: Mosby.

Pedretti, L. W., & Pasquinelli, S. (1990). A frame of reference for occupational therapy in physical dysfunction. In L. W. Pedretti & B. Zoltan (Eds.), *Occupational therapy practice skills for physical dysfunction* (3rd ed.). Philadelphia: Mosby.

Reed, K. L. (1984). *Models of practice in occupational therapy.* Baltimore: Williams and Wilkins.

Roots and Shoots. (1998). *A Curriculum Packet to Connect Los Angeles Youth With Their Community, Environment and Wildlife.* Printed and distributed by the Los Angeles Zoo.

Schkade, J. K., & Schultz, S. (1992a). Occupational adaptation: Toward a holistic approach to contemporary practice. Part 1. *American Journal of Occupational Therapy, 46,* 829–837.

Schkade, J. K., & Schultz, S. (1992b). Occupational adaptation: Toward a holistic approach to contemporary practice. Part 2. *American Journal of Occupational Therapy, 46,* 917–925.

Schmidt, R. A., & Bjork, R. A. (1992). New conceptualizations of practice: Common principles in three paradigms suggest new concepts for training. *Psychological Science, 3,* 207–217.

Toglia, J. P. (1992). A dynamic interactional approach to cognitive rehabilitation. In N. Katz (Ed.), *Cognitive rehabilitation: Models for intervention in occupational therapy* (pp. 1,041–1,043). Boston: Andover Medical Publishers.

Trombly, C. A. (1995). Theoretical foundations for practice. In C. A. Trombly (Ed.), *Occupational therapy for physical dysfunction.* (4th ed., pp. 15–27). Baltimore: Williams and Wilkins.

CHAPTER 8

Staffing: Who Will Do It?

Learning Objectives

1. To learn to connect the program goal and related objectives to staffing needs
2. To consider direct and indirect services required to meet the needs of the service population
3. To understand the relationship between the nature of services offered and the selection of staff to meet the needs of the program
4. To become familiar with the many potential roles of occupational therapy practitioners
5. To become familiar with the guidelines for supervision of occupational therapy personnel
6. To develop the job description for the occupational therapy practitioner(s) who will be hired for your program
7. To draft a sample advertisement to include the tasks to be performed (job description) and the credentials and experience desired for your proposed hiree

Key Terms

1. Staff/Staffing/Personnel
2. Direct Services
3. Indirect Services
4. Registered Occupational Therapist (OTR)
5. Certified Occupational Therapy Assistant (COTA)
6. Supervisor/Supervision
7. Consultant
8. Entrepreneur
9. Advisory Board
10. Job Description

121

Many of you probably read this chapter heading and thought, "Of course, *I'll* do it." Certainly you might wish to start the program and perhaps stay directly involved indefinitely; but would your program better (and perhaps more economically) serve the needs of the community after start-up if you functioned as a consultant or as an on-site or off-site supervisor of other staff? Although you do not necessarily need to address these questions now, they are worth considering for your long-range planning. You might feel a bit overwhelmed with the demands of the initial planning process, but try to extend your thinking to first a one-year plan, then a two-year plan, and finally a three-year plan. Make your plans for controlled growth or perhaps for stability. While growth seems to be the "American way," you should always ask yourself *why* before you decide to *grow*. Decide if there is a need, and most importantly, consider what will be necessary to maintain quality if growth is in your long-range planning. Chaos planning in response to emergencies is not the way to operate a program or to ensure balance in the life of the programmer.

MEETING THE NEEDS OF YOUR PATIENTS/CLIENTS/MEMBERS

The term **staffing** refers to the process of identifying, finding, and hiring those persons who will assist in providing the services to your population of choice. In some settings, these persons might be referred to as *personnel,* and in other settings they might be referred to as **staff.** Often in the language of the community, they are referred to simply as *the people who work here.* When anticipating your staffing needs, there are several considerations. First, what are the occupation-centered services you wish to provide? To answer this question, return to your initial planning. What is your goal? And what are your objectives for the program? In developing your goal and the accompanying objectives, you have carefully assessed the needs of the community and your population. Through this process, you have defined what services you will need.

However, you must also consider the number of clients/patients/members you can accommodate while offering quality services, and several things will impact that decision. Certainly the funding for your program and the physical space where you will operate your program must be considered. It is possible that you will not have the answers to funding and space when you begin; rather, you might focus on designing a program that is somewhat conservative but yet responsive to the need. You might then seek funding and space with a strong and well-planned program design. When seeking grant funding, the initial "pilot" program often is purposefully small so that it can be well controlled to ensure that outcomes are met. An adequate funding amount can then be requested based on these early results.

We will want to know *how* services are offered to our population. We think of **direct services** as those services we provide that *directly* support the goal or goals of our clients/patients. These services might consist of assessment and/or inter-

Volunteers bring their skills, expertise, and caring to many programs, which might be realized in the making and sharing of a banana split.

vention offered by a therapist. The term *direct* is more important when used to determine the costs of billing for professional services. **Indirect services** likely are less costly and include those services we provide through our programming that *supports* our direct services. In the community programs described here, the distinguishing characteristics between these two kinds of services are not nearly as significant as they might be in a more traditional fee-for-service practice. Certainly you will want to identify the nature of the services you wish to offer because this will significantly impact who you hire and why. When considering staff to provide direct and indirect services, it will likely be the direct services that require specific and sometimes specialized knowledge and skills. While more indirect services may be designed and coordinated by a practitioner with specialized skills and knowledge (perhaps as a consultant), the day-to-day program may be conducted by someone with more generalized skills. As you make your decisions regarding the kinds of services needed to facilitate the goal achievement of your population, it would be helpful to review the description of the occupational therapy process provided by Rogers and Holm (1991) and Moyers (1999).

In addition to knowing how our services will be offered, we will also want to know *when* our population is available to receive services. This information was likely obtained in the Phase II needs assessment and must be considered now. The following case example describes the reasoning that led to *when* this particular program was offered:

When parents in the parent-child program were surveyed during the Phase II needs assessment, it became clear that all were working and would not attend a program that occurred immediately after school. Weekends were preferred for other things (such as shopping, laundry, and household chores). Early evening seemed the best time, although a potential conflict with dinner began to emerge. The solution was found through the inclusion of a shared meal as one aspect of the program that could then meet a number of the objectives.

Finally, we must decide on the configuration of our service delivery; that is, will we provide direct and indirect services to individuals or to groups? If you choose a group model, the size of the groups will be determined by whether your population consists of children or adults and the nature of their needs.

For example, goal attainment for adolescents with behavior/conduct disorders requires the configuration of a smaller group size than might be successfully managed with a gardening group of individuals who are homeless. Likewise, a different level of staff expertise and supervision might be required for the two populations to meet the goal of their program.

Direct group services to the adolescents in our example would likely require the education, skill, and experience of an intermediate or advanced practitioner (perhaps an entrepreneur). Although it would be designed and supervised by an intermediate or advanced practitioner/consultant, the gardening program could be conducted by an entry-level occupational therapist (OTR) or by an intermediate certified occupational therapy assistant (COTA) supervising occupational therapy aides, volunteers, and both occupational therapy and occupational therapy assistant students (and in the case of the entry-level OTR, perhaps a COTA).

Therefore, to determine staffing needs, you must determine the following:

1. The needs and availability of the service population
2. Potential funding sources and estimated funds available to support the program
3. Physical space where the program is likely to be provided
4. The nature of services needed—direct or indirect
5. Configurations of service delivery—individual or groups

Occupational Therapy Practitioners
The Registered Occupational Therapist (OTR)

Our purpose is to design community-based programs that are occupation-centered, and at the *center* of all these programs will be one or more occupational therapy practitioners. Although they may not always be on-site, they will always be responsible for maintaining *occupation* as the central organizing theme of the program. Other personnel may be hired to support the multiple functions of the program, but occupational therapy practitioners are the gatekeepers of occupation and the ones to ensure that programs remain occupation-centered.

Our next task will be to consider what practice skills are required to provide quality services to our population and, further, what occupational therapy practitioners can best provide these services. For our purposes in this chapter, we are most concerned with those documents that describe the roles and supervision requirements of occupational therapy personnel as determined by the American Occupational Therapy Association, or AOTA (1998, 1999a). At some level, the program will require the skills and knowledge of one or more registered occupational therapists (OTRs), perhaps to design and develop the program, to provide direct or indirect services, or to supervise COTAs or other personnel.

According to the "Roles and Functions Papers" included in the AOTA's 1998 reference manual, OTRs may be considered to be practicing along a continuum from entry level to intermediate level to advanced level based on their level of education, their experience, and their demonstrated practice skills (pp. 267–299). For each category of role (for example, practitioner, supervisor, or administrator), major functions are described, the scope of the role is defined, and key performance areas are outlined. For all categories of occupational therapy personnel, the OTR carries the responsibility for service supervision (AOTA, 1999a, pp. 592–594). Whether your program will require the expertise of an entry-level, intermediate, or advanced practitioner will again depend on your goal and objectives and the services you wish to provide. You will want to review the AOTA's guidelines to match the service needs of your population to the skills and experience of the practitioner you wish to employ. Refer to the Appendix for an example of staff selection for a pediatric camp program.

To summarize, the program goal, objectives, and planned services determine

1. the necessary level of education,
2. the level of experience, and
3. the required skills and knowledge of the occupational therapy practitioner.

The Certified Occupational Therapy Assistant (COTA)

The Certified Occupational Therapist (COTA) may also demonstrate the three categories of ability—entry level, intermediate, and advanced—based on the same considerations that were applied to the OTR. For both of these key categories of occupational therapy personnel, the "Roles and Functions Papers" delineate performance areas according to skills level and qualifications for practice. Requirements for supervision are also provided in the "Guide for Supervision of Occupational Therapy Personnel in the Delivery of Occupational Therapy Services" (AOTA, 1999a). As the levels of role performance increase (from entry to intermediate to advanced), the COTA requires less intense supervision. Clearly the occupational therapy program planner (either new or experienced) should keep these documents as well as the state practice act and licensure requirements and any other regulatory documents that might affect the hiring and supervision of professional personnel where they easily can be accessed.

The Occupational Therapy Aide

Another category of occupational therapy personnel, the Occupational Therapy Aide, is described in the "Guidelines for the Use of Aides in Occupational Therapy Practice" (AOTA, 1999b). According to this document, "the term aides refers to those individuals who provide supportive services to the occupational therapy practitioner" (p. 595). The role of occupational therapy aides is described as well as the supervisory relationship, accountability, statutory requirements, training, and reimbursement.

SUPERVISION OF PROFESSIONAL PERSONNEL

Collaborative **supervision** of numerous levels of personnel is the key to operating a successful occupation-centered program. According to the AOTA official document, "Guide for Supervision of Occupational Therapy Personnel in the Delivery of Occupational Therapy Services," supervision may be classified as close, routine, general, and minimal (1999a, pp. 592–594). Of course, the continuum of supervisory classification depends on the experience and skills of the supervisee; there is closer and more supervision for the entry-level practitioner (OTR, COTA, or Aide) and less supervision for the intermediate to advanced practitioner.

The *COTA Information Packet: A Guide for Supervision* combines all of the AOTA information delineating the OTR/COTA collaborative relationship (AOTA, 1995) and specifies that all levels of occupational therapy practitioner (OTR and COTA) are qualified to supervise some level of personnel. Both the entry-level OTR and the entry-level COTA can supervise aides, technicians, care extenders, and volunteers; in addition, the entry-level occupational therapist may supervise all levels of COTAs and Level 1 academic fieldwork students. Other levels of practitioner from intermediate to advanced can assume more levels of supervision. You will not want to delimit your programming by failing to carefully research the roles, supervisory options, and requirements of occupational therapy personnel. All of the references listed at the close of this chapter are strong companions to what is noted here.

OTHER PERSONNEL

It is likely that you also will want to staff your program with other personnel to assist in the provision of direct and/or indirect services or to offer other support to the program. Office staff may be necessary, particularly in a for-profit venture where billing and receipt of payment for services is an integral part of the success of the program. The multiple roles of reception will also be important to many settings. Clients/patients must be greeted, phones must be answered, messages must be received, records must be updated, and so on. The decision to either employ these persons or to employ an external service will need to be made based on your mission and your volume of services. If your service is offered under the umbrella of another agency or agencies, they may provide these services.

As your program develops, you might want to add opportunities for volunteers and/or interning students. If you expect to consider adding interning students to your staff, again refer to the "Guide for Supervision of Occupational Therapy Personnel in the Delivery of Occupational Therapy Services" to determine who may offer supervision and at what level (AOTA, 1999a, p. 594). You may also want to refer to the AOTA *Fieldwork Evaluation for the Occupational Therapy* and *Fieldwork Evaluation for the Occupational Therapy Assistant Student* (AOTA, 1983, 1987) as well as other documents describing levels of fieldwork for occupational therapy and occupational therapy assistant students available from the AOTA.

If you are designing and developing a community-based program as an experienced occupational therapy practitioner, you might want to contact the occupational therapy academic programs in your area to discuss their curricula and specific service learning/fieldwork/internship requirements. The costs of providing opportunities for students as opposed to the benefits has been a long-standing debate in the profession, particularly in recent "cost-crunching" times. However, in community-based programs, particularly those that are not-for-profit, students can learn while providing much needed services. This is also true for volunteers. Volunteers offer a wealth of skill and experiences and are a valuable addition to a program. But a program cannot expect to exist based on volunteer services or student services (volunteer, service learning, or interning) alone. There are two obvious reasons. First of all, both students and volunteers are time-limited. Since volunteers provide services because they want to not because they have to, often they move on to other things, just as students will. Secondly, both groups are adjunctive intended to enhance professional services, and both groups must be closely supervised. Although this second reason of supervision is not prohibitive, it must be considered. While there is always some cost involved in supervision, the richness of an educational environment added to the community mix far outweighs any dollar cost.

OTHER PROFESSIONAL PERSONNEL

Depending on your goal and your objectives, your program can also benefit from the services of other professionals, including speech therapists, physical therapists, special education teachers, and others. Similar to occupational therapy personnel, if you wish to involve the services of other therapy specialists, then you will need to carefully research their roles and requirements for supervision. The national organizations of other professions also publish documents describing service provision and supervisory requirements. If you plan to hire professional personnel in addition to occupational therapy practitioners, it would be helpful to contact these organizations.

Keep in mind, however, that the kind of programming that would require the consideration of multiple personnel at professional levels is more along the lines of a community-based, free-standing or extended practice rather than much of the programming described in this text.

You will also need to become familiar with the credentialing of those personnel you intend to hire so that services are provided by properly credentialed and trained individuals. Academic standards for occupational therapy education are maintained by the Accreditation Council of the American Occupational Therapy Association according to the guidelines provided by the *Standards for an Accredited Educational Program for the Occupational Therapist* (1999c, pp. 575–582) and a separate but similar document for occupational therapy assistants titled *Standards for an Accredited Educational Program for the Occupational Therapy Assistant* (AOTA, 1999d, pp. 583–589). Initial certification for occupational therapists and occupational therapy assistants is provided by the National Board for Certification of Occupational Therapists and Occupational Therapy Assistants (NBCOT). You must also be familiar with the further requirements of your State Licensure Board; you can access that information through the NBCOT Web site (http://www.nbcot.org).

ACCREDITING AGENCIES

If there is to be further credentialing/accrediting of your organization/program, then you must become familiar with those agencies who provide this credentialing and you must know their requirements as well (not only for staff but also for other aspects of your program). Some examples of agencies that set standards for operations of health care provision include the Commission on Accreditation of Rehabilitation Facilities (CARF) and the Joint Commission on Accreditation of Healthcare Organizations (JCAHO). Whether or not you will be required to meet the standards of these organizations or others will depend on the kinds of services you expect to provide and where they will be provided. You will need to explore this further when you initiate the early process of developing a program. If you are affiliating with another organization or agency, they can help you explore your role in any accreditation or credentialing procedures.

THE CONSULTANT AND THE ENTREPRENEUR

Let's consider two other roles for the experienced occupational therapy practitioner that are both very appropriate to many kinds of community-based programs in terms of both required expertise and affordable costs. First let's consider the role of the **consultant.** The AOTA (1998) "Roles and Functions" document describes the consultant as one who provides occupational therapy consultation "to individuals, groups, or organizations" and does so within the systems related to "practice, education, administration, or research" (p. 272). This role is not restricted to the OTR. The experienced COTA also may consult within his or her area(s) of expertise with the appropriate OTR supervision to meet all levels of regulatory and professional standards. Programming examples in this text span a broad arena of systems where a consultant with appropriate knowledge, experience, and expertise could first design and develop a program and then consult through the continuing phases.

Hanft and Place (1996) provide an example of the role of the consultant in the school system. They provide a model for consultation that includes the development of a *strategy,* which is followed by the development of a *method* according to the therapist's *style* (p. 77). This model is very appropriate for those who might wish to consult in other systems as well as the school system, and it is not unlike the process of community program development advocated in this text.

A consultant has the opportunity—and, we presume, the ability—to see the "whole picture." When entering an agreement with an organization, the consultant is obligated to provide the best advice/plan possible to assist the organization to meet the needs of its service population and the needs of the organization as expressed through its mission and philosophy. The consultant is able to do this without becoming enmeshed in the day-to-day operations of the organization; therefore, his or her vision for the organization can remain unclouded.

The consultant's practice and programming experience permits him or her to provide the very best strategies and methods to accomplish the goals of the organization. In fact, the consultant along with the members of the organization may have assisted in establishing the goals. In our discussions of program development, it is possible that the consultant would be hired to do all aspects of development described in this text, including the recommendations for the personnel to operate the program(s). The consultant might then stay on to consult at regular intervals. This role of consultant is not to be confused with the role of supervisor. In fact, the consultant might wish to supervise on-site professional personnel, but this would not be one of the expected roles of a consultant.

Hanft and Place mention "style" as one of the elements in their consulting model. They suggest that "style," or how you present yourself and your information to the organization, may include the following choices: "tell, sell, teach/advise; and encourage or support" (1996, p. 77). When you function as a program planner/consultant in the community, you must engage in all of these behaviors and more. The skills and information drawn from your intellect, education, and experience must be matched with the strong qualities of leadership; you must have the ability to have a vision, to exude a sense of ethical responsibility (and as such, to merit trust), and to model a belief in the therapeutic and formative potential of occupation. And, perhaps most importantly, you must be convincing in the belief that *community* is integral to our professional strength and must be encouraged and protected as an ideal.

The role of the occupational therapy **entrepreneur** is also very appropriate to our discussions. This is another potential role for occupational therapy practitioners described by AOTA in "Roles and Functions" (1998, p. 272). Modestly, the entrepreneur is a partially or fully self-employed occupational therapy practitioner who provides occupational therapy services. Of course, the consultant may fit this description as well, but we may think of the entrepreneur more as the "independent contractor and private practice owner and/or operator" (1998, p. 271). As an independent contractor, the entrepreneur offers services *independently.* As opposed to *employees,* independent contractors' work is task driven; they often set their own hours, and they are paid by the job. They also supply their own resources to do the job, including any health insurance or benefits. These "resources" may also include employees.

Jesierski and Gauch (1996) and The Occupational Therapy Association of California (1999) offer suggestions for the entrepreneur to include the management of multiple employees. Foto (1999) discusses competence and the entrepreneur. Because of the growing numbers of practitioners assuming this role, she notes that the future stature of the profession may depend on the competency of these practitioners.

In her view, competency of these independent practitioners will likely be judged by marketplace success (1999, pp. 765–769). As a private practice owner and operator, the entrepreneur may select from a number of business options. He or she may choose to enter into a partnership, group practice, corporate organization, a joint venture, or may operate a sole proprietorship. A partnership simply means that you are going into business with at least one other person and likely more than one. Ryan, Ray, and Hiduke (1999) describe the arrangement as "psychologically comforting," while legally it is little more than an accounting entity (pp. 196–198). Joint venture means somewhat the same thing but is less a business term than one to describe a shared "adventure." A sole proprietorship, of course, is the opposite of these. You start the business on your own, without partners. A group practice likely means that you will be practicing fairly independently in the company of other professionals. Most often support services (that is, billing, supplies, equipment, reception, and so on) are shared by the group, along with cost. You may elect to incorporate your business. Corporations are often a way that a small business can limit liability, channel heavy expenses, guarantee continuity, improve the tax circumstances, upgrade the business's image, and perhaps offer employees internal incentives (Ryan, Ray, & Hiduke, 1999, pp. 201–202). It is certainly recommended that none of the above enterprises be entered into without first completing some substantial research, consulting a business attorney, and consulting a certified public accountant.

THE ADVISORY BOARD

The one other category of persons we should consider in the process of program development is the **advisory board.** An astute programmer will recognize the advantages of appointing a group of persons from the surrounding community to assist in providing expertise and in offering "links" to those in the community who may be of assistance as we develop and market our program. This group generally consists of professionals from occupational therapy or other disciplines, laypersons, consumers, and/or caregivers. It is unusual that they are paid; however, travel expenses may be reimbursed if they must come from some distance for meetings, and as a courtesy, a meal is often provided along with the meeting. Experienced members of this group may also provide mentoring to the programmer, which is particularly useful if the programmer does not share in the culture of the community.

▮▮▮ EXERCISE 1 ▮▮▮
Developing Your Staffing Plan

In the previous chapters' exercises, you developed the goal and objectives for your community-based service population, you selected a frame of reference to guide the selection and provision of services, and you began to develop your ideas for programming that would enable your population to meet the goals. Continue to develop your program by answering the following questions and noting your responses in the space provided.

1. What, if any, direct service(s) will your program provide?

_____

_____

_____

_____

_____

2. If you intend to provide direct services, what level of occupational therapy practitioner will you require (review the "Roles and Functions Papers" and the "Guide for Supervision of Occupational Therapy Personnel")?

_____

_____

_____

_____

3. What, if any, indirect service(s) will your program provide?

_____

_____

_____

_____

_____

4. If you are providing indirect service(s), who can best provide these (again, consider the above documents)?

_____

_____

_____

_____

Although we will more carefully develop the volume of services and anticipated service configuration when we consider costs, these things will impact staffing in a number of ways, and you might wish to consider them now. For example, offering services in less traditional time slots such as evenings and weekends might appeal to many patients/clients/members as well as staff who wish to work full-time during the days at another facility (perhaps another facility where benefits are paid). Such a schedule might also appeal to fieldwork students who seek part-time or nontraditional options.

If you intend to supplement your program with volunteers, the day and time services are offered will likely affect the age and experience of your volunteers. Retired adults may wish to volunteer during weekdays; students, on the other hand, might prefer to help after school and on weekends.

A combined volunteer model is recommended to supplement services for a community gardening program. In our gardening program, for example, retired gardeners preferred the early morning hours for working in the gardens as did some of the members; other members, some retired volunteers, some working adult volunteers, and younger (working or in school) volunteers preferred the late afternoon and early evening. Still others were available on weekends. Service-learning students balanced out the options. On the surface, this might seem problematic; but with a continuous thread of direction and supervision, these options invite creativity and flexibility with tasks such as tilling, planting, weeding, and watering in the early mornings; picking, cleaning, preparing, and socializing under the trees in the afternoons; and viewing seed and equipment catalogues, researching options (such as a "taco" garden and an "early native american" garden), building benches and ponds, and attending community meetings in the evening or on the weekend!

The community garden was restricted by the fact that gardening space was at a premium. In order to involve as many members as possible, it was necessary to operate on a broad seven-day schedule. The garden also dictated this kind of attention. Thus, a wide array of personnel over a broad programming schedule was required. The two important requirements for the occupational therapy practitioners were 1) advanced supervisory skills and experience and 2) skills and experience in program management and coordination. There were other requirements, but the preceding were of most importance. For example, interest and experience in psychosocial practice and an interest in gardening were advantages but were not critical.

Watering a garden project in the early morning hours is enjoyed by a garden–club volunteer.

5. Considering the gardening example, what is your present planning with regard to how and when you will provide services? How will these plans dictate the paid and perhaps volunteer staff that you will require?

_____

_____

_____

_____

_____

6. Consider what you will want your occupational therapy practitioner(s) to do. Make a list of the tasks that will make up the job (separately if you anticipate hiring more than one).

Some examples for the occupational therapy manager of the community garden program include the following:

1. Management of the gardening program to include staff, supplies, materials, equipment, scheduling, and budgeting
2. Hiring, training, and supervision of staff
3. Training and development of volunteers
4. Supervision of students to include service-learning, level 1, and level 2 fieldwork students
5. Monitoring program objectives and revising and updating as needed
6. Monitoring all aspects of program evaluation
7. Preparing statistics and documentation for funding reapplication or for new funding

Overlooking the city, an urban pocket garden can bring many pleasures to all involved—members, staff, students, and volunteers—while achieving significant goals for the participants.

While in other kinds of programs, expertise and experience with a particular service population might be the most important factor, in this example it was not. Make your list of tasks below:

_____

_____

_____

_____

_____

In the development of the above list, you have created the **job description** for the occupational therapy practitioner, or practitioners that will provide services for your program. *If you are the one who will do this, can you do the job that is required?* From the job description, you can identify the credentials and experience that will be required to perform the job, and an advertisement can be written. You may wish to review examples of job listings in the official news magazine of the American Occupational Therapy Association, *OT Week* (www.otweek.org).

7. Following your review of examples in *OT Week* or other professional sources, try writing a draft advertisement for the position you described above (the advertisement also markets your program, so you will want to describe it in the most positive way):

_____

_____

_____

_____

_____

You might choose to place your advertisement in national sources or local ones or sometimes both. This choice is substantially influenced by cost and by what you believe to be the local/regional availability of qualified therapists. If you already anticipate funds to be limited, you might circulate a job description and advertisement in the form of a flyer to academic programs (for recently certified practitioners) or to State Association Chapter Newsletters for more experienced practitioners. A well-designed, strategically placed flyer is also a good way to attract volunteers.

SUMMARY

Finding well-prepared, ethical, and creative staff may be one of the most complex challenges to developing new programs. Once you have developed the goal, objectives, and ideas for the program, it is usually not difficult to write a job description for the occupational therapy practitioner(s) and other staff; the task then is to market your program to potential staff through carefully placed and well-written advertising. When considering the staffing of a new or extended program, you must consider the match between the needs of the service population and the expertise and experience of the practitioner. If supervision of other personnel or students will be expected, then the experience and practice credentials of the occupational therapy practitioner must be carefully considered. A thorough review of the *Reference Manual of the Official Documents of the American Occupational Therapy Association*, will provide the foundation for first advertising for and then selecting the appropriate practitioner or practitioners to provide the program. Chapter 11 will offer additional discussion of considerations for hiring and retaining staff.

REFERENCES

American Occupational Therapy Association. (1983). *Fieldwork evaluation form for the occupational therapy assistant student.* Bethesda, MD: AOTA.

American Occupational Therapy Association. (1987). *Fieldwork evaluation for the occupational therapist.* Bethesda, MD: AOTA.

American Occupational Therapy Association. (1995). *COTA information packet: A guide for supervision .* Bethesda, MD: AOTA.

American Occupational Therapy Association. (1998). *Reference manual of the official documents of the American occupational therapy association, Inc.* (7th ed.). Bethesda, MD: AOTA.

American Occupational Therapy Association. (1999a). Guide for supervision of occupational therapy personnel in the delivery of occupational therapy services. *American Journal of Occupational Therapy, 53*(6), 592–594.

American Occupational Therapy Association. (1999b). Guidelines for the use of aides in occupational therapy practice. *American Journal of Occupational Therapy, 53*(6), 595–597.

American Occupational Therapy Association. (1999c). Standards for an accredited educational program for the occupational therapist. *American Journal of Occupational Therapy, 53*(6), 575–582.

American Occupational Therapy Association. (1999d). Standards for an accredited educational program for the occupational therapy assistant. *American Journal of Occupational Therapy, 53*(6), 583–589.

Foto, M. (1999). Competence and the occupational therapy entrepreneur. *American Journal of Occupational Therapy, 52*(9), 765–769.

Hanft, B. E., & Place, P. A. (1996). *The consulting therapist, A guide for OTs and PTs in schools.* San Antonio, TX: Therapy Skill Builders.

Jesierski, R., & Gauch, P. (Eds.). (1996). *On your own: An introduction to private practice and self-employment.* Ottawa, Ontario: The Canadian Association of Occupational Therapists.

Moyers, P. (1999). The guide to occupational therapy practice. *American Journal of Occupational Therapy, 53,* 247–322.

Occupational Therapy Association of California (Sponsors). (1999). Growing in size: Employment law, employee retention, and employee records. *Branching Out: Private Practice and Beyond.* Sacramento, CA: Author.

Rogers, J. C., & Holm, M. B. (1991). Occupational therapy diagnostic reasoning: A component of clinical reasoning. *American Journal of Occupational Therapy, 45,* 1,045–1,053.

Ryan, J. D., Ray, R. J., & Hiduke, G. (1999). *Small business: An entrepreneur's plan* (5th ed.). Fort Worth, TX: The Dryden Press.

Related Web Sites and Telephone Numbers

OT Week:

http://www.otweek.org

NBCOT:

http://www.nbcot.org

Occupational Therapy Products:

http:// www.aota.org

AOTA Educational Standards:

http://www.aota.org/students/standot.html

Developing a Small Business:

www.lectlaw.com

www.awsource.com

www.hg.org

www.cnnfn.com/smbusiness

U.S. Small Business Administration:

www.sba.gov

(1-800-U-ASK-SBA)

EEOC Guide: Reasonable Accomodation and Undue Hardship Under the ADA:

www.eeoc.gov/docs/accommodation.html

(1-800-669-3362)

Equal Employment Opportunity Commission:

(1-202-663-4900)

Pacific Disability and Business Technical Assistance Center:

http://www.pacdbtac.org

(ADA Hotline: 1-800-949-4232)

The Job Accomodations Network:

(1-800-526-7234)

Space: Where Will It Be Done?

Learning Objectives

1. To understand the distinction between *space* and *environment*
2. To learn to project space/environment needs from program goal(s) and objectives
3. To determine square footage needed to provide intervention and support services to meet program objectives
4. To determine the need for utilities, plumbing, and safety to support the objectives of the program
5. To compare the characteristics of service provision to the characteristics of available space to determine where negotiations may occur without compromising program goals

Key Terms

1. Space/Dedicated Space
2. Environment
3. Negotiation

You now have taken your early idea, and either alone or with your classmates or colleagues, you have developed a brief profile of the agency, the community, and the population. You have assessed the need for services both from those in the agency and/or the community and from the population to be served. You have reviewed developing trends that may impact this program (such as growing populations of homeless mothers and children, increases in funding for school, home-based services, and so on). From the results of this work, you have selected a goal or goals and supporting objectives for the program.

Considering the goal(s) and the objectives, you have identified specific directions for programming that will meet the needs of the agency or organization, the community, and the service population. You have determined your staffing needs, including the levels of skill, knowledge, and expertise that will be required to meet your goal(s). You also know what levels of supervision will be needed. To review, you have done the following:

1. Profiled the agency, community, and service population
2. Assessed the need from the community and/or agency and the service population
3. Reviewed trends that might impact your program
4. Selected a goal or goals for your program
5. Selected objectives to support your goal or goals
6. Designed programming to meet the objectives of your service population
7. Identified the staff that will be needed to meet the range, volume, and nature of programming required to meet the goal(s)

You are now ready to identify the remaining resources needed to conduct the program according to your design and plan.

PLANNING THE UTILIZATION OF EXISTING SPACE

Let's consider space. Actually, that statement is a bit vague; what we are really doing is not just considering space but analyzing, designing, and engineering environments. **Space** happens to be where we complete these activities; it defines our parameters. Before you begin this process, think about **environments** and how they impact outcomes. Space denotes emptiness; think of it as a blank canvas on which we paint images. Just as you transform a blank canvas, you can transform the space designated for your program into a positive environment with color, light, and contours.

The same *space* can invite entirely different outcomes when the *environment* is created with the needs of the population in mind. For example, consider the choice of classical music and stimulating color for an older adult population or cartoon favorites and subdued color for a population of potentially hyperactive children (or perhaps the reverse depending on the theoretical framework selected by the planner).

Now let's return to the tracing of our progress. If you have initiated planning at the invitation of an agency or organization, it is likely that the agency or organization has identified some space it thinks would be suitable for the proposed programming. While this offered space often is small and less than ideal, it is usually adequate to begin. Remember that the space, in part, will structure the volume and design of service offering. Initially you should be conservative until you have matched your objectives to outcomes, so a small space is not necessarily restrictive.

If space is offered by the facility, it probably is not presently in priority use; for example, it might be a storeroom (to be emptied); a garage (to be cleaned out); a partially covered patio; or the sharing of a dining room, a classroom, or a church basement. If you will have **dedicated space** (used for your purposes exclusively), you will have much more flexibility in programming; if not, you will need to negotiate the sharing of space around other programming that may already exist. Occasionally part of the **negotiation** process includes the need to revisit your objectives and the structure of your program as well as the volume of services you wish to provide. You might not be able to realistically meet the needs of either the facility, community, or the service population as they originally were assessed. If you are an inexperienced planner, this is an extremely challenging juncture, for you want to meet *all of the need*. It is likely that if your program evaluation results indicate that you were successful with a smaller component of the population, you can negotiate for more (and maybe more desirable) space. If your initial work was accurate, then your goal or goals do not change, regardless of what negotiations you must make along the way.

Before you begin to actually identify and acquire space, revisit the work you already have accomplished, including your goal(s), your objectives, the nature of services you wish to provide, and the volume of services that you will provide to meet the identified needs. You cannot negotiate until you know what you want— *the best case scenario.*

■ EXERCISE 1 ■

Identifying the Required Space to Meet the Needs of Your Program Design

Square Footage

Consider the space/square footage required for each participant served (that is, an area that is a 2-foot square will contain 4 square feet). Remember that many service models can be considered, including rotating groups or individuals and weekday, weekend, or evening scheduling.

The earlier example of the day camp to promote movement and socialization through play could be offered in a number of different ways to accommodate the needs of the community. For example, you could offer two groups a day, each for one-half day; four groups a day for shorter periods; groups that rotate on one or two-week schedules; or after-school groups. Depending on space and staffing, perhaps concurrent groups could be accommodated. Neville-Jan, Fazio, Kennedy, and Snyder (1997) describe an elementary to middle school occupation-centered transition program that utilized scheduling concurrently with the children's academic day (pp. 144–157).

1. Note below your anticipated program schedule and the square-footage space needs (both indoor and outdoor as required by your program):

_____

_____

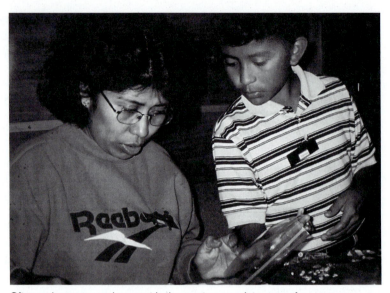

Often a classroom environment is the most appropriate space for programs centered around the occupations of the "student."

_____

_____

_____

Consider the space/square footage for any equipment your goal(s) and objectives require.

The planner of the day camp, for example, intended to access the objectives and goal primarily through the sensory-integrative frame of reference. Both indoor and outdoor space was considered in accommodating equipment such as the flexible crawl tube and a ball-crawl for a program providing service to six children between the ages of four and five.

The parent-child program mentioned earlier blended integrated community sites with classroom-style table-and-chair work space for both a parent and a child of middle-school age that took into consideration the varying heights and weights of the participants.

2. Note below your anticipated space needs for equipment:

_____

_____

_____

_____

_____

3. Will your program require space for files, office equipment, and office supplies? Note below what will be needed and the approximate square footage required:

_____

_____

_____

_____

_____

Consider any additional equipment/supplies for your program (including what was noted above) such as assessments, arts and crafts, and so on. What kind of storage will be required? Also consider office supplies. Will your supplies/equipment require secured (locked) storage? If you need to move supplies from place to place (programming in more than one location), do you need storage for supply carts?

For example, the space for the community garden was dictated by the size of the ground plots available to the program (later negotiation permitted the acquisition of additional space). The acquisition of a secured storage shed for equipment/tools and supplies, however, was not negotiable.

4. Note below your anticipated storage needs:

_____

_____

_____

_____

_____

▬ EXERCISE 2 ▬
Utilities and Plumbing

Again consider the design of your program and the anticipated nature and volume of services to be offered. Consider the toilets, sinks that you will need, and the location. What will be the needs of your population for adaptations, for accessibility, and for structural changes to the fixtures? Do you need a bathroom in the intervention area, or will one dual-purpose bathroom serve both the intervention area and perhaps reception? Does the bathroom need to be large enough for diaper/clothing changes? Will you need a tub and/or a shower?

1. Note below your needs for bathrooms:

_____

_____

_____

_____

_____

Will you require water sources and/or sinks in the intervention areas? Will you need a water source/sink for arts and crafts? Will you have specialized needs such as over-sized sinks for paper making with the addition of a clay trap in the sink drain? Will you include orthotics or other treatment procedures requiring plumbing? An outdoor faucet is a necessity for filling inflated swimming pools and for cleaning up children after a day camp activity.

2. Note below your additional needs for water/sinks:

_____

_____

_____

_____

Consider your needs for dedicated telephone lines, computer access (for intervention and/or staff needs), and utilities. Will you require heavy-duty electrical wiring for equipment? Specialized lighting? Wall and/or floor outlets? Outside outlets?

3. Note what you will require below:

_____

_____

_____

_____

_____

▬▬▬ EXERCISE 3 ▬▬▬
Safety

Consider any special requirements to ensure the safety of your service population and your staff. Will you require security for the building and/or the parking lot? If you are working with a facility, you might not be able to control this; but it is certainly a question to ask, particularly if your staff will be working evening or weekend hours when other employees might not be present. Will outside areas require security walls or fences (for example, are you servicing potential "runaways")?

1. Note below your needs with regard to the above considerations:

_____

_____

_____

_____

Do you anticipate facility-specific safety requirements with regard to space design (such as codes or restrictions)? If so, what might be the potential impact on your program? When you survey the existing space, make note of any safety concerns you may want to have addressed.

2. Note your responses below either now or after you have surveyed the proposed space:

_____

_____

_____

_____

_____

▇ EXERCISE 4 ▇
Space and Environment

What kind of environment do you wish to create? Will your intervention require individualized space that is free from distractions? A large space for group intervention that might include games, exercises, and maybe dancing? A patio area? A room for parent/family conferences? A waiting area for clients/patients/ families? A formal reception area?

Consider color, furnishings, windows for natural lighting or more subdued artificial lighting, sound (such as distracting noise), and privacy.

1. Note below your needs with regard to the creation of an environment that will facilitate the achievement of objectives:

_____

_____

_____

_____

_____

TAKING A FIRST LOOK AND THEN ANOTHER

If you have not already done so, it is time to take a critical walk-through of the space where you will be providing your program. Before this visit, carefully consider your responses to the exercises you just completed with regard to the space requirements deemed necessary to meet the objectives of your program. If necessary, make a second visit; walk the space and determine the exact square footage that is available to you for intervention and storage. Compare these figures with the results of your earlier exercises. Spend time envisioning how the space will be laid out and how people will get in and out of it. While you are there, also draw a rough floor plan and note the details of the space, including placement of doors/exits, windows, closets, electrical outlets, lighting, telephone lines, and anything else that presently exists in the designated space. For exact square footage, use graph paper to scale (for example 1/4" = 1 foot). See Figure 9–1 for an example of a floor/space drawing for a pediatric intervention program.

▆▆▆ EXERCISE 5 ▆▆▆

Comparing Your Rough Space Drawing to Your Original Plan

With your group or colleagues, carefully compare your drawing of the available space with the results of the previous exercises. Discuss any discrepancies you might find. On another sheet of graph paper, note any *additions or alterations* that meeting your program goal will *require.* What compromises are you willing to make? Remember that you might be willing to negotiate the mode of service delivery and you might also reconsider your objectives, but you cannot alter your goal and still meet the needs of your service population and the community.

In the planning of the elementary to middle school transition program mentioned earlier, the most desirable space (one without distraction) was thought to be a small classroom or meeting room adjacent to the regular classroom. Although it was added later when the program was expanded, such a space initially was not available. The format for programming was redesigned and negotiated to blend and flow with actual classroom and playground activities during the course of the daily round of activities supporting the occupation of "just going to school"/education. The goal of the program accurately reflected the need; thus, negotiation was possible. Without such preliminary work in assessing the need, the assistance of the school administrators and teachers would not likely have been forthcoming (Neville-Jan, Fazio, Kennedy and Snyder, 1997, pp. 144–157).

1. After you have made your comparisons, note below any additions or alterations in the existing space that *must* be negotiated in order for your program to meet the goal(s):

_____

_____

_____

_____

_____

FIGURE 9–1 Example of a Floor/Space Drawing for a Pediatric Intervention Program

IDEAL SPACE

You might want to draft what could be described as an *ideal* or *most desirable* space plan to keep in your file for future planning; for now, however, you will need to negotiate from what you *require* to meet your goal(s), not necessarily from what might be ideal. Space is a desirable and scarce commodity for most agencies and organizations, particularly if they are not-for-profit. However, if you have followed through on the previous exercises and have an accurate and detailed assessment of needs, then you will have an informed position from which you can negotiate. Do not settle for less than what you require to satisfy your goal(s). If you must negotiate for less space (reduced square footage) or less desirable space than you intended (inadequate storage, no windows, and so on), then you may need to alter your objectives and the volume of services you can offer. You will need to be clear about this in your negotiations. Also consider your bottom line for negotiation. There is always a point from which you might decide that you cannot meet the expected need or cannot do so while offering quality services. Negotiation does not mean compromising ethics, integrity, or quality. If it comes to this, you know to step away and perhaps broker your plan elsewhere in the community.

Designing New, Remodeled, or Renovated Space for a Private Practice

If you are designing space for inclusion in a grant application or for a private for-profit practice, you can be more creative in the expression of your needs. However, even if you have substantial freedom in space design, it is critical that you always be realistic in what you must have to meet your goal(s) and objectives. If you are successful as you initiate programming and if your outcome measures demonstrate this success, then you will be in a position to negotiate for additional and perhaps more desirable space.

Assuming careful planning and good business savvy (or advice), it is likely that private practices will soon outgrow their space and will find the need to expand into other existing space. It would be advisable to keep this in mind if you anticipate leasing space for a free-standing practice. Consider a business building that is zoned appropriately for your practice, with easy access, elevators to upper floors, adequate parking, and with *potential to lease adjoining space* when the practice grows. This will help in the future to avoid the time, potential client loss, and expense of having to move everything to a new address.

If you are starting a private practice, then the space plan must be detailed, accurate, and comprehensive. This is also true if you are "shopping" for existing space to remodel or if you are able to design your space as a building is being constructed. As a culture, occupational therapy practitioners seem to have a good sense of space, environment, and design; however, the design of a practice space from the ground up requires the services of an architect and perhaps other design professionals. Certainly you must carefully collaborate from your area of expertise, which is knowledge about the characteristics and needs of the community, the service needs of your population, and the characteristics of adapted environments. Occupational therapy practitioners can and do create positive environments, but they need the assistance of a good architect in this circumstance.

There are a few other points to consider if you intend to design and plan a private practice. Just as we discussed previously, conduct all steps of the programming process, including the needs assessment, trends analysis, and the community profile. Although you might believe that you know the community, it is likely that you only know it from your own perspective (that is, the environment that supports your chosen occupations). Of course, place your practice within the community you wish to serve, with consideration for the round of activities that your targeted client/patient population engages in daily and weekly. If your program's targeted population includes children with learning and/or emotional disorders who are seen after school or on Saturdays, consider the daily occupations of the parents and families, and place your practice close to areas such as schools, athletic fields, and shopping.

If a mother or father is able to first drop off one child for soccer practice, another for an after-school music lesson, and another for therapy then shop for dinner, your practice will be more successful than one that is located outside of (his or) her round of daily activity. Convenience is also a factor for adults who come for therapy before or after work or during their lunch hours. "Mapping" your community and the daily occupations of your targeted population and their families and using this "map" to locate your practice and develop your programming hours will be a long-standing advantage to you. While it might seem to be common sense, placing your practice convenient to the occupational routines of your client/patient population is also a sophisticated marketing strategy.

The above considerations also hold true for the planning of day camps for differently abled children. Again, parents may have to balance the needs of other children, their own work schedules, and the needs of a differently abled child. In the case of a day camp, offering low-cost transportation is a real plus, but sometimes simply offering a small space for parents and caregivers to have a cup of coffee, chat with others, and relax is enough to get children there when otherwise they might not have been included. Anticipating and addressing the needs of a caregiver while providing intervention to the client/patient/camper permits the planner to meet several objectives. In addition, if our camp example also includes the siblings of the service population, several needs may be satisfied. Additional programming for these caregivers through focused "help" sessions while their children are receiving services might be a wise marketing tool or, in some cases, another point of potentially profitable service.

The wise utilization of space—whether a room, a building, or a location within a community—is often key to the success of a program. As stated by Ryan, Ray and Hiduke, "one of the most important decisions an entrepreneur has to make is where to locate his or her business . . . location, location, location" (1999, p. 119).

SUMMARY

Anticipating space needs by matching them closely to program goal(s) and objectives will place the planner in an excellent position to prepare for the necessary negotiation that will take place in the process of locating or sometimes being assigned space for program operations. A detailed analysis of the size and nature of space required for intervention, the plumbing and utilities needed, and considerations for safety place the planner in a good position to review available space with a careful eye toward what negotiations may be made without compromising the goal(s) of the program. In the process of designing and planning a program, objectives and/or service delivery patterns may be negotiated; however, goals are not. Although somewhat different than the space considerations of the planner working in cooperation with an agency/facility, the space needs of those who anticipate initiating a free-standing practice continue to be based on the community and service profiles, the comprehensive assessment of needs, and on-going reviews of trends that might impact the success of the program.

REFERENCES

Neville-Jan, A., Fazio, L. S., Kennedy, B., & Snyder, C. (1997). Elementary to middle school transition: Using multicultural play activities to develop life skills. In D. Parham and L. S. Fazio (Eds.), *Play in occupational therapy for children* (pp. 144–157). St. Louis, MO: Mosby-Yearbook.

Ryan, J. D., Ray, R., & Hiduke, G. (1999). *Small business: An entrepreneur's plan* (5th ed.). Fort Worth, TX: The Dryden Press.

CHAPTER **10**

Furnishings, Equipment, and Supplies: What Do I Need to Do It?

Learning Objectives

1. To understand the relationship between the program goal, the nature and volume of services to be provided, and the furnishings, equipment, and supplies that will be required to operate the program
2. To distinguish between furnishings, equipment, and supplies
3. To understand the distinction between capital and noncapital equipment
4. To identify the characteristics that determine the categories of expendable and nonexpendable supplies
5. To develop a list of furnishings, equipment, and supplies needed for your anticipated program along with accompanying suppliers, quantities, and costs
6. To develop a short-term and long-term cost projection for the furnishings, equipment, and supplies needed to support the goal(s) of your program

Key Terms

1. Volume of Services
2. Furnishings
3. Capital and Noncapital Equipment
4. Supplies (Expendable and Nonexpendable)
5. Direct and Indirect Costs
6. Cost Projections

149

Now that you have accomplished your preliminary planning and have identified your space/programming environment, it is time to furnish it. Again, revisit your goal(s) and objectives. It seems redundant by now, but your well-crafted and informed goal(s) and objectives structure every plan and every decision that you make as you develop your program. We have all witnessed programs where there is an apparent lack of planning, direction, and structure. Consider, for example, treatment rooms filled with laundry lists of supplies and equipment because they were assumed to be important to an occupational therapy practice. This particularly happens when a planner solicits donated items without a clear sense of the program's direction. To avoid making a list of, for example, twelve reachers or five boxes of raffia or five inflatable swimming pools or four computers with cognitive retraining software, let's begin by defining exactly what we want to accomplish.

As we have already noted, our first consideration is our goal, our accompanying objectives, and our target population. In Chapter 7 you developed the frame or frames of reference that you would use to structure your intervention. The **volume of services**—or how many clients/patients/members you would see in the course of a day, week, or month—was established as you considered the needs of your population and the number of staff, their qualifications, and their skills. These considerations also helped you select and plan the space where the program would take place. As summarized in the following equation, all of these considerations form the pieces of a puzzle that will lead you to the furnishings, equipment, and supplies that you will need to operate the program.

goal/objectives + target population + frame of reference + staff + space +
service volume = furnishings, equipment and supplies

Let's examine how all of these considerations come together to result in our recommended inventory of furnishings, equipment, and supplies.

Case Example

You may recall that in Chapter 9 we reviewed the space needs for a day camp example. The goal of that program was to promote movement and socialization through play, and the sensory-integrative frame of reference was selected to facilitate the objectives designed to accomplish the goal. The available space could easily accommodate the program design to offer services for six children between the ages of four and five, four days a week from 10:00 A.M. to 3:00 P.M., for two weeks. This service model was then repeated for new groups of children. Children require attention both to facilitate the achievement of intervention objectives and to guarantee safety. For the six children, there were two occupational therapists, one occupational therapy assistant, and two student volunteers. In addition to direct service, administrative tasks and marketing/promotion were shared by the two occupational therapists.

The program was conducted both indoors and out-of-doors. The out-of-doors area combined a large sand strip with a grassy area for sensory-integrative games and activities. An awning covered four picnic tables for lunch, snacks, and arts and crafts. A smaller indoor area was available for rainy days and was used primarily for storage.

This service-delivery model could be expanded if the children came to camp for only half-days or if two camps were run simultaneously. Such decisions would require that the planners revisit their objectives and their goal. Could the campers meet their objectives in only half-day visits? How would this decision affect the staffing pattern? And what would happen if two camps were run simultaneously? Would more space be required? More supplies and equipment? How would this decision impact the staffing pattern? And could the objectives continue to be satisfied? Would new objectives be required to meet the goal? Would these potential changes in the service-delivery model continue to meet the needs as expressed by referring community therapists, teachers, and parents? (See Appendix at the back of the book for a partial supply list for this program.)

This example demonstrates several things. The equation we have offered to take us to our decision of what equipment and supplies we will need to provide the program is certainly not linear. With each option we might consider, there are pros and cons. It is our developing clinical reasoning that permits us to integrate all of these potential choices into a *best-case scenario* for the child/camper. Certainly adding more children to the camp while hiring fewer staff and not increasing supplies or equipment has the potential to "make more money." Or, does it? Can we consider that offering the very best services (that through our evaluation process we can guarantee are effective) may be more lucrative over time?

How Do You Find What You Need?

We have mentioned several service items in our example that will have to be purchased, including picnic tables, games and activities, and arts and crafts. The picnic tables and perhaps the games will be a one-time purchase, but the supplies for arts and crafts will require continuous replacement. If you are a practicing therapist, choosing the furnishings, equipment, and supplies for your program will not be difficult. On the other hand, if you are a student, you will first need to peruse the catalogues of suppliers that occupational therapy practitioners use to furnish their practices. Although some of the supplies and equipment probably surround you in your classrooms, until now you probably were not aware of how and where they were obtained or how much they cost. (See the partial list at the end of this chapter for companies that provide equipment and supplies.)

This issue of cost brings us to another important consideration: we have not yet established a budget for our program (that will come in the next chapter). Depending on how you have become accustomed to handling your personal budget, you might be a little confused about designing a program without knowing what you can afford. If you are a student, you should use what might be described as *optimistic budgeting,* or designing the best-case scenario of what the program *should be.* When you know what you want and what it will cost, then you target the funding. If you are unable to acquire enough financing to run the program exactly the way you want, you can make reductions in a number of areas (such as volume of services, staff, equipment, and supplies) before start-up and during the first year, while still meeting your needs/goal. As you become a more experienced planner, you will always have a funding source and a "ballpark" figure for funding in mind. You then will match each step of the process to the anticipated source and potential amount for funding.

FURNISHING YOUR PROGRAM

The term **furnishing** refers to the furniture we will need to provide the program that will help our clients/patients/members meet their objectives and the goal of the program. What will be required to furnish a welcoming environment? Will you require work tables, chairs, lamps, a television set/VCR, a radio, a sofa, a bed, and so on? Many of the programs described in this text have operated on little more than the above list. Most have required minimal supplies, and a few have required some equipment; however, equipment for therapeutic purposes has seldom been included. From our examples, you might think that community-based programs are always low-budget, "shoe-string" ventures that seldom, if ever, require expensive furnishings or equipment. However, keep in mind that the furnishings, equipment, and supplies are dictated by your goal, your objectives, and the needs of your target population, not by their placement in the community. While not *intended* to be therapeutic, a riding garden tiller that would permit several of the community gardeners with physical disability to be central to the development of new garden space was a fairly high-end expense.

If you are designing a private practice, the way you furnish it will be extremely important to how you market and promote it to your targeted population. While the primary aim in some of our community examples was a comfortable, inviting, and safe environment, the private practice will certainly provide all of these things and more. A well-appointed reception area and intervention environment, for example, contributes more than comfort to a practice setting; it must appeal to the senses of the consumer, and it enhances the quality of the intervention. Consider how much the environment and furnishings contribute to your acceptance of practicing professionals (such as your doctor, dentist, counselor, or therapist), assuming that the quality of services is equal.

■ EXERCISE 1 ■

How Will You Furnish Your Program?

1. Consider what furnishings you will require to meet the set objectives and goal of your program. Consider the volume of services and the age and differing abilities of your target population (for example, will adaptations be required in furnishings?). List below the furnishings you will need along with costs from your catalogue sources (such as Sears, J.C. Penney, or others of your choice):

Furnishings	Source	Anticipated Cost

EQUIPMENT

Equipment is categorized in terms of cost. Although this may vary from one agency or institution to another, for our purposes we will consider any equipment needed to support the programming at a cost of $1,000 or more to be in the category of **capital equipment.** Equipment may be intended exclusively for therapeutic purposes (such as adaptive playground equipment or work hardening equipment), but our garden tiller is also equipment that would fall into this category even though its intended purpose is not to provide therapy. Standard playground equipment and many kitchen appliances would also be considered as capital equipment (unless the umbrella agency places such things in the category of *furnishings,* which is something you will determine when you actually do your budget). We consider most equipment to be nonexpendable; that is, we will expect to use it many times and for many clients/patients/members. Of course, eventually the equipment will wear out and will need to be replaced, and such replacement costs will be anticipated in our long-range budget planning. Any equipment below the cost of $1,000 is considered **noncapital equipment** but is also included in the category of nonexpendable.

EXERCISE 2
Selecting Equipment for Your Program

1. List below all of the equipment you will need for your program (if you will not need equipment, simply indicate *none*):

2. When you have completed your equipment list, refer to the catalogues and determine the source and the cost of each piece of desired equipment. Note these items below, and place an asterisk beside the equipment that is in excess of $1,000 (capital equipment):

Equipment   Source   Anticipated Cost

_____

_____

_____

_____

_____

_____

3. You can now make two lists of equipment—one for capital equipment and one for noncapital equipment:

Capital Equipment   Noncapital Equipment

_____

_____

_____

_____

_____

_____

In fact, you might not have to purchase all or any of the furnishings or equipment for your program. If the agency is providing a space, it might also provide the loan of furnishings and equipment. In many of our examples, the tables, chairs, computers, and kitchens of the facility/agency were used. However, it is always good to know all of the costs should you wish to recreate the program elsewhere. Some facilities/agencies will also expect that you replace any equipment that is stolen or damaged because of negligence or misuse by you or your clients/members. Although we would expect that this would not occur, knowing the cost sometimes helps programmers to be more aware of security and maintenance.

SUPPLIES

Now consider **supplies** needed to support the services provided by your program (such as computer software, arts and crafts, paper, pencils, toys, garden seeds, cooking ingredients, and so on). Consider supplies needed per client/patient on a daily/weekly basis. Also consider what supplies are **expendable** (such as masking tape or plant fertilizer, which must be replaced when they are used) or **nonex-**

pendable (such as scissors, gardening forks, or inflatable wading pools, which can be used several times without replacement). If you have used wading pools in your practice, you know that they are a good example of an item that could be considered either expendable or nonexpendable. (They are, in fact, listed as a non-expendable supply item, but if you purchase the cheap ones, they are extremely vulnerable to rips and punctures and might not last the course of one day.) Over the long haul, spending a little more for equipment and nonexpendable supplies is very wise. Again, make your lists from what you want, and decide later where you can cut some corners without jeopardizing your goal and the quality of your program.

Assessments/screening instruments also generally are listed under nonexpendable supplies (except for paper forms, of course). These will be considered in Chapter 12 and will be included in the combined supplies selected to support your client/patient/member services in the development of the total budget.

■■■ EXERCISE 3 ■■■
Selecting Supplies for Your Program

1. Consider now what *nonexpendable* supplies you will need to begin your program. To determine the number of items needed, consider the number of clients/patients you will service, the daily or weekly time schedule, and the specific supplies required to provide the program. Consider the following examples:

six campers serviced *daily* (=) *six pairs of right-handed scissors and (to be on the safe side) three pairs of left-handed scissors.*

six campers serviced *daily* (=) *two "quality" inflatable wading pools (three children to each pool with no hard edges to encourage safe movement as well as socialization).*

twelve community gardener/members attending daily (=) *twelve pairs of gardening gloves.*

twelve community gardener/members attending daily (=) *four spading forks, four long-handled hoes, and four short-handled hoes.*

Using the above formula to help determine quantity, note below the *nonexpendable* supplies you will need for your program, the source, amount, and anticipated cost (remember that *if* you have sufficient storage, sometimes it is substantially cheaper to order in bulk even though it may be more than you require at the present time). Write your formulas below:

Nonexpendable Supplies	Source	Quantity	Anticipated Cost

_____

_____

_____

_____

2. Decide now what *expendable* supplies you will need to start your program and to operate it for one cycle of clients/patients/members. Consider the following examples:

two four-day weeks (=) *eight one-hour arts and crafts sessions* (×) *six day campers* (=) *12 1.7 fl. oz. nontoxic, nonflammable glue sticks* (estimated that gluing would be involved in 1/3 of the arts and crafts activities, assumed one stick would be used per child per week, and anticipated little waste and better product with the glue stick as opposed to a bottle of less expensive glue).

on-going community garden supplied (expendables) in "gardening cycles" (planting, maintaining, harvesting, and clearing):
planting cycle (=) *area of garden* (×) *twelve gardeners/members* (=) *72 packets of assorted seeds, twelve spools of row-marking string, 100 row-marker sticks, and five large bags of fertilizer* (estimated planting of some individual and some group choices, including annual flowers, herbs, and vegetables for future saleability; assumed that row-marking string and sticks are cheaper in quantity and are easily stored; and assumed that supplies are donated or purchased locally).

Using the examples as guidelines, note your formula below for determining the expendable supplies that you will need:

_____

_____

_____

_____

_____

List below the *expendable* supplies you will need to provide your program for one cycle:

Expendable Supplies	Source	Quantity	Anticipated Cost

EXERCISE 4

Long-Term Budgeting

Most budgets will be based on three-month, six-month, one-year, and three-year cycles. This may be referred to as *short-term budgeting* (what you require to operate one cycle of your program) and *long-term budgeting* (what you require for several cycles of your program, usually up to three years). Long-term budgeting requires that you make **cost projections,** including a percentage increase for inflation. For our purposes in this chapter, we are only considering the costs associated with furnishings, equipment, and supplies. We will consider other costs in the chapter to follow.

Consider the equipment noted in the previous exercise. Will any of it require replacement over the course of a three-year period? When we figure the final budget later, we will include **indirect costs** such as the costs of service and maintenance contracts and overhead (electricity, telephone, Internet, and so on). For now, however, we are only considering some of our **direct costs,** or those costs for equipment and supplies that will directly support the client/patient/member services.

1. Note below any equipment (capital or noncapital) that you anticipate may need to be replaced during the first three years of your program:

Replacement of Capital Equipment   Anticipated Cost (consider inflation)

_____

_____

_____

_____

Replacement of Noncapital Equipment   Anticipated Cost (consider inflation)

_____

_____

_____

_____

2. Now consider your *nonexpendable* supply list. How often will you need to replace these supplies?

For our earlier examples, the gardening gloves and the wading pools probably would be the most vulnerable to "short lives." For example, a good pair of gardening gloves with rubber or leather palms would be expected to last the home gardener for perhaps a year or more with proper care. Twelve pairs of such gloves would cost about $30 *each, or $360 out of a 12-month budget. It is not likely that all of our gardeners/members will wear out gloves equally, so we could cut some corners and spend $7 for a pair of good (but not the best) gloves and anticipate that they would probably last a year for some of our less enthusiastic gardeners and six months or three months for others. We could then anticipate glove replacement in increments over three months, six months, and a year. In reality, gloves are items that gardening-supply stores might donate, but we want to know what they will cost in the event that we must pay for them.*

A durable, inflatable wading pool might last through a summer of two-week camper rotations or approximately six eight-day cycles (with each of two pools meeting the needs of three children each and with the combined pools sheltering some 288 small bodies over the course of a summer). Although it is possible that these pools will last all summer, it is likely that at least one will require replacement at a cost of around $42 to $45 during the three-month interval.

Make your calculations and note below what *nonexpendable* supplies you anticipate replacing, how often, and the anticipated (plus inflation) costs:

Nonexpendable Supplies   Replacement Cycle   Anticipated Costs

_____

_____

_____

_____

_____

_____

3. What will be your replacement cycle for *expendable* supplies? Will you bring in new groups every two weeks like our day camp example? Or will your cycle be every month, three months, or six months? Or will you have new members/patients/clients cycling through your program all the time? Or will your expendable supplies be exhausted in cycles like the community garden example?

For the community garden, the most expensive season was the first one—the planting season. Seventy-two packets of seeds cost from $.50 to $2.10 per packet depending on the quantity of seeds per packet (100–8,000) and how exotic the potential plants were considered to be. The hemp twine for row marking sold for $8.95 per 200-foot ball, and the wooden markers were $5.00 for 100. The program later received a donation of nonexpendable metal row markers that would have cost $22.95 per 50 if purchased and ten flats of live seedlings that would have cost approximately $15.00 per flat.

Although starting up the garden each season appeared to be expensive, for most of the year, costs were substantially reduced. Therefore, the budget for the year was heavily influenced by the planting season and was less influenced by the maintenance (fertilizer and mulch) and the harvest and clean-up. The garden was organic so there were no chemical pesticides to purchase; this also enhanced marketing for produce and floral sales.

Note below your anticipated *expendable* supplies and when you will anticipate replacement along with your projections of cost (consider that inflation will also impact your expendable supplies):

Expendable Supplies　　　Replacement Cycle　　　Anticipated Costs

_____

_____

_____

_____

_____

SUMMARY

In preparing to initiate a program, you will need to obtain (and likely purchase) a number of items to facilitate the achievement of objectives and, ultimately, the goal of the program. These items fall under the categories of furnishings, capital and noncapital equipment, and expendable and nonexpendable supplies. Furnishings are those things that we would describe in our households as *furniture*, including tables, chairs, sofas, lamps, beds, and dressers. They may be considered part of our indirect services in some cases (such as providing a comfortable reception area) and direct services in others (such as tables and chairs for activities or perhaps a bed for activities of daily living practice). In program design and development, many of these items are intended to add comfort and style to the space where we will carry out our intervention rather than to directly support the intervention itself.

Equipment may be intended for therapeutic purposes such as playground equipment designed to facilitate the sensory-integration aspects of a child's development. On the other hand, it may be used for purposes not necessarily considered to be therapeutic in intent. An example of this kind of equipment would be a riding tiller or tractor for the community garden. In most settings, equipment is categorized by cost. Although the amount may differ depending on the setting, generally those items over $1,000 are considered to be capital equipment, and those under this purchase amount are considered to be noncapital equipment.

Supplies are also categorized but not usually by cost. They may fall into the category of expendable, or those things that are "used up" by participants in the course of their direct-service program. Items that have a longer life, or are not "used up" in the process of intervention, are termed nonexpendable items. Even though they may be purchased in large quantities, such things as glue, masking tape, paints, and splinting materials are expendable, for they are "used up" and are not recycled to be used again in the same form. On the other hand, brushes, scissors, rulers, and gloves are considered to be nonexpendable even though they will "wear out" over time. All of these items cost the program money, and they are considered to be a substantial part of the budget process—both short-term and long-term. Assessment and screening instruments utilized in direct-service provision may also be included under supplies; sometimes they are considered to be expendable and sometimes nonexpendable.

Of course, there are other indirect and direct costs to programming, which will be considered in detail in Chapter 11. In this chapter, we will consider all of the costs to operate our program and, further, how we will pay these costs.

COMPANIES THAT PROVIDE EQUIPMENT AND SUPPLIES APPROPRIATE FOR OCCUPATION-CENTERED PROGRAMMING

Attainment Company, Inc.
P.O. Box 930160
Verona, WI 53593-0160
800-327-4269
(multiple options/supplies for children
    and adults with special needs)

Best Priced Products, Inc.
P.O. Box 1174
White Plains, NY 10602
800-824-2939
(rehabilitation supplies and equipment
    for adults and children)

Childswork/Childsplay
P.O. Box 1604
Secaucus, NJ 07096-1604
800-962-1141
email: care@GenesisDirect.com
(social and emotional needs of children and
    adolescents)

Communication Skill Builders
3830 E. Bellevue
P.O. Box 42050-CS4
Tucson, AZ 85733
602-323-7500
(communication supplies for adults and
    children)

Communication/Therapy Skill Builders
(A Division of the Psychological Corporation)
555 Academic Court
San Antonio, TX 78204-9941
800-211-8378
(pediatric and adult assessment and
    intervention)

Dick Blick Art Materials
P.O. Box 1267
Galesburg, IL 61402-1267
800-828-4548
www.dickblick.com
(arts and crafts supplies)

Eastman
Northwest District Headquarters: Denver
303-576-1000
Southwest District: Phoenix
602-269-3131
(office furniture and products)

Enrichments (for Better Living)
P.O. Box 579
145 Tower Drive
Hinsdale, IL 60521
800-323-5547
(adult and pediatric rehabilitation
    supplies and equipment)

Flaghouse
601 Flaghouse Drive
Hasbrouck Heights, NJ 07604-3116
800-793-7900
email: info@flaghouse.com
http://www.flaghouse.com
(adult and pediatric rehabilitation
    supplies and equipment; physical
    education and recreation supplies and
    equipment; furniture—for school,
    office, institutions, and health care
    facilities)

Imaginart
307 Arizona Street
Bisbee, AZ 85603
800-828-1376
email: imaginart@aol.com
(therapy supplies for pediatrics, physical
    rehabilitation, and mental health)

Lilypons Water Gardens
6800 Lilypons Road
P.O. Box 10
Buckeystown, MD 21717-0010
800-723-7667
www.lilypons.com
(supplies, equipment, plants for water
    gardening, fish, and frogs)

NorthCoast Medical, Inc.
187 Stauffer Blvd.
San Jose, CA 95125-1042
800-821-9319
(adult rehabilitation and fitness supplies;
    hand therapy supplies)

PCI Educational Publishing
2800 NE Loop 410 Suite 105
San Antonio, TX 78218-1525
800-594-4263
(supplies for cognitive and emotional
    independence)

Sammons Preston AbilityOne
P.O. Box 5071
Bolingbrook, IL 60440-5071
800-323-5547
http://www.sammonspreston.com
(supplies and equipment for adult
    rehabilitation)

S & S Opportunities
P.O. Box 513
Colchester, CT 06415-0517
800-937-3482
(adult and pediatric rehabilitation
    equipment, supplies, and furniture)

S & S Healthcare
P.O. Box 513
Colchester, CT 06415-0517
800-243-9232
http://www.snswwide.com
(arts, crafts, games, and exercise for
    therapy and rehabilitation)

Sears Home Health Care
20 Presidential Drive
Roselle, IL 60172
800-326-1750
(adult rehabilitation equipment)

Shepherd's Garden Seeds
30 Irene Street
Torrington, CT 06790-6658
860-482-3638
www.shepherdseeds.com
(garden seeds—ordinary to the exotic—and
    gardening supplies)

Smith and Nephew, Inc.
One Quality Drive
P.O. Box 1005
Germantown, WI 53022-8205
800-558-8633
(adult rehabilitation supplies)

Tandy Leather and Crafts
TLC Direct
1400 Everman Parkway
Fort Worth, TX 76140-5089
888-890-1611
www.tandyleather.com
(leathercraft, Indian Lore; leather hides for
    the craftsperson and hobbyist)

Wellness Reproductions, Inc.
23945 Mercantile Road, Suite KM
Beachwood, OH 44122-5924
800-669-9208
(supplies and resources for mental health
    facilitators and educators)

Whole Person Associates
210 W. Michigan
Duluth, MN 55802-1908
800-247-6789
http://www.wholeperson.com
(stress management, wellness-promotion,
    and emotional self-care resources)

What Will It Cost, and How Will It Be Funded?

Learning Objectives

1. To recognize the important features of program evaluation and cost determination in maintaining program viability
2. To appreciate the importance of maintaining occupation and quality of life in the outcome measures of programs while managing costs
3. To understand the various cost structures for programs to include those that are for-profit and those that are intended to be not-for-profit
4. To become aware of the multiple considerations when hiring and retaining an employee
5. To explore the possibilities for funding a program or practice
6. To learn to figure costs for your program and anticipate funding needs

Key Terms

1. Overhead
2. Budget/Cost Sheet
3. Benefits
4. Insurance
5. Employee/Employer
6. For-Profit/Not-For-Profit
7. Fee for Service
8. Malpractice/Professional Liability
9. Private Payer/Pay Out-Of-Pocket/Cash Flow
10. Capital
11. Business Plan

12. Collection Agency
13. Revenue/Funding

There are two critical dimensions of the community programming proposal. While they are no more or less important than other aspects of the proposal, when it comes to anticipating long-term success of the program, *carefully determining the cost and evaluating the effectiveness of the program* make the difference in its staying power. Frequently the programmer least favors developing these two areas, but they also are the areas that separate the daydreamer from the true proactive planner.

If we could maintain our excitement and momentum through the processes of budgeting and evaluation-planning, then we would find evidence of many more successful and long-running programs. Sadly, many programming efforts are like sparklers on the 4th of July; on July 5 they have disappeared into the land fill. The idea that will last, on the other hand, is supported by sound money management and careful evaluation of outcomes. How do we deal with our budgetary concerns? What will this program cost? And how will it be funded? What does it mean to manage the finances of a program?

Smith (1996) outlined the key categories that an occupational therapy financial manager must be alert to in light of the external environment within which health care organizations function. Her discussions describe the multiple levels of financial accounting and management known to most occupational therapy managers. Focusing largely on service billing, her categories included such tasks as establishing prices and pricing policies and the negotiation of reimbursement contracts with third-party payers and individual payers (pp. 63–100). Of course, there are many other functions of the financial manager, which include the multiple and complex interfaces between manager and therapist-employee and between therapist and patient. Although Smith's information may be more suited to what we might describe as a clinic or hospital-based, treatment-focused practice, her words also ring true for many free-standing practices. Her considerations of certain aspects of cost accounting such as strategic planning and monitoring productivity and efficiency are critical to all programming, whether it be treatment-based intervention, wellness promoting, or prevention. And these considerations apply, whether the administrative structure is a private practice or a program operated under the umbrella of another agency or agencies.

Logigian (1994) and Thomas (1996) discuss cost management as well as additional roles of the financial manager. Accountability is the key word in financial management, whether it be in health care or the business sector. In terms of accountability in occupation-centered, community-based programs, the linkages between occupation, quality improvement, and program evaluation must be supported and encouraged alongside the present-day concerns for efficiency and cost-effectiveness. We cannot afford to let the current payment systems restrict our creativity, diminish our goals, or compromise our ethics.

Edwards (1997) supports the measurement of quality of life that goes beyond our usual parameters for quality improvement and medical measures of outcome. Certainly meaning and life quality are outcome measures to be pursued in our programming efforts, even in the face of cost reductions and downsizing. Although difficult to accomplish, we should not minimize the need to consistently and accurately define and measure these characteristics of carefully planned and truly occupation-centered programming as we work to anticipate and manage costs.

COSTS AND BUDGETS

Figuring costs, budgeting, and anticipating resources is always a bit of a dance—forward and backward but hopefully well syncopated and with all participants well coordinated. Some program planners prefer to plan big and scale back; other planners like to start small and expand their thinking later. Starting with a "big" plan is a way of encouraging excitement and creativity, and in many ways it widens the scope of opportunity. However, the "big" plan is seldom obtainable in the early efforts. As long as the planner is prepared for this and is willing to grow in increments (postponing the larger version for somewhere later on the three-year time line), planning can progress smoothly. Thus, good management ensures the reality, and for both the conservative and the aggressive approach, a long-range plan is critical.

Regardless of the nature of the intervention, all programs have expenses that must be funded. In previous chapters, you began the process of outlining your programming costs to include furnishings, supplies, equipment, space, and personnel. These items begin to form lines in your **budget.** Even though you might not actually keep one, the word *budget* is probably quite familiar to you. *Webster's Dictionary* (1975) defines *budget* as "a financial statement of estimated income and expenditures covering a specified future period of time." We will approach the budget process a bit backwards by first drafting a list of all of our anticipated expenses and then making a projection of our needed income from these expenditures. This needed income may come from a number of sources, including **revenues** generated by payment for services, revenues from program-generated products or services, or what we will describe as general funding (comprehensive funds for programming from an agency or foundation). For those who are anticipating initiating a private practice, this list of costs first becomes part of your start-up worksheet and then your business plan.

Before we begin to draft such a cost sheet in the initiation of our budget, however, there are some additional categories of expense that we have not yet considered, including overhead, insurance, and benefits for employees. Whether or not you are responsible for these expenses will depend on what kind of program you are planning. In all of the areas of financial management, our level of responsibilities and specific tasks will fall along a continuum depending on the nature of the program. There are obviously fewer fiscal (money-related) management responsibilities for the planner/manager who works under the umbrella of another agency or agencies than there would be for the planner who is establishing a business/ private practice. Of course, someone must assume the responsibilities—and perhaps liabilities—of financial management, but in many cases, it will be someone other than you. Whether you are responsible or not, it is important that you thoroughly understand the process so that you can anticipate what will be required to ensure the financial success of the program.

THE NATURE OF YOUR PROGRAM

Occupation-centered practitioners may offer their services under many different administrative structures. It is important to distinguish between those kinds of practices we are describing as independent and private versus those programs that are established under the administrative umbrella of another agency or facility. If you are an **employee,** then the contents of this chapter are generally the concern of your **employer** (the agency/facility). Of course, you would be expected to maintain a budget for your program and generally provide administrative services, but it is not likely that you would be responsible for funding the collective costs of your program.

Although it does not have to be, a private practice is usually **for-profit;** in other words, it expects to have money left over after expenses are paid. These practices are much different from those that are **not-for-profit.** Not-for-profit programs intend to pay expenses, but they do not intend to make money. Not-for-profit programs may be eligible for numerous grants and gifts that a for-profit program would not be. Although both kinds of programs may charge their patients/clients fees, the intent to make a profit or not to is the difference. Whether a program is for-profit or not-for-profit does not necessarily impact the salaries of employees. In fact, salaries may be higher in not-for-profit programs than those in for-profit programs, and benefits may be better. Many of the programs described in this text, for example, are not-for-profit and do not charge a **fee for service** (that is, the clients/members are not charged for the therapist's services). In fact, these programs are supported through grant funding and indirectly through student tuition for *service learning* or *fieldwork.* In these ways, a preceptor can be paid, any needed equipment and supplies can be purchased, and overhead is paid. In some cases, there is some revenue generated (for example, through the sale of garden produce or hand-made paper products); however, these monies are funneled back into the program for the purchase of supplies. Sometimes these programs require a trial period—several months or maybe longer—in order for the program staff and participants to establish a firm rapport with the community and to evaluate the effectiveness of the program. A small start-up grant may be appropriate during this period of becoming established. After this pilot period (assuming the program is effective in achieving its goal), there will likely be other funding appropriate to the target population that may be accessed to support the program (for example, from state and federal sources such as the Department of Child Welfare or Department of Corrections). Even though a program is not-for-profit, it is important to remember that no program is "free." Someone pays, but how much and in what way can be very convoluted.

If you are a student, it is important to remember that everything is accounted for in your program cost sheet and budget, from the needs of your employees to each piece of paper and pencil that you will use to provide your program. Whether you have assured funding before you begin or you intend to seek it as part of the planning process, nothing will happen unless you know exactly how much money will be required. See the Appendix at the back of the book for a sample cost sheet developed for a variation of our earlier day camp example.

THE OFTEN TAKEN-FOR-GRANTED OVERHEAD

Overhead is a term that refers to cost items such as utilities (electric, gas, water, telephone, and Internet access) that collectively support your program. In the start-up process of a private practice or another such entrepreneurial venture, there also may be expenses such as a security deposit on a lease, first and last month's rent, insurance, and perhaps a security system. Also, such ventures would incur costs to obtain a standard business license with the city. In addition, expenses might be associated with licensing, certification, or accreditation, depending on the nature of your services. If you are starting a private practice, overhead has to be carefully accounted for and usually begins immediately when you obtain space. When you apply for grant funding to start a not-for-profit program, overhead costs generally are grouped and included as a percentage of costs in the amount prescribed by the particular granting agency. You would be able to obtain this information from the granting agency and the prospectus for the specific grant.

REDUCING RISKS: INSURANCE

For occupation-centered community-based programs, at least three kinds of **insurance** must be considered. The private-practice planner generally will be responsible for all of these. The first is the insurance for your practice or company. Insurance, which is always about managing risk, can protect your practice from loss due to fire, public liability, and crime, among other things. When considering insurance for your company, you must first decide on the type of insurance you will need, and then you must decide on the amount of coverage. As a general rule, do not risk more than you can afford to lose. You should also talk to several insurance agents who are accustomed to offering policies to similar practices.

The second type of insurance is **malpractice** or **professional liability** insurance. Malpractice insurance covers against claims from clients/patients who suffer damages as a result of services you or your employees perform. You may wish to offer employees this insurance coverage as part of their "employee benefit package," although many companies require that employees provide their own malpractice insurance. Students are already familiar with malpractice or professional liability insurance since all receive this coverage when they enter their occupational therapy clinical program. Some people mistakenly believe that malpractice insurance is only appropriate when you are "learning" to be a practitioner and that when you actually become a practitioner, you no longer require it. However, the reality is that in todays' litigious climate, the more you know, the more you acquire responsibilities—and the more malpractice coverage you require!

The third category of insurance is also the responsibility of the private practitioners or those who will be responsible for employees. There are three categories of insurances that help employees manage risk and therefore help employers maintain their businesses. Providing *health insurance* for yourself and for your employees may seem to be a big expense when you are establishing your business plan, but consider how much work might be lost if you do not provide it. You can always offer a better insurance package than your employees could find on their own, and they may choose not to provide their own. In order to keep their employees healthy and to help them balance life at home with life at work, many small businesses offer incentives such as limited child care, exercise programs, and weight management/substance abuse programs. Occupation-centered practitioners who own businesses should be the first ones to consider these benefits for their employees.

You will also want to include *disability insurance, life insurance,* and *worker's compensation* insurance. If you are the owner of the business, disability insurance is critical, and you may also wish to offer it to employees. Ryan, Ray, and Hiduke (1999) suggest that disability for a business owner is a much greater risk than death. While life insurance may not offer a direct advantage to the owner of a practice, it is a service to the employee and the employee's family, and it is generally not as costly as the other insurances. Worker's compensation protects employees if they are injured while on the job. Again, occupational therapy practitioners are generally aware of ergonomics and should ensure that the workplace does not provide risks to the safety and well-being of employees.

THE POTENTIAL COSTS OF EMPLOYEES

There are several questions that come to mind when we hire employees to assist with our program. In Chapter 8 we discussed the various roles of the professional and nonprofessional staff you might wish to hire to support the services of your program. We also discussed how to develop a job description and an advertisement to initiate the employee search. This was the easy part. The hiring and retention of employees make up a large part of your anticipated labor and budget. We have already discussed the insurances and other benefits you may wish to provide, but there are additional considerations that will impact your finances as an owner of a practice.

First you must decide *when* you will hire your employees. Will you hire them before your first client or concurrently? If they are hired concurrently with the arrival of clients, how will the preparation and final planning be accomplished? Will you do it? Perhaps you can hire some temporary or part-time employees. In this case, you are able to delay paying benefits during the preparation phase. Although the percentages vary, many employers provide certain benefits only to employees who work more than 80% of a full-time work schedule. However, consider that you might require a high level of professional experience and expertise to assist with the final preparations—perhaps expertise that you do not have; in this case, you will want to offer all of the potential options you can to attract the person you need. If you are starting a for-profit practice, you may wish to offer this first employee stock options or profit sharing as an incentive to help with the final preparations. Hiring and then keeping good employees is the key to a successful private practice. All of these questions must be considered *before* you run your ad. In addition, you must budget the cost of placing employment advertisements and any costs that may be incurred for recruitment. Not only is this true in the beginning, but this also must be anticipated as the program begins to grow. Of course, salary must be considered, as well as employment taxes (social security, unemployment, and Medicare) and additional benefits such as retirement, vacation, and sick leave.

The best way to determine professional salaries is to talk to other managers in your area to obtain a range for the kinds of services you wish to provide. This is another reason to network and to belong to your professional organizations. The professional organizations may also be able to provide you with salary ranges but will not likely be as current as your colleagues. For other staff, you can find salary comparison data on the Internet at http://recruitmentextra.com/salarysurveys.html and at www.wageweb.com. When you have decided exactly what kind of employees you want and when you wish to hire them, it is time to place the advertisement and to begin the screening and interview process.

Pre-Employee Screening, Interviews, and Hiring: Maintaining Compliance

As with many of the planning tasks we have discussed, this is yet another area where you may have differing levels of responsibility depending on whether you are starting your own practice or whether you are only assisting the company you work for in the employee hiring process. Screening may include a number of measures to verify that your potential employee has provided you with truthful information. A careful review of the resume initiates the process, which is followed by contacting references and verifying state and national certifications and licenses. The next steps can include pre-employment medical examinations and perhaps drug screenings. One or more in-person interviews are employed, and in addition to standard interview questions, role-playing of intervention scenarios particular to your program might be appropriate.

If hiring is your responsibility, you should review legal and illegal pre-employment inquiries before you schedule an interview. You can obtain these from http://www.nolo.com. Also contact the civil rights office for your state and the Department of Industrial Relations for guidelines they may provide. Refer to the list at the close of this chapter for other sources that may be helpful.

When you have completed the interview process and are prepared to make an offer, you should check to see that your new employee can legally work in the

United States and have that person complete an Employment and Eligibility Verification Form (I-9); you must also be familiar with the requirements for complying with the Americans with Disabilities Act (ADA). As occupational therapy practitioners you should be familiar with the *ADA Title I: Employment provision* and may, in fact, have encountered it in the workplace. As an employer your responsibilities are even greater. Refer to the ADA and also to Regulations to Implement the Equal Employment Provisions of the Americans with Disabilities Act.

As the owner of a practice, you also must be compliant with all labor laws and all tax laws with regard to employees. It is recommended that you become familiar with the U.S. Department of Labor Statutes, the Fair Labor Standards Act, the Immigration and Nationality Act, the Occupational Safety and Health Act (OSHA), and the Employee Retirement Income Security Act (ERISA). (See the references at the close of this chapter for more information.)

If you find it necessary to dismiss an employee, it may be equally problematic. Consider the above resources should firing become necessary, and spell out all procedures in an employee handbook.

Employee Records

If you are the owner or soon-to be owner of a practice, you must maintain records for all employees. These include all of the basic information (such as name, address, social security number, and so on) as well as the original application and the results of any pre-hire inquiries. As the employee continues with your company, you add performance reviews, continuing education, and notations of any disciplinary action. Your state Fair Employment Office can provide you with additional information for what must be maintained in an employee's file and for how long. Human resource files are considered legal documents and may be requested in any malpractice suit or other legal action, so it is best to be proactive by being sure that they are complete.

Summing Up Costs

Now that we have considered expenses related to employees, we have covered the standard cost items. As you think of other items that are indirectly or directly related to client/patient services, remember to consider all associated costs. For instance, perhaps you anticipate the need to lease a van for transportation. Remember that if you transport clients/patients, you will need additional insurance coverage and an appropriate driver's license. An occasional trip might be accommodated less expensively by hiring outside vans or buses.

Once you have listed your start-up costs and the costs for one cycle of your program, you can project these for lengthier periods of time. These extensions of time from one year up to three years will include areas where you wish to grow (such as more or different staff, perhaps more space, or additional equipment).

The next section is intended to provide you with some direction for how your services might be paid for or how to seek funding. It is not intended to provide you with specific directions for who and how to bill for services or exact resources where you might find loans for a private practice or a grant to initiate a program, but enough information is provided to guide you to the specific information and resources that you will need to make these decisions. If you are a student, you will have (or presently have) coursework complementary to this text. This coursework will guide you in the specifics of such management responsibilities as determining costs for services, anticipating and projecting revenue, developing an actual bill, and determining how to interface your interventions with appropriate payment services. The following section will describe the configuration of the "money trees"; you will have to figure out which ones you wish to shake!

POTENTIAL FUNDING SOURCES
Public and Private Funding Sources

At the close of this chapter, you will find a number of resources that can help you make your way through the confusing maze of anticipating and covering your costs. While these resources describe structurally sound systems, specifics are usually a bit behind what is actually happening in the rapidly changing world of today's health care.

What might be described as public **funding** for occupational therapy services includes both insurance and grant-based programs. Federal and state insurance programs such as Medicare, Medicaid, and worker's compensation require constant attention to updated policies and procedures. Examples of grant-based programs include the Individuals with Disabilities Education Act (1990) and the Older Americans Act (1965). We also must remain attentive to the policies of private insurance benefit programs such as Blue Cross/Blue Shield, managed care organizations, and other commercial insurers. If you plan to bill Medicare or private insurances as an independent practitioner, you should work as an employee within a system that receives their compensation from these agencies before you try it on your own. Once you understand the systems and know the correct coding for billing required by the particular carrier or agency to facilitate payment, you can likely do it on your own. You can also contact the Web sites of your particular carriers for the latest updates. The American Occupational Therapy Association's Fax-on-Demand provides updates regarding the latest summaries of frequently utilized CPT codes and Medicare fee schedules (the AOTA Fax-on-Demand number is listed at the close of this chapter).

Even though a lot of homework is required to receive payment for services through public and private insurances, many occupational therapy practitioners who engage in community programming wish to fit their services into the more conventional payment models just described. There are many ways to access funding options. The clinical psychologist Patrick Vega (1998) notes what he describes as a developing trend toward interest in behavioral disease management, which is also an area of interest to occupation-centered practitioners. He encourages clinical psychologists who wish to engage in this kind of programming to go directly to local hospitals with their well-developed educational programs targeting the facility's wellness programs and cardiac units. There is a message for occupation-centered practitioners here as well, for we also promote education/skills-based wellness programming. Vega goes on to propose that disease management, whether somatic or behavioral, will target those diseases that have high cost, high frequency, and high chronicity (such as cancer, diabetes, heart disease, asthma, and HIV). Cost savings for purchasers of insurance coverage is the key to the future, according to Vega. He suggests the following strategies, which are appropriate for our consideration as well (p. 3):

1. Consider case managing a population via capitated or subcapitated contracts.
2. Be flexible in the way you offer programming.
3. Propose what you think you can do, based on what you've done (programming effectiveness, yours or that of others before you).
4. Be willing to work as part of a team.

If these ideas match your interests as an occupation-centered program planner, you can tailor the development of your proposal(s) toward these ends. Few of the caregiving professions really "own" anything today; the market share goes to those who have the skills and information to do the job cost-effectively and to those who demonstrate that they can do what they claim. None of the health-oriented professions have a secure foothold in todays' market; and they all are searching for opportunities. In many instances you must be your own ethical gatekeeper; and in light of competition for resources, this is a continuing challenge.

Private Payers

Although not explicitly mentioned earlier, if you anticipate operating a practice as a business, the first professional relationships you must establish are with an attorney and/or a financial planner. The next and most lasting relationship is with an accountant/bookkeeper. You will likely need help in setting up monthly profit and loss statements and certainly to keep track of accounts payable and receivable. There are computer software programs (such as *QuickBooks*) to help you if you decide to handle your own finances, which you may want to consider, at least in the early stages. How will you know whether you can make it on your own? Consider the size of your start-up practice, and look at how you manage your personal finances; these two things will help you make the choice of whether to try to manage the "business" side of your practice or to hire someone to assist you.

This bring us to another form of payment for services in which the client/patient, or **private payer,** "pays out of pocket." In many of the developing community-based practices, it is not uncommon that clients/patients/parents pay directly for the services that are provided. Many parents are accustomed to paying for special classes, music lessons, and camp fees, so paying for occupation-centered intervention for their children is seen as being of very little difference. Older clients are accustomed to paying for classes, sports club memberships, and prevention programs (such as *Weight*

Watchers). Many occupation-centered wellness and prevention programs are similar in structure. Oftentimes, such as in a camp program, there may be many forms of payment, including private pay for those who can, donation-based "gift tuitions" for those who cannot, and public and private funding for those who are eligible.

Regardless of the kinds of payment you expect to receive, you will likely require the services of a **collection agency.** For a fee, these people will help you retrieve payment from clients who are past due. For a specified time, your bookkeeper will follow those who are delinquent (usually past 30 days), then the bill is turned over to a collection agency. Sometimes insurance companies take a period of time to pay for a service, but usually you can anticipate receiving payment; that may not be the case with private payers. Depending on the volume of services you offer, this could present a substantial problem for your **cash flow.** Cash flow is the actual money you have on hand to operate your business. Remember that you can be turning a profit in a private practice but still have no money on hand—another reason to hire an accountant.

PUBLIC AND PRIVATE GRANT FUNDING
Federal Grants

Although extremely competitive, federal granting agencies are an excellent way to obtain a substantial amount of funding for three years or more of programming, associated research, and/or student training. The Federal Register lists opportunities appropriate for community-based programs from the Department of Education and the Office of Special Education and Rehabilitative Services. For example, opportunities may be in the areas of training and technical assistance for Centers for Independent Living, independent living services for older adults who are blind, and research and innovation to improve services and results for children with disabilities. (For more information, see http://ocfo.ed.gov/fedreg.htm, http://www.ed.gov/news.html, http://www.nih.gov/grants/guide/index.html, or *Federal Grants and Contracts Weekly.*)

Other federal departments also have opportunities appropriate to community-based programming. For example, the *Children and Youth Funding Report* (1998) noted that Human Services had dollars for "out-of-school" youth pilot demonstrations, empowerment zones, and enterprise communities; and at the time, Juvenile Justice was interested in applications targeting youth offender demonstration projects. This Washington-based newsletter also noted opportunities in private and regional funding and described in "news format" successful programs. In synthesizing and summing up granting opportunities, it provides a shortcut to helping you select programming that may be fundable through federal monies. There are certainly *trends* in funding based on the *trends* in politics and social issues, but if you are tracking the trends that may influence your programming, then you can anticipate where funding is available now and where it will likely be in the future.

All federal agencies are interested in programs that "work"; many have a specific research component written into their description, and all of them expect a strong outcome-based research design. Therefore, the program-evaluation component of your proposal must be developed to provide viable measures of the success or failures of your programming.

Federal agencies have specific guidelines for applications, but if you have developed your full proposal as outlined in this text, you will have the bulk of your work already accomplished.

Private Funding

Although private funding agencies may offer smaller dollar amounts, generally their application process is much less rigorous than the federal agencies. Those that do offer larger amounts of money are generally more competitive, and their application process is equally rigorous. As an example of a private funding organization, the Pfizer pharmaceutical company's corporate philanthropy includes, among many other agendas, maternal and child health programs to help low-income, high-risk parents get prenatal and well-baby care and information. Occupation-centered community nonprofit programs such as those targeting skills for teen mothers, those designed to encourage nurturing mother-baby shared occupations, or those providing screening for developmental milestones in infants and children would be appropriate for this organization (Children and Youth Funding Report, 1998, pp. 10–11).

Wherever your community is located, it is likely that a Wal-Mart retail store is somewhere at the heart of it. If you are looking for a small amount of matching money (up to $2,000 to double what you already have) for your children and youth program, consider this organization. Information, applications, and deadlines may be obtained at your local store or by writing the company (Children and Youth Funding Report, 1998, p. 11).

If you are particularly interested in private funding to provide the "seed money" to get your program up and running, visit your local library or arrange to purchase *The Foundation Directory*. This directory reports on foundations with assets in excess of $2 million or annual giving of at least $200,000. The *Foundation Directory, Part 2* provides the same kind of descriptive information of private and community foundations in the United States but for those holding assets from $1 million to $2 million or with annual granting programs from $50,000 to $200,000. Together these two volumes constitute the standard reference work for information on the country's largest 12,824 active grant-making foundations (*The Foundation Directory*, 1999; *The Foundation Directory, Part 2*, 1999, Introduction). A companion document, *Guide to U.S. Foundations, Their Trustees, Offices, and Donors*, provides brief data on foundations with assets below $1 million and giving programs of less than $50,000 annually.

We sometimes speak of private granting agencies, but in this category we are generally referring to a foundation. The Foundation Center defines a foundation "as a nongovernmental, nonprofit organization with its own funds" (*The Foundation Directory*, 1999, p. vii, Introduction). The funds most often are from a single source, either an individual, a family, or a corporation. The purpose of the foundation may be to maintain or support educational, social, charitable, religious, or other activities serving the common welfare, primarily by making grants to other nonprofit organizations.

The Foundation Directory describes four categories of foundations: independent, company-sponsored, operating, and community. The nature of the foundation is, in part, determined by the tax codes of the Internal Revenue Service. For example, the Independent Foundation is designated under the law as a private foundation with the primary function of the making of grants. The assets of most independent foundations are derived from the gift of an individual or family, whereas the community foundation is publicly supported and makes grants in a specific community or region. Community foundations are usually classified under the tax code as public charities (*The Foundation Directory, Part 2*, 1999, p. ix, Introduction). Other directories published by the Foundation Center include *The Foundation 1000, National Directory of Corporate Giving, Guide to Greater Washington D.C. Grantmakers, Foundation Grants to Individuals*, and numerous others. (See the complete list at the end of this chapter.)

It is important to read the descriptions of the funding agencies—federal or private—and to write your application appropriate to the descriptions. Many disciplines, occupational therapy included, have worked hard over the course of their history to set themselves apart and to provide themselves with an identity composed of idiosyncratic jargon that others outside the profession do not share (although it has been ostensibly useful in uniting our profession).

The International Classification of Impairments, Disabilities, and Handicaps—2 (ICIDH-2) provides us with a shared language not only to broaden our relationship to others in the health professions and to collaborate more effectively for the good of the patient/client but also to be more competitive in seeking funding as well. The World Health Organization published the first version of ICIDH in 1980. For the past twenty years, the meanings associated with the terminology have been debated by occupational therapists and many others, and many valid arguments were proposed regarding the early usage of the terms *disability* and *handicap*. These terms have now been replaced by perhaps less controversial terms such as *activity* and *participation*. The term *impairment* has been retained for the present Beta-1 Field Trials of the document.

The components of the ICIDH-2 that lend themselves neatly to our views of occupation without lengthy debate are those of activity, participation, and context. As we continue to reinvent who we are as occupational therapists, we also might be required to reinvent our language to describe what we have always done and continue to do. A skillful bridging of occupation, impairment, activity, participation, and context will further solidify our shared thinking of how we provide services and why—while permitting us to be paid/funded for what we wish to do.

BANKS AND LENDING AGENCIES

If you are planning a for-profit program/practice, then some of your funding needs may fall into the category of a loan. It is generally expected, however, that you have your own **capital.** If you have other sources of income and collateral (home equity, stocks, or bonds), you would be in a position to borrow funds in addition to your own. Of course, there's always some risk that must be considered if the practice struggles. A solid **business plan** with good projections and supporting data is a prerequisite to requesting a start-up loan. Ryan, Ray, and Hiduke (1999) suggest the following outline for developing a business plan appropriate for seeking funds from a lending agency (you will recognize in their suggested plan many of the components you have already prepared during your planning process):

1. Cover sheet
2. Statement of purpose
3. Table of contents
    I. The Business
        A. Description of business
        B. Marketing
        C. Competition
        D. Operating procedures
        E. Personnel
        F. Business insurance
        G. Financial data
    II. Financial Data
        A. Loan application
        B. Capital equipment and supply list
        C. Balance sheet
        D. Break-even analysis
        E. Proforma income projections (profit and loss statements)
            Three-year summary
            Detail by month, first year
            Detail by quarters, second and third years
            Assumptions upon which projections were based
        F. Proforma cash flow
            Follow guidelines for letter E
    III. Supporting Documents
        Tax returns of principals for last three years
        Personal financial statement (forms supplied by lender)
        If franchised, a copy of the contract
        Copy of proposed lease or purchase agreement for space
        Copy of licenses and other legal documents
        Copy of resumes of all principals
        Copy of letters of intent from suppliers, etc.
                                            (Ryan, Ray, & Hiduke, 1999, p. 6)

These authors also suggest the following Web site to assist in the preparation of this plan: www.sba.gov/starting/indexbusplans.html. Clearly, going this route is not for the "faint of heart," and you still should seek the services of an accountant. It should be comforting to know, however, that the planning you already have accomplished is the foundation upon which you can attach the additional pieces.

■ EXERCISE 1 ■
What Kind of Program Do You Have?

1. Discuss with your classmates, colleagues, or partners whether your program is free-standing or is under the management umbrella of another agency or agencies. Is your program intended to be for-profit, not-for-profit, or a service-learning component of an academic program or community agency?

To help you define your responsibilities, you must decide if you will be the planner and manager of a program as an employee of an agency or institution or if you will be owner and manager.

Note below what kind of program you have and why you believe this to be the case:

_____

_____

_____

_____

2. With regard to the characteristics of your program as noted above, write below what your responsibilities will likely be with regard to selection, hiring, and retention of employees; purchase and maintenance of furnishings, equipment, and supplies; the marketing of the program; management of the budget; and obtaining funding:

Selection, hiring, and retention of employees:

_____

_____

_____

_____

Purchase and maintenance of furnishings, equipment, and supplies:

_____

_____

_____

_____

Marketing of the program (to the community and potential consumers):

_____

_____

Managing the budget for the program:

Identifying a funding source and obtaining funds for some or all of the program:

EXERCISE 2

Developing a Cost Sheet for Start-Up, One Year, and Three Years of the Program

You already have accomplished a large part of the task of developing a cost sheet in the exercises you completed for Chapter 8 and Chapter 10. When you have completed Chapter 13, you will have all of the projected costs for the program. You may wish to revisit the Appendix for a cost sheet example.

Return to your lists of furnishings, equipment, and supplies and your staffing requirements. Using the structure provided by the example define your costs in the following exercises.

Start-Up, One-Month, and Yearly Costs

Our first consideration will be the professional and nonprofessional staff that we will require to run the day-to-day programming. Revisit the discussion in Chapter 8. To first determine your staffing needs, you must consider the needs and availability of the service population, the physical space where the program will be offered, the nature of the services you expect to provide, and the configuration of service delivery. Because professional staff can be expensive, you should also begin to give some attention to your anticipated budget and your potential funding, although you must first consider your program goal and the needs of your target population. Although you must be able to justify your costs, it is always important that you do not jeopardize the quality of your program by seeking to reduce costs too soon.

1. Consider your costs for staffing (including the cost of advertising, salary, and benefits for full-time employees). For company-paid benefits, you can estimate approximately 20 percent of the salary figure, but realize that this can vary substantially):

Staff Position	% of time	Monthly/Yearly Gross Salary	Benefits

Total cost of staff salaries and benefits:

For one month _____ For one year _____

Total costs of start-up hiring: _____

Total staff associated costs (advertising positions, salaries, and estimated benefits): _____

2. Return to the exercises in Chapter 10 for your estimated cost lists for furnishings, equipment, and supplies. Finalize all estimated costs (including shipping) for start-up and for one cycle of your program (for example, one month, three months, and so on); note below your total costs for each of these categories:

Total cost of capital equipment for start-up: _____

Total cost of noncapital equipment for start-up: _____

Note any replacement of equipment that may be required over a three-year period and anticipated cost:

_____

_____

_____

Total cost of furnishings for start-up: _____

Note any replacement of furnishings that may be required over a three-year period and anticipated cost:

_____

_____

_____

Total cost of nonexpendable supplies for start-up: _____

(Remember to include any assessment materials here or in the question that follows.)

Note any replacement of nonexpendable supplies and the estimated cost (what are the anticipated cycles for replacement—six months? one year? more?):

_____

_____

_____

_____

Total cost of expendable supplies for one programming cycle: _____

What is the anticipated cycle for replacement of supplies? _____

What is the resulting 3-month, 6-month, and/or yearly total costs of supplies:

_____

3. Note below your estimated overhead for one month and for one year (carefully consider how you will operate your program, seasonal changes, anticipated fluctuations in service volume, and how this may impact overhead):

Utilities (gas, electric, water, trash, other)   Monthly Estimate   Yearly Estimate

_____

_____

_____

Other overhead costs you may anticipate (such as equipment maintenance contracts, security, transportation, and so on):

_____

_____

_____

Total estimates of overhead for: One month _____
                                   One year _____

4. A detailed marketing plan will be developed in Chapter 13, and you will wish to return to this exercise to record specific costs. For now provide a rough estimate of what you may wish to spend for such things as brochures, business cards, yellow pages, and so on. You can finalize the costs later. Record your estimates below.

Marketing Methods   Cost for Start-Up   Yearly Cost

_____

_____

_____

_____

5. Carefully review your developing program proposal for any anticipated costs that you may have forgotten to include. If you find additional costs, record them in the appropriate categories.

6. Add all of the above totals to determine an estimated figure of operating costs for your program for one year and for three years.

Total operating costs for one year: _____

Total operating costs for three years (remember that this figure will reflect inflation and will not necessarily include all of the categories in your start-up and one-year costs): _____

EXERCISE 3
Identifying Funding Sources

Now that you know what your program will cost, where will you get the funding? Your responses to Exercise 1 have already answered some of this question. Will you investigate public and private funding that may be appropriate for your target population and your program? Will you bill insurances? Will you combine these resources with private pay? Will you seek funding from your umbrella agency (such as through United Way, City Programs, and so on)? Perhaps you will research federal or private granting agencies to initiate your program, or maybe you will initiate a thorough investigation of how you may qualify for a small-business loan.

This is the place your *proposal* comes to the forefront—whether you present it in person to an umbrella agency, to your employer if you are designing a satellite program, or to a private granting organization. Perhaps you will glean from it the information you will need to apply for a loan. The strength and accuracy of the proposal will likely make the difference in whether or not you receive funds. If you are relying on external payers to fund your program, then the organization and content of the proposal will prevent any surprises. You will know what information you must have, what you have to do, and when you need to do it.

1. Discuss the previous descriptions of funding options with your classmates, colleagues, or partners to determine which ones seem most appropriate for your program. Note your selections below:

_____

_____

_____

_____

2. You may find that you need more information to make your decision. If so, go to the resources at the end of the chapter and further investigate the options that interest you. You may wish to talk to practitioners who are administering programs similar to the one you are planning, or you can use resources in addition to the ones listed here. When you have completed your research, note below your plan for funding your program:

_____

_____

_____

_____

_____

_____

Some sources (such as federal and private grants and lending agencies) require a fairly lengthy application process. When you prepare your time line in Chapter 14, be sure to include the funding process.

3. Following your research, will you need to develop your proposal further to comply with the requirements for your identified funding source? Do they require information that you may not have? If so, list below what additional steps you will need to take and your plan for doing so:

_____

_____

_____

_____

_____

_____

SUMMARY

The strength of your program evaluation plan and the accuracy of your cost sheet are critical to the funding success of your program. Through this process of planning program evaluation and anticipating costs and funding, you must maintain the importance of occupation and the more qualitative aspects of meaning in your program design and plan. In the potentially restrictive environments of todays' health care, it is important to not lose sight of the goal and purpose of your program.

This chapter has proposed numerous resources for you to explore as you develop your budget, your financial plan, and your proposed resources for initial or ongoing funding. You have completed a brief review of your plan, and you have decided exactly what you hope to accomplish and how you aim to do it. Your careful analysis of what will be needed to operate your program in previous chapter exercises has now resulted in the combined estimated costs of your program. You have identified the characteristics of your program and, in that regard, have come to some decisions about potential funding sources. If your venture calls for external funding either through grants or a loan, then you must anticipate that early in your planning. Select the direction you wish to go, and utilize the resources at the close of this chapter to obtain the additional information that you will require.

REFERENCES

Children and youth funding report. (1998, November 4). Silver Spring, MD: CD Publications.

Edwards, D. (1997). The effect of occupational therapy on function and well-being. In C. Christiansen & C. Baum (Eds.), *Occupational therapy enabling function and well-being* (pp. 557–572). Thorofare, NJ: Slack.

The international Webster new encyclopedic dictionary of the English language.(1975). Chicago: The English Language Institute of America.

Logigian, M. (1994). Cost management. In K. Jacobs & M. Logigian (Eds.), *Functions of a manager in occupational therapy* (pp. 99–121). Thorofare, NJ: Slack.

Ryan, J. D., Ray, R., & Hiduke, G. (1999). *Small business: An entrepreneur's plan.* Philadelphia: The Dryden Press.

Smith, N. (1996). Financial management. In M. Johnson (Ed.), *The occupational therapy manager* (pp. 63–100). Bethesda, MD: American Occupational Therapy Association.

Thomas, V. (1996). Evolving healthcare systems: Payment for occupational therapy services. In M. Johnson (Ed.), *The occupational therapy manager* (pp. 577–602). Bethesda, MD: American Occupational Therapy Association.

Vega, P. (1998, October). Industry trends. In *Practice strategies, A business guide for behavioral healthcare providers.* Washington, D.C.: American Association for Marriage and Family Therapy.

Recommended Readings

American Occupational Therapy Association, Inc. (1994). Uniform terminology for occupational therapy, 3rd edition. *American Journal of Occupational Therapy, 48,* 1,047–1,054.

American Occupational Therapy Association, Inc. (1996). *Managed care: An occupational therapy sourcebook.* Bethesda, MD: Author.

Federal grants and contracts weekly. (1998, September 28). Alexandria, VA: Aspen.

Jackson, L. (1998). Idea 97. *O.T. practice.* Bethesda, MD: American Occupational Therapy Association.

Kannenberg, K., Fine, S., & Lang, S. (1996). Reimbursement guidelines. In M. Brinson & K. Kannenberg (Eds.), *Mental health service delivery guidelines* (pp. 63–74). Bethesda, MD: American Occupational Therapy Association.

Occupational Therapy Association of California. (1999). *Branching out: Private practice and beyond.* Sacramento, CA: Author.

Regulations to implement the equal employment provisions of the Americans with Disabilities Act (1998). 29 CFR 1630.2(5). Washington, DC: U.S. Government Printing Office.

Internet Sources

Business Plans: www.sba.gov/starting/indexbusplans.html

ICIDH-2: http://www.who.ch/programmes/mnh/mnh/ems/icidh/icidhtrg/sldoo1.htm

Legal and Illegal Pre-Employment Inquiries: http://www.nolo.com

Federal Register: http://ocfo.ed.gov/fedreg.htm or http://www.ed.gov/news.html

National Institute of Health: http://www.nih.gov/grants/guide/index.html

National Association of Women Business Owners (NAWBO): www.nfwbo.org

General Business Salary Comparisons:

Recruitment Extra!: http://recruitmentextra.com/salarysurveys.html
 Wage Web: www.wageweb.com

Occupational Safety and Health Administration (OSHA): www.osha.gov

Equal Employment Opportunity Commission (EEOC) (202-663-4900):
 www.eeoc.gov/smallbus.html

Department of Labor: www.dol.gov

Internal Revenue Service (IRS): www.irs.gov

U.S. Department of Justice, Americans with Disabilities (800-514-0301; 202-514-0301):
 www.usdoj.gov/crt/ada

Immigration and Naturalization Service:
 www.ins.usdoj.gov/employer/index.html

The American Occupational Therapy Association (FAX-on-request) 800-701-7735

The Grantsmanship Center: http://www.tgci.com

Grantwriting Resources: http://www.fundsnetservices.com/grantwri.htm

Publications and Services of the Foundation Center, 79 Fifth Avenue, New York, NY 10003-3076 (1-800-424-9836); Foundation Center's World Wide Web site: http://fdncenter.org

General Research Directories

The following are published by the Foundation Center, New York, 1997:

The foundation directory, Michael Luller and Nicole Luman, eds., published annually

The foundation directory Part 2, Michael Luller and Nicole Luman, eds., published annually

The foundation directory supplement, Michael Luller and Nicole Luman, eds., published annually

Guide to U.S. foundations, their trustees, officers, and donors, published annually

The foundation 1000, published annually

National directory of corporate giving, published biennially

Corporate foundation profiles, published biennially
National directory of grantmaking public charities, 1st edition
Guide to greater Washington D.C. grantmakers, 2nd edition
New York State foundations: A comprehensive directory, published biennially
Directory of Missouri grantmakers, 1st edition
Foundation grants to individuals, published biennially

Subject Directories

AIDS funding: A guide to giving by foundations and charitable organizations, 4th edition
Guide to funding for international and foreign programs, 3rd edition
Funding in aging: A guide to giving by foundations, corporations, and charitable organizations
National guide to funding in arts and culture, 4th edition
National guide to funding for children, youth and families, 4th edition
National guide to funding for community development, 1st edition
National guide to funding for elementary and secondary education, 4th edition
National guide to funding for information technology, 1st edition
National guide to funding for the environment and animal welfare, 3rd edition
National guide to funding in health, 5th edition
National guide to funding in higher education, 4th edition
National guide to funding for libraries and information services, 4th edition
National guide to funding in religion, 4th edition
National guide to funding in substance abuse, 1st edition
National guide to funding for women and girls, 4th edition

Grant Directories

Grant guides, series published annually in October
The foundation grants index
The foundation grants index quarterly
Who gets grants: Foundation grants to nonprofit organizations

Guidebooks, Manuals, and Reports

AIDS fundraising
Arts funding
Arts funding revisited
The foundation center's grants classification system indexing manual and thesaurus, revised edition
Foundation fundamentals, 5th edition
The foundation center's user-friendly guide: A grantseeker's guide to resources, 4th edition
Foundation giving: Yearbook of facts and figures on private, corporate and community foundations
The foundation center's guide to proposal writing, 2nd edition
Program-related investments: A guide to funders and trends

Bibliographies

The Literature of the nonprofit sector: A bibliography with abstracts, volumes I-VIII

Other publications available through the Foundation Center that may be of interest:

Berstein, P. (1997). *Best practices of effective nonprofit organizations: A practitioner's manual.*

Booth, M. (1995). *Promoting issues and ideas: A guide to public relations for nonprofit organizations, revised edition.*

Cohen, L, & D. Young. (1989). *Careers for dreamers and doers: A guide to management careers in the nonprofit sector.*

Firstenberg, P. (1996). *The 21st century nonprofit.*

Freeman, D., and the Council on Foundations. (1991). *Handbook on private foundations.*

Kibbe, B., & Setterberg, F. (1992). *Succeeding with consultants: Self-assessment for the changing nonprofit.*

New, A. (1991). *Raise more money for your nonprofit organization: A guide to evaluating and improving fund raising.*

O'Connell, B. (1993). *The board member's book, 2nd edition.*

O'Connell, B. (1994). *People power: Service, advocacy, empowerment.*

Olenick, A., & Olenick, P. (1991). *A nonprofit organization operating manual: Planning for survival and growth.*

Salamon, L. (1992). *America's nonprofit sector: A primer.*

Seltzer, M. (1987). *Securing your organization's future: A complete guide to fundraising strategies.*

Skloot, E. (Ed.). (1988). *The nonprofit entrepreneur: Creating ventures to earn income.*

Young, D., & Steinberg, R. (1995). *Economics for nonprofit managers.*

CHAPTER

Program Evaluation: How Will Outcomes Be Measured?

Learning Objectives

1. To understand the purpose of program evaluation in achieving and maintaining quality services
2. To identify various methods that may be used to measure program effectiveness
3. To understand the link between the goal(s) and objectives of the program and the evaluation of outcomes
4. To consider the formative and summative measurement of individual progress to facilitate the measurement of program outcomes
5. To explore the rationale for selecting both quantitative and qualitative measures to evaluate program outcomes and to ensure quality
6. To develop an evaluation plan for the program you are designing and developing

Key Terms

1. Program Evaluation
2. Program Success
3. Program Effectiveness
4. Program Outcomes
5. Quantitative Measures of Outcome
6. Qualitative Measures of Outcome
7. Pretests and Posttests
8. Formative and Summative Measures of Outcome

What is program evaluation and why should it be done? C. MacDonell (1996) describes **program evaluation** first of all as a "system" that is put into place "to provide information that an organization can use to improve performance to an agreed-on level that meets desired **outcomes**" (p. 398). Therefore, we know that program evaluation is intended to improve programming performance and that it does so in the process of meeting our desired outcomes (our goals and the accompanying objectives). If we meet our desired outcomes, then we can at least partially assume that our programming is effective.

For occupational therapy practitioners and other health care providers, the impetus for scrutinizing the effectiveness of our services began some thirty years ago with the newly developing social programs, but it has only been in the last ten years that evaluation has become imperative for programs to continue. Certainly through our unfolding history we have placed the provision of quality patient care at the top of our priorities, and in providing that care we have focused our attentions on the *process* of therapy. In many ways this attention to process at the exclusion of outcome has created inefficiency in our treatment styles and a tendency to "trust" in the effectiveness of our services rather than devise ways to effectively measure those outcomes.

The field of physical rehabilitation was perhaps most effective in the 1970s and 1980s in the refinement of outcome measures, but effective measurement of outcomes did not quite happen for psychosocial practices—and we now see the results with shrinking service provision for the mentally ill. Since much of our work in the community considers the needs of those persons with mental illness, it is imperative that we work to refine outcome measures and determine the most efficient programming to obtain results. If our future is to include occupation-centered community-based programs in the areas of prevention and health maintenance, we will have an even greater challenge as we design and implement outcome measures.

METHODS OF EVALUATION

Let's investigate further the different ways to evaluate **program effectiveness.** Forer describes outcome evaluation as the method of evaluation that "concentrates on the *results* of services, programs, treatments, or intervention strategies" (1996, Introduction). Our primary goal in all of our programming efforts is, of course, the evaluation of the effectiveness of our *program*—the full component of services. Weiss (1972) emphasizes that program evaluation is a broader concept than outcome evaluation and suggests that the components of *program* evaluation be expanded beyond outcome evaluation to include the following: needs assessment, process evaluation, program efficiency, program effectiveness, impact of the program, and outcome evaluation.

If you have worked with the guidelines of The Commission on Accreditation of Rehabilitation Facilities (CARF) or the Joint Commission on Accreditation of

Healthcare Organizations (JCAHO), you know that these organizations place a great deal of emphasis on outcomes. CARF documents define program evaluation as "a systematic procedure for determining the effectiveness and efficiency with which results are achieved by persons served during the service delivery phase and following program completion . . . as well as the individual's satisfaction with them" (1995).

The programs' performance is always measured against the goals and objectives established by the planner or planning group. Therefore, the careful and accurate expression of the goal and the objectives coupled with a well articulated and comprehensive plan to achieve them will not only provide accurate guidelines for measurement of outcomes but also will ensure that those outcomes compare favorably with the intent of the planner.

WILL YOU EVALUATE INDIVIDUAL CLIENTS?

Certainly one cannot design a program with accompanying goal and objectives without considering the needs of the client/participant. Those needs collectively provide the basis for the program. All programs deliver services to a client/participant group, and for most programs monitoring individual process and progress provides us with incremental measures that ultimately contribute to our evaluation of the program's effectiveness. These measures contribute to the **formative** evaluation process that is occuring at intervals throughout the program. These measures allow us to know how the group is responding to the objectives and goal of the program. Formative evaluations can identify where changes may be required. These formative measures are then coupled with **summative** measures that occur at the end of a programming cycle. You may wish to develop your own evaluation instrument(s) based on the goal and the objectives of your program. In some cases, you also may choose to purchase evaluation instruments for individual participants that are designed to accompany the frame or frames of reference you have selected to guide your programming.

You may need to research what is available for your population and your frame of reference and what will meet the needs structured by your objectives and your goal. Some assessments can be copied from texts or articles, while others are restricted. Hinojosa and Kramer (1998) have provided an excellent resource for client evaluation in their text, *Occupational Therapy Evaluation: Obtaining and Interpreting Data*. Another excellent resource is Asher's (1996) *Occupational Therapy Assessment Tools: An Annotated Index, 2nd edition*. You may wish to review both of these texts should you consider individual evaluation of clients/patients as part of your formative and/or summative program evaluation process. You may also want to review the extensive list of studies utilizing various outcome measures in Moyers' (1999) "The Guide to Occupational Therapy Practice" as well as your occupational therapy textbooks for lists of assessments appropriate to particular populations. For assessments that may be conducted by the Certified Occupational Therapy Assistant (COTA), refer to the "Roles and Functions Papers" of the AOTA *Reference Manual of the Official Documents* for guidelines (1997, pp. 208–210) as well as the *COTA Information Packet: A Guide for Supervision* (1995).

Your decision regarding individual assessments will be based on what the results of these will tell you about the effectiveness of your *program*. Your *program evaluation* is linked to the progress your individual clients make, so some consistent baseline measure of their performance must be made. In some instances that measure will be made by other agencies/practitioners, and you will need to access the information.

For example, if we are providing day camp services for children who are presently being seen by other therapists, then we might assume that these children have already been evaluated. There is no need for us to further evaluate each child (at least not in the same way). Certainly we would collaborate with the therapist who is continuing to see the child or perhaps sees the child through a school year; we would have initiated this process with the needs assessment. The camp will provide intervention to "enhance" the treatment the child is receiving from the referring therapist and to assist in meeting the therapist's goals for the child. In addition, the camp experience might "supplement" the child's individual therapy with opportunites to learn socialization through structured group play.

In this example you might wish to go further and consider establishing baseline measures and continuing formative and summative measures around the goal of socialization/group play. Certainly your marketing efforts for such a camp would be enhanced if you could demonstrate indicators of success in addition to what you expect the child's primary therapist might identify.

In some kinds of programs a structured interview also is used to establish a baseline assessment. You would likely establish the interview format yourself, which certainly would be based on your goal and on your chosen frame or frames of reference.

OTHER MEASURES TO CONSIDER

In many of the programs described in this text, there is not individual measurement of progress as we may be accustomed to in our traditional models of evaluation and intervention, but we are always aware of the progress of individuals and that their goal and objectives are reflective of and companion to those of the program. For example, a program goal may target the development of moral judgment in adolescents as they transition to young adulthood. The goal may specifically target the development of skills to negate law-breaking in the community. Accompanying objectives may focus on skills to find work and a residence or perhaps the provision of opportunity to explore and engage in alternative meaningful occupations. All of these objectives are measurable, and all are related to outcomes. But not all of the adolescents participating in such a program may be successful in the attainment of each objective, and they may not all accomplish the goal; however, it is important to remember that a *program* may still be successful even if all of the participants are not.

The best way to evaluate the objectives and ultimately the goal of your program is to ask yourself the following questions: How will I know if that actually happens? *and* When and how will I measure it? All programs must be able to evaluate effectiveness in order to justify their continued existence. Such evaluation will not only justify their continuation but also will provide the information that is needed to continue to improve the match between the goal, the objectives, and the programming. This is the function of formative evaluation. The day-to-day program *enables* you to meet the program objectives and ultimately the goal. If objectives are not being met, then alterations, adjustments, and fine-tuning may be made in day-to-day programming. If the goal is not satisfied, then likely these adjustments are required in the objectives as well.

There are several dimensions or tiers of measurement needed to fully evaluate a program. We begin program evaluation by determining the dimensions within which we will establish measures of **program success.**

Case Example: Measuring Outcomes in a Head Start Program for Children

To provide an example of outcome measurement in an occupation-centered community-based program, we will highlight a program established to support the mission and goals of Head Start. As you may know, Head Start is a federally mandated program designed to aid preschool children in the attainment of skills that have been determined to be necessary for successful achievement when they enter school.

Children who qualify for Head Start programs are those considered to be "at risk" with regard to lower economic status, some level of involvement with social services-child protective services, or physical and/or emotional disabilities.

As with all program design, the Head Start program was initiated with the community and population profiles followed by the needs assessments. The mission and philosophy of the Head Start program was discussed with the director and teaching staff of the selected site. In this first phase of needs assessment, which also included teachers in the district schools these children would attend, several unmet needs were identified that were appropriate for occupation-centered programming. The teachers expressed a strong desire to assist parents in assuming the role of prime educator of their child; through this process they would help to identify potential problems the child might be experiencing. They specifically identified the need for fine-motor/prewriting skill development and the additional need for early screening to determine which children might require more specific intervention before they entered school as opposed to those who might benefit from a little extra help in school or at home. In the focus group utilized for Phase II and performance skills deficits assessment, parents were concerned that they did not know what behaviors they should look for in their child that might present problems in school; if they did suspect problems, they did not know what to do about them. All parents concurred that they would like to help their child be ready for school if they knew what to do.

The goal of the program was essentially the same as that of the larger organization: To enhance the children's successful entry into school through parent-teacher-child teamwork.

The objectives to enable the accomplishment of the above program goal were:

1. *The parents and teachers will be provided with information and activities to assist them in identifying deficits in the child's development that may indicate potential problems in school.*
2. *The parents and teachers will be provided with games and activities to engage in with children to encourage the development of fine-motor/prewriting skills.*
3. *Early developmental screening by occupational therapy practitioners will be conducted to assist in determining which children may require more extensive assessment and intervention.*

The *program* provided a number of training sessions to parents and to teachers. Materials were developed to meet the needs of both groups in their efforts to help their children prepare for school. In addition, home and Head Start program visits and observations by occupational therapy practitioners and occupational therapy students assisted both parents and teachers in learning to identify potential problems. These visits were coupled with developmental screening of each child in the Head Start program. This program provided what might be considered both indirect and direct services. In community programming—perhaps in all occupation-centered programming—it is important to provide services that will empower the recipient and the family to share in meeting the responsibilities required to satisfy the program goal.

EVALUATING THE PROGRAM

Now that we have our goal and our objectives and we have conducted the program for a period of time, we must ask ourselves the following questions: Is the program effective? Does it do what we think it does? Did we satisfy our objectives? Did we meet our goal? Were we successful? There are several steps to be accomplished before we can answer these questions and determine whether or not we are successful in meeting our goal. First we must measure the objectives we have established to permit us to meet our goal. If our objectives are accurate in their expression of our goal and if they are measurable, we will have no problems in accomplishing this task.

To return to our case example, there were three objectives for the Head Start occupation-centered program. All three objectives are measurable:

1. *Parents and teachers **will be provided with information and activities** to assist them in identifying deficits in the child's development that may indicate potential problems in school.*

2. *The parents and teachers **will be provided with games and activities** to participate in with children to encourage the development of fine-motor/ prewriting skills.*

3. **Early developmental screening by occupational therapy practitioners will be conducted** *to assist in determining which children may require more extensive assessment and intervention.*

Regardless of the parameters of time established (such as one month, six months, one year, and so on), we should be able to measure these objectives. Did we provide the parents and teachers with information and activities to assist them in identifying deficits in the child's development that may indicate potential problems in school? Did we provide parents and teachers with games and activities to participate in with children to encourage the development of fine-motor/prewriting skills? And did we provide early developmental screening by occupational therapy practitioners to assist in determining which children may require more extensive assessment and intervention?

Even though we always begin by measuring the objectives established for our program, this alone is not enough. Even if we can clearly answer yes to all of the above objectives, we really know nothing about the effectiveness or success of our program. We simply know that our program has provided the services that we promised. A positive evaluation of an objective that is designed to measure the dissemination of information and materials is only as meaningful as the *quality of the materials* and the *mode of dissemination*. Our professional knowledge, skills, and experience contribute to our clinical reasoning in helping us to provide the programming (the information and materials) that will be effective.

Recall our case example of the Denver sanctuary program. The goal of encouraging self-efficacy was enabled through an objective of providing developmentally appropriate information and skills with which to make informed choices about practiced sexual behaviors. As was mentioned previously, this is very different than simply offering condoms. The success of this program is contingent on all of the embedded "clues" known to occupation-centered practitioners. By linking efficacy to cognitive and moral development and to sexuality as occupation, our clinical reasoning guides us to arrive at a program that is far more than providing information and skills; rather, we can provide information and skills that result in the program's success.

■ EXERCISE 1 ■

The First Step in Program Evaluation: Measuring Objectives

1. Considering the previous examples, discuss with your classmates or colleagues ideas for how you will measure the program you are designing. Revisit your goal and your objectives. In the space provided, write the goal or goals for your program, your objectives to support your goal, and the time you have established for measurement:

Your goal:

_____

_____

_____

Your objectives:

_____

_____

_____

_____

Consider whether or not you will use individual assessments and, if so, what you will use. Will you be able to obtain baseline assessment data for your population from other sources?

For each of your objectives noted above, determine the quantitative measures that you will utilize:

_____

_____

_____

_____

_____

Clearly the first step in evaluating any program is to meet the objectives we have established as our first line of measurement. These first measures are **quantitative;** that is, we determine who received the services and how often. Without first knowing that everyone has received the services specified in our objectives we cannot go further to determine the **qualitative** measures necessary to evaluate whether or not our services met our expectations and therefore were effective.

By carefully logging contact hours with parents and teachers and by videotaping the informational meetings, it was clear that the foundation (the quantitative measure) of the first two objectives for the Head Start program had been satisfied (27 parents and 4 teachers had received the information).

Over the course of six weeks, all of the children (23) had been screened to determine if any of them might require more extensive assessment and intervention. Following review of the screening results, 6 children were referred for further occupational therapy assessment.

Following review of the three objectives that were established, it was determined that the third objective required no further evaluation. There were no qualitative measures required to further assess this objective as it was written. In fact, it is arguable whether or not this objective relates to the goal for the program, which was "to enhance the children's successful entry into school through parent-teacher-child teamwork." Though nothing in this objective directly relates to parent-teacher-child teams, there is certainly an assumption that early screening and any resultant intervention will enhance the child's successful transition to school. In any further work with this program and to ensure funding for this objective, it would be necessary to evaluate this assumption through extensive literature review and by following each child's progress in school either by single case or compared to children who did not receive assessment and intervention.

However, the question of how we measure the outcomes to determine whether or not the program is effective still remains. There are several methods—both quantitative and qualitative—we can use to accomplish this task.

PRETESTS AND POSTTESTS

When we use the term *outcome*, we are referring to the results that were obtained at the completion of our program. However, one cannot measure the result of a program, or a treatment for that matter, without first obtaining a base measurement. If we were to use this method in our Head Start example, at the first meeting of parents, teachers, and occupational therapy practitioners, a brief **pretest** or questionnaire would be administered to determine how much the teachers (one group) and parents (one group) knew about the developing child generally, how much they knew about the identification of potential deficits, and how much they knew about the development of fine-motor skills related to prewriting specifically.

For our example, the pretest would ask specific questions regarding the developmental markers for fine-motor coordination in children between the ages of 3 and 4 (the ages of the children in the program). A video might be used in conjunction with the questionnaire to provide examples of motor skills.

The same questionnaire/test (a **posttest**) would be given following the in-service or series of in-services. The comparison of responses to the pretests and posttests provides a further marker for how successful the intervention (the in-service) was in meeting the objective of providing information, games, and activities. Our posttest will also provide us with information as to how *effective* we were in developing materials that were appropriate to the needs of each group—parents and teachers. From this information we could return to the materials and the way they were provided to make necessary changes to enhance their receptivity.

Since the first objective of our example suggests that the information we provide will assist the parent and teacher to identify any deficits in the child's development that may indicate potential problems in school, we would want to evaluate whether this happened or not in order to further ensure the effectiveness of our program. We might do so by asking the parents and the teachers to note any deficits they observe on a chart or check-sheet. This information might then be correlated with the results of the occupational therapy practitioner's screening. Positive correlations would add further strength to the results provided by this objective. If these correlations were not found, then we might wish to return to our programming to determine how we might be more effective. Stronger and more definitive research designs might also be employed to measure the effectiveness of this program (see the reference list at the end of this chapter for examples of such measures).

Meeting the second objective goes beyond the quantitative measure of providing games and activities and assumes participation by parent-teacher-child to encourage the development of fine-motor prewriting skills. To provide a valid measurement of this objective, each child's fine-motor prewriting skills would need to be measured before the program (pretest) and again following the program (posttest). Although these tests would not provide enough information to definitively say that our program supported improvement in these skills, such test results could strongly suggest such a finding, particularly if we had measures of normative parent-child or teacher-child participation in our suggested games and activities.

REVISITING GOALS

It is wise to continue to revisit our goal to be sure that our evaluation of objectives has not caused us to become blind to our purpose. Although the objectives for our case example are sound and do relate clearly to the goal, it is likely that we will want to have one or two more. None of the objectives truly address the idea of *teams* mentioned in our goal, and as has been indicated in earlier chapters, *teams* can be empowering. Teamwork assumes a sharing of responsibility and equal distribution of rewards. Without a specific objective, we do not know whether we have established programming that will encourage the formation of teams or the philosophies and ideas that support teamwork. Without such an objective, the child appears to be the targeted "problem" in this program rather than a shareholder in the outcome. Although not formally tied to an objective, videotaping all aspects of the program offered a potential opportunity to qualitatively evaluate the formation of teams from the early stages of program design through actual programming, and the elements of teamwork did emerge. You might like to write an objective that would target the development of parent-child-teacher teams to help us more fully support our goal. Our goal also uses the subjective term *successful* to describe the desired transition from Head Start to school. Our objectives translate the results of our needs assessment into the skills we believe to be necessary for this transition to successfully occur. The results of the needs assessment also identified the need for children to be socialized to the school environment before actually entering; although we did not develop an objective to meet this need. Can you suggest one?

▬▬ EXERCISE 2 ▬▬

Going Beyond Quantitative Measures to Measure Quality

1. Again review your objectives and your goal(s). Are there further measures you will need to make in order to determine the effectiveness of your program? How will you measure the quality of your program? First consider other quantitative

measures then more qualitative ones. Note what additional measures you will require below:

_____

_____

_____

_____

_____

2. Do you have a mode of measurement for every aspect of your objectives? Will
the results of these measures determine whether or not you have met the goal(s)
for your program? Will they help you determine if changes in programming
may be necessary? Make notations below for any alterations you may need to
make now:

_____

_____

_____

_____

_____

Continuing program evaluation at whatever interval you've determined—
three months, six months, yearly (or all of these)—will also be the time you reevaluate your goals. Even a year is likely too soon to alter the original goals and
certainly too soon to throw them out and start over, but it is not too soon to make
changes in objectives and/or programming. This will also be the time to evaluate
staffing, costs, and the program environment. How do these factors impact the
quantity and the quality of your intervention? Most federal granting agencies expect at least yearly outcome reports and provide the program a two- or three-year
running period before reapplying for continuation. This offers a reasonable time to
measure outcomes and make minor alterations in programming. Consider, too, re-
peating your phases of needs assessment as a way of evaluating the connection between need, your goal(s), and your program design. You may wish to conduct a
focus group as a qualitative measure of program effectiveness whether or not you
used this technique in assessing need. Such a group can provide a strong measure
of how you are doing. A focus group of parents and one of teachers would be extremely useful as a formative or a summative measure for our Head Start example.

Outcomes Over Time

It is often of interest and/or critical to determine if your program has lasting effectiveness—effectiveness *after* the program has been terminated for the participant.
We have alluded to this in our Head Start case example with the recommendation

that the children be followed through their school experience to effectively determine whether or not we have enhanced their progress and success. Evaluation over time is more difficult to achieve and will require more manpower and financial resources than formative and summative in-house evaluations. A long-term follow-up evaluation will require a system to track participants and a set of measures related to your original goals. If follow-up effectiveness seems critical to what you want to achieve, then your original goal(s) should state the follow-up outcomes as well as the immediate measures of success.

If you intend to manage numerous outcome measures, particularly over time, then you will need an effective data management system to do so. Forer (1996) also offers a substantial reference section that provides a list of publications describing programming in a variety of disability areas as well as outcome evaluation techniques appropriate to differing kinds of programming. Review the discussion of programs in Part III for examples of program evaluation plans and instruments.

SUMMARY

This chapter has provided the rationale for program evaluation. The reader is reminded to always link the goal or goals of the program and the objectives to the evaluation of outcome. Not only is program evaluation necessary to determine the effectiveness of a program, but it also can provide a measure of the quality of the programming. Both measures of effectiveness and quality are necessary to enhance the successful future of a program and often are necessary to guarantee its continuation. These measures will also provide information with regard to the effectiveness of your staffing and the impact of your intervention environment and may also help you reevaluate costs.

This chapter completes the process of program design. The next chapter offers some ideas for marketing, and the following chapter will demonstrate ways to establish a time line for the tasks you will need to accomplish in order to actually begin. You are almost there!

REFERENCES

American Occupational Therapy Association, Inc. (1995). *COTA information packet: A guide for supervision*. Bethesda, MD: Author.

American Occupational Therapy Association, Inc. (1997). Roles and functions papers. In *Reference manual of the official documents* (pp. 208–210). Bethesda, MD: Author.

Asher, E. (1996). *Occupational therapy assessment tools: An annotated index* (2nd ed.). Bethesda, MD: American Occupational Therapy Association.

Commission on Accreditation of Rehabilitation Facilities (CARF). (1995, January). *Survey standards for medical rehabilitation*. Tuscon, AZ: Author.

Forer, S. (1996). *Outcome management and program evaluation made easy: A toolkit for occupational therapy practitioners.* Bethesda, MD: American Occupational Therapy Association.

Hinojosa, J., & Kramer, P. (Eds.). (1998). *Occupational therapy evaluation: Obtaining and interpreting data.* Bethesda, MD: American Occupational Therapy Association.

MacDonell, C. (1996). Program evaluation. In AOTA (Eds.). *The occupational therapy manager* (pp. 398–410). Bethesda, MD: American Occupational Therapy Association.

Mandel, D., Jackson, J., Zemke, R., Nelson, L., & Clark, F. (1999). *Lifestyle redesign: Implementing the well elderly program.* Bethesda, MD: The American Occupational Therapy Association.

Moyers, P. (1999). The guide to occupational therapy practice. Appendix F: Outcomes. *American Journal of Occupational Therapy, 53*(3), 298–322.

Weiss, C. (1972). *Evaluation research: Methods for assessing program effectiveness.* Englewood Cliffs, NJ: Prentice-Hall.

CHAPTER

Marketing: How Will I Let the Consumer Know?

Learning Objectives

1. To learn the components of a marketing plan
2. To determine the characteristics of a promotional mix
3. To identify the pros and cons associated with the different elements of a promotional strategy
4. To conceptualize the program you are designing and developing
5. To develop the marketing plan and promotional mix for your program

Key Terms

1. Marketing
2. Advertising
3. Public Relations
4. Publicity
5. Direct Selling/Personal Selling
6. Sales Promotion
7. Promotional Mix
8. Press Release
9. Free Ink/Free Air
10. Networking
11. Marketing Logic

As the title of this chapter indicates, in the simplest terms **marketing** is the process of letting your potential consumers know that you have services that may be of interest to them. However, marketing also includes an intent to "sell" the services to them (even if the services are free). This marketing aspect of selling is often referred to by the more aggressive term **sales promotion,** and those areas that are selected to promote your services are referred to as the **promotional mix.** In her discussions of marketing yourself as an occupational therapy practitioner, Gilkeson (1997) describes this promotional mix to include the three areas of advertising, publicity, and personal selling. Gerson (1991) utilizes a more conventional list preferred by business to include advertising, public relations, direct selling, and sales promotion. Writing for the potential small business entrepreneur, on the other hand, Ryan, Ray, and Hiduke include all of these areas in their promotional mix. In their words, *mix* "refers to all the elements that are blended to maximize communication with the target customer or population" (1999, p. 99). An important aspect of promotion for these authors is the advancement of the "image" of your practice, or displaying for the potential consumer the "quality" of your services.

Advertising, of course, includes all of those marketing methods we have come to take for granted in our lives, such as visual media (television), print media (magazines and newspapers), radio, and now the Internet. We hardly notice media ads, billboards, or bus signs, yet we are influenced by their messages. **Publicity** may be positive or negative and is usually not targeted by the marketer; rather, it is received by the marketer. The receipt of positive publicity, for example, could be in the form of responses to a public presentation we have done or to a community service event we have organized and/or in which we have participated. Of course, there is also the negative potential of such publicity as the announcement of a malpractice suit or other legal sanctions having to do with unethical or unsafe practices. **Public relations** describes the direct intent of interfacing with your public in such a way that the image of you and your service delivery remains positive.

Personal selling has been emphasized in earlier chapters, but let's examine it in consideration of our marketing mix from the perspective of personally going out to make others aware of our program. Peter Drucker (1973) has long been a compelling voice in the wilderness of business management. He suggests that if the marketing process has been well organized and carried out effectively, personal selling might not be necessary. For our purposes, however, personal selling is a critical—perhaps the most critical—part of health promotion, intervention, and the extensive scope of most of the program development described in this text. A few minutes taken to meet the pediatricians, teachers, and parents in your community coupled with the delivery of a well-appointed brochure describing your pediatric occupational therapy services is well worth the time.

Although your new program or practice may represent one of those circumstances where you will open your doors and they will come, this is not likely. If others in the community have a vested interest in your program (such as our examples of the cooperative gardening project for the mentally ill who are homeless or the sanctuary program for runaway adolescents), then they will likely assist you in attracting clients and in getting them to you. Anytime you have the enthusiasm, interest, and support of an agency or organization, you will have less marketing to do in order to get your clients through your doors.

As we mentioned earlier in the text, your first marketing task was to *sell yourself* to the people who required a planner. If they were not yet aware that they needed a planner, then you sold them on the idea. We assume that you already have done this, but the process of selling yourself never quite ends. Even if you have the support of an agency to start the program, you will have to continue "selling" the idea and, more importantly, making people aware of how effective your programming is. As described by Gilkeson (1997), this is **marketing logic,** or the representation of an attitude that supports the principles of *selling* yourself and the belief in your ideas. It is the belief that *you* are the *program* and that the program is an extension of you. It represents your beliefs, your ideas, and your ethics.

If you are developing a new program under the sponsorship of your employer, then the marketing task will not be yours alone. It is likely that you have already proven your worth or you would not have been invited to develop a new program. In addition, assuming the development is responsive to an expressed need, part of the marketing/promotion probably already has been accomplished. In a case such as this, the primary marketing task—as it is for all programs—will be one of proving effectiveness weighed against cost.

Sometimes a program is initiated because someone else has recognized the need but does not have the expertise or perhaps the interest to provide it. That person might come to you, or you might hear of it and go to them: the marketing task then is to *sell yourself* as the best one to do the job.

Let's consider the following scenario. You are attending an open house of a new cardiac care unit and happen to overhear one of the attendees ask if there would be a cardiac "wellness" program to complement the surgical practice. You are an astute marketer/planner and later ask one of the cardiac surgeons if you could meet with him or her regarding your ideas for supplementary services organized around occupation; after all, you are an occupational therapy practitioner (or "therapist" if that is a more marketable term in this environment). Needless to say, after some planning, promotion, and negotiation with the corporation, you will develop a maintenance and wellness program that may include providers of information and skills in the areas of balanced lifestyle, nutrition, relaxation (maybe yoga), graduated exercise, and sexuality; and you have further marketed this program to other cardiac caregivers and surgeons. This is an example of a "success" story.

Of course, you are not finished; you must keep careful formative and summative outcome data to market your program's effectiveness in lengthening life and in enhancing quality of life. The goal of a program such as this could be not only the promotion of longer lives but also the assurance of longer *meaningful* lives. This is a burgeoning area of interest and research in occupational therapy, so part of your task is to keep abreast of all of the work that is being accomplished to support the establishment of *meaning* in one's life and to provide potentially *valued* options for how one chooses to live, perhaps to include the *redesign* of one's life (Mandel, Jackson, Zemke, Nelson, & Clark, 1999).

The most challenging marketing task may be for the private practice. Many therapists who initiate private practices do so a bit cautiously while still being employed by other organizations. As we said earlier, a private practice is a business, and there are risks to be considered. If you were an entrepreneur as a child or adolescent and started a successful business (a lemonade stand, babysitting service, or anything else), you know something about marketing and promotion. You may have been selling a product or a service or maybe both.

For example, neighborhood children might collaborate to climb trees, retrieve mistletoe, package it, and sell it door to door during the holiday season. The mistletoe was likely hanging on the trees of most of the people who purchased it. The marketing mix would include an attractively wrapped product and a service (retrieval of the "product" from the trees), and most people would probably buy it. There is little doubt that known neighborhood children are a strong component of the promotional mix, regardless of what they are selling. Consider how many subscriptions, packages of candy, and holiday cards you have purchased from a child at your door. This example may seem a bit remote from our interests as occupation-centered practitioners, but it clearly shows how an effective promotional mix is developed, and it is not unlike what you will do.

You will be selling a product and a service—thoughtful, skilled intervention that is well packaged in a comfortable and welcoming environment. In addition, you can and will prove that this particular intervention makes a difference. Your clients/patients/members may be able to do for themselves some of what you do but certainly not as effectively or as efficiently. Consider why people go to clubs to exercise when they could exercise at home. Could some of their reasoning also apply to your clientele? You are the professional skilled in understanding and utilizing meaningful occupation, so your marketing brochures and your business card should reflect this. If you find that people misinterpret what you do as an occupational therapist or as an occupational therapy assistant, include a meaningful explanation of your services on a brochure or an explanatory phrase on your business card. You may want these materials to be focused toward the population you wish to serve. For example, a pediatrics program might be described as providing "supportive play through small-group interactions."

THE PROMOTIONAL MIX

What are the choices available to us as we prepare to let others know about our program, and how do we select the options that will be most advantageous? Consider the following possibilities adapted from Ryan, Ray, and Hiduke (1999):

Promotional Element	Pros	Cons
1. Paid media advertising (radio, television, Internet, newspapers, and magazines)	Quick, effective	Expensive
2. Direct mail (to your potential consumer)	Affordable, efficient	Can be wasted if you have a fragmented market; difficult to write

(continued)

Promotional Element	Pros	Cons
3. Professional literature (become a source of information in your specialty and an expert in your field, and write about it)	Little or no cost; respected by colleagues and consumers	Will take work and experience
4. Free ink and free air (reviews, features, interview shows, press releases, newspaper columns to talk about what you do)	No cost and effective	Takes time to "market" to media
5. Promotional products (products with the name of your program, such as key chains, pencils, mugs, shirts, etc.)	Targeted and effective; can be very creative	Can be costly
6. Working visibility (develop and maintain a positive presence in the community; stand out from the competitors because you are better)	Common sense	You have to be good!
7. Personal selling and networking (business cards distributed at events, meetings); displays	Personal and effective	Takes time and can be costly

Consider these alternatives as you develop your promotional strategies. For most nonprofit community programs, the planner will rely on those with low cost. Communicating with others in the community about your program is known as **networking,** or getting to know others in the community who can and will help you remain a viable community resource. Sometimes this is accomplished through very informal means such as going to the same coffee shop as those you wish to know, and living in the community is certainly a plus. Networking also might be more formal and can include attending professional meetings or town meetings, or if you have a private practice, you may wish to join the Chamber of Commerce. Getting free media coverage, or **free ink/free air,** by providing a news item or story is excellent advertising. Writing a human-interest story about one of your clients or a client's family and then sending the story along with a photo to the media in the form of a **press release** will not only let the potential consumer know about your services but also will let those who may be able to offer financial assistance know as well. Always keep in mind working visibility and the process of becoming a professional authority in your specialty; certainly these are substantial facilitators to a successful private practice. Consider offering to do presentations, workshops, or seminars to Parent-Teacher Associations, Lions or Kiwanis Clubs, and church groups. These are excellent ways to market your program and to give the potential consumer a way to see how you work and to know whether or not they wish to engage your services. You may also target some referrals in this way as well. Public service activities such as community health fairs are yet another way to interface with potential consumers and those who may wish to refer consumers to your program.

PROMOTIONAL PRODUCTS AND ADVERTISING

Regardless of the nature or size of your program, you will likely wish to develop a logo with accompanying business cards and letterhead/envelopes and perhaps a brochure. You may also want to place your logo on a t-shirt for campers, on the side of a transportation van, or on "Halloween" candy that your clients give to local businesses in a marketing "reverse trick or treat."

Business cards (always carried with you) and brochures (distributed where your potential consumer or family/friends of the consumer will see them) always should be professional. In many ways, these may be considered as print advertising, and they are a representation of your practice. If they are less than serious, your practice will be assumed to be less than serious. In addition, your informational materials (flyers/brochures) should not be overly dramatic, and never make claims you cannot support.

Some therapists put advertisements in the telephone yellow pages and in newspapers (particularly neighborhood or community newspapers). Again, these must be professional. Brochures, pamphlets, or flyers made available directly to the consumer, to consumers' family members, and to other professionals from whom you may get referrals is sometimes enough to initiate a practice, particularly when start-up funding is limited. Physicians will often permit other practitioners to place brochures in their reception area (after marketing to them and with their approval, of course). A marketing/networking visit to teachers, psychologists, ministers, and other therapists and a brochure or business card left behind may also generate referrals. Of course you would not try to advertise in the offices of competitors, but consider whether your services can supplement or complement those of other occupational therapy practitioners (for example, day camps to complement pediatric practices).

Once you have established programming, consider sending holiday greetings with your logo on the cover. A holiday greeting may be coupled with an end-of-the-tax-year "invitation" for dollars to support programming (such as tuition for camp attendance). If you and your clients/members go into the wider community either as part of your services or to do exhibits and community fairs, a logo on a shirt can go a long way to make your services known. If you choose to do this, you may wish to remind your clients/members that they are your best advertisements—a very persuasive enabler for a goal of personal efficacy.

See Figure 13–1 and Figure 13–2 for examples of marketing flyers, brochures, and logos.

EXERCISE 1
Conceptualizing Your Program

1. Think about the program you are designing and developing. How would you like to represent it to potential consumers or other professionals? Referring again to your goal(s) and your objectives, write down a few words or phrases that sum up your program in user-friendly terms. Consider *what* you will do for the client/patient/member, *how* you will do it (your programming), and *who* will do it (the expertise of your staff):

_____

_____

_____

_____

_____

2. Consider now what your marketing mix will be. Will you use direct mail and/or personal distribution for brochures? Will you and your employees carry business cards? Will you create some kind of specialty advertising/promotional products? Will you use paid media advertising? Will you rely on free ink/free air? In what ways will you ensure visibility in the community? Note your ideas below:

_____

_____

_____

_____

_____

Now that you have selected your marketing mix, you may find it helpful to collect advertisements from the telephone book or newspapers or a few brochures or promotional items from organizations or professional offices that you visit in your weekly round of activities. Most professionals are finding it necessary to advertise these days. How do they conceptualize the services that they offer? Which ones do you like and why? Which ones do you not like and why?

FIGURE 13–1   Examples of Promotional Logos and Brochures

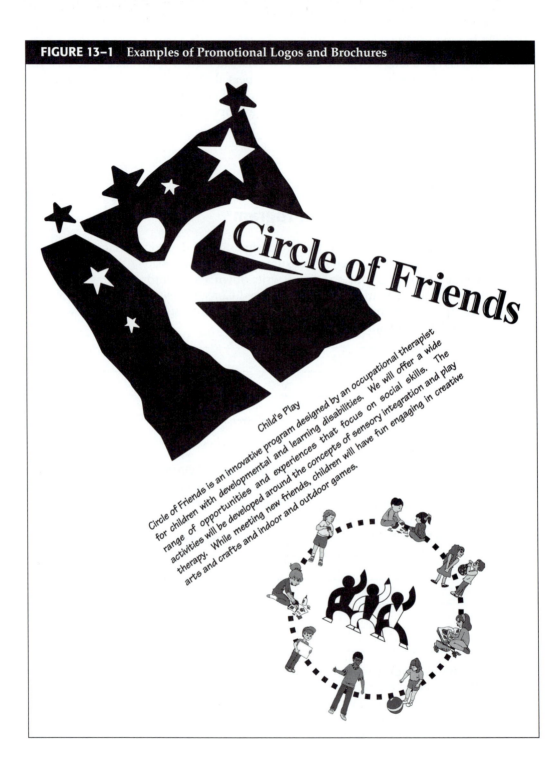

Child's Play

Circle of Friends is an innovative program designed by an occupational therapist for children with developmental and learning disabilities. We will offer a wide range of opportunities and experiences that focus on social skills. The activities will be developed around the concepts of sensory integration and play therapy. While meeting new friends, children will have fun engaging in creative arts and crafts and indoor and outdoor games.

FIGURE 13–2 Examples of Promotional Flyers

REGISTRATION

PLEASE FILL OUT AND RETURN TO: _____

Phone: _____ Camp Voice Mail: _____ Fax: _____

Name of Child: _____ Name of Child: _____
Birthday: _____ Birthday: _____

Phone: _____

Session Preferred: _____

✂ -

Each week will offer a theme around which the activities, games, arts, and crafts are designed and organized. A field trip complementing the theme will offer children and their parents the chance to share a fun experience in the community.

PLAY AWAY YOUR DAY!! A SUMMER DAY CAMP FOR CHILDREN

PLAY AWAY YOUR DAY! is a day camp offered from 10:00 A.M. to 3:00 P.M. for children with special needs between the ages of four and seven (and their siblings of the same age range).

Through arts, crafts, games, and activities, the campers will be encouraged to actively play and learn together.

Each camp group will be staffed by an occupational therapist, an occupational therapy assistant, and volunteers to ensure that each child's needs are acknowledged and respected.

Dates: Session 1   May 31–June 11
        Session II   June 14–June 25
        Session III   June 28–July 9
        Session IV   July 12–July 23
        Session V   July 26–August 20

Location: Sunset Park in Alta Vista Ranch

FIGURE 13–2 Examples of Promotional Flyers —continued

PLAY AWAY YOUR DAY!!

...... a summer day camp for children with special needs and their siblings.

Sponsored by: "We Care" Therapy Services

TO:

PLAY AWAY YOUR DAY!!

Fill out and return the attached registration form along with your $25.00 deposit. Priority will be given to children who are currently receiving services in our clinic or are clients of a regional center.

Camp fees:

$600.00 per 2-week session

Funding options:

* Private pay (may be considered day care for tax purposes)

* Regional center (consult with your caseworker)

* Some scholarships (based on financial need)

▬ EXERCISE 2 ▬▬▬▬▬▬▬▬▬▬▬▬▬▬▬
Developing Marketing Materials for Your Program

Based on the previous exercise, think about a logo that will symbolize your programming. Consider how it will be expressed on your letterhead, envelopes, and business card. Before you begin, collect some examples, and with your group or colleagues note why some appeal to you and why some do not. Is there too much information? Not enough? Do you consider the font, color, and paper quality to be professional? What might you do differently?

1. Sketch some ideas for your logo in the space below or on another sheet of paper:

2. Now consider your letterhead and envelopes and your business card. How will you use your logo? Will you use any terms or phrases to define your services? In the space below, sketch how you would like the letterhead, envelopes, and business card to look:

3. On a separate sheet of paper, sketch ideas for a brochure highlighting your program (consider color, photos, font style, as well as the information you will include). Keep it simple, but include everything your potential consumer will need to know.

When you have formulated your ideas, go to your computer and complete the brochure.

SUMMARY

We have explored the elements of marketing a program to the community and to the potential client/consumer. Our first interests are in the "selling" of ourselves as program planners, developers, and practitioners. From this stance of personal selling, we have then gone on to identify ways we might promote our program. Several elements of the promotional mix have been identified, which include paid media advertising, direct mail, promotional products, and free ink/free air. We have also described low-cost ways we might promote our program, including doing the job well and letting others see what we do (or working visibility). Promoting ourselves as authorities on a particular element of practice following the development of our expertise and some accumulated experience through the professional literature is also recommended as a further way to legitimatize our programs and our practices. We have also developed a marketing/promotional plan that includes a logo, business card, and a brochure to describe our program. With the completion of our marketing plan, we are now ready to firmly establish our time line for the initiation of our program.

REFERENCES

Drucker, P. F. (1973). *Management, tasks, responsibilities, practices.* New York: Harper and Row.

Gerson, R. F. (1991). *Writing and implementing a marketing plan.* Los Altos, CA: Crisp Publications.

Gilkeson, G. (1997). *Occupational therapy leadership: Marketing yourself, your profession, and your organization.* Philadelphia: F. A. Davis.

Mandel, D., Jackson, J., Zemke, R., Nelson, L., & Clark, F. (1999). *Lifestyle redesign: Implementing the well elderly program.* Bethesda, MD: American Occupational Therapy Association.

Ryan, J. D., Ray, R., & Hiduke, G. (1999). *Small business: An entrepreneur's plan.* Fort Worth, TX: The Dryden Press.

Internet Resources

Information on Web advertising and building a Web site: www.e-land.com

Information on Direct Mail Advertising: www.dmworld.com

SCORE, a nonprofit association of retired and active business owners and executives providing education for entrepreneurs and to encourage small companies, is located in Washington, D.C. and is sponsored by the U.S. Small Business Administration. Volunteers offer counseling in the areas of writing a business plan, managing cash flow, and obtaining capital. Workshops are offered around the country. Contact SCORE at www.score.org or at 1-800-634-0245 (for SCORE chapter information).

Developing a Time Line: How Will I Be Ready on Time?

Learning Objectives

1. To appreciate the importance of a time line in the accomplishment of program design, implementation, and review
2. To define the three phases of program development to include: 1) the design and planning phase, 2) the preparation and implementation phase, and 3) the review and evaluation phase
3. To identify tasks associated with each phase of the program-development process and to develop a time line to reflect these tasks

Key Terms

1. Time Line
2. Design and Planning Phase
3. Preparation and Implementation Phase
4. Review and Evaluation Phase

The final step of the program design and development process is to establish a firm calendar of what is to be done in order to accomplish the program and when it must occur in order to initiate the program on time. This calendar, or **time line,** ensures that nothing is forgotten and that there are no surprises that cost time and often add expense.

There are many ways to develop a time line, and much of the design and detail depends on the organizational style of the individual. For planners who are sufficiently organized in their work routines, a sketchy time line is generally enough to permit them to maintain a schedule; those individuals who are less organized, on the other hand, will need to include everything.

Designs for Time Lines

Time lines may be organized according to the full process of designing and developing a program. For example, one might prefer to develop the time line according to the three phases of program development:

1. Design and planning phase
2. Preparation and implementation phase
3. Program review and evaluation phase

The Design and Planning Phase

The **design and planning phase** can include the following: 1) organization and selection of the planning team or group (unless you are working alone, of course), 2) research of established and existing programs similar to the one you are designing, 3) analyses of trends that may impact the program, 4) developing the community profile, 5) developing the service population profile, 6) consideration of a tentative goal or goals for the program, and 7) conducting Phase I and Phase II assessment of need.

This preliminary phase would include the detailed calendar for interviews and on-site visits to collect needed information such as the mission and philosophy of the sponsoring facility, data for the community profile, and the needs assessment. You should also block out time for the research that may be needed to develop the service population profile and perhaps to explore other established and existing programs that may be similar to the one you are designing. In addition, scheduled time to review and chart trends on a daily or weekly basis would help to ensure that this program will likely be viable now and in the future. If you are a practicing clinician and you find that you will need to obtain new practice skills or knowledge, then you must anticipate this on your time line as well. For those working in a group or as part of a team, a coordinated time line/calendar will balance the workload.

The Preparation and Implementation Phase

The **preparation phase** will include: 1) review of all data collected in the preliminary phase; 2) establishment of a firm goal or goals and accompanying objectives; 3) selection of a frame or frames of reference to guide the development of the programming; 4) development of detailed, day-to-day program plans to enable goal achievement; 5) matching of potential staff, furnishings, equipment, supplies, and space to the goal and objectives; and 6) selection of program-evaluation methods.

Although there may be some blurring between the preparation phase and the **implementation phase**, knowing that some of the planning has already occurred, our time line for the implementation phase will include the following: 1) detailed budgeting, 2) hiring of staff, 3) acquisition of all equipment and supplies, and 4) active marketing. The completion of this phase would then signal actual start-up and continuation of the programming.

The Program Review and Evaluation Phase

The program **review and evaluation phase** would normally occur at about six months; for some programs, however, it can take place after one year. This phase would include critical review of all data collected, including data provided by any individual assessments that may have been done as well as formative and summative assessments of the program. This data would then be evaluated against the program's goal or goals and objectives. The results of these evaluations would prompt the examination of program content and mode of delivery to determine if either or both would require change to better satisfy the goal(s). Finally, resultant changes might be initiated in the actual measurement of the goal or goals and the objectives, objectives might be altered (we would assume goals would not be), and programming content or delivery might be changed.

At the one-year review it would be appropriate to again review the ongoing collection of trends, to update the community profile, and perhaps to revisit the assessment of need. At earlier intervals—perhaps monthly and certainly at three-month intervals—the budget, staffing, furnishings, equipment, supplies, space, and marketing would require scrutiny.

For the above phase planning, some program planners prefer to keep a large, lined calendar where they record what has to be done each month and each week of the month for the full length of the process. If they were also the recipient of grant funding, they would include any reporting and resubmission deadlines on this calendar. It should be noted that your funding sources may require program evaluation and review on differing schedules.

Other planners who may not require a detailed calendar might prefer to develop lists of what must occur each month. For example, if a planner wishes to establish a private practice, a monthly list calendar might look something like the following:

Month 1:

1. Investigate trends.
2. Meet with financial planner and/or small business attorney.
3. Conduct market analysis.
4. Complete community profile.

Month 2:

1. Investigate site location.
2. Network the professional community.
3. Initiate Phase I needs assessment with professional community .

Although the style you choose to form a time line will depend on personal preference, some form of time mapping must be included to ensure that nothing is forgotten.

Some sites will require inspections by fire and safety personnel or perhaps licensure or credentialing before a program is permitted to open. Both of these requirements could take months, so they must be anticipated. Another consideration is equipment, which could arrive in a matter of days but sometimes can take six months. If it only takes a few days for delivery, then it cannot be ordered until you have a space for it. Finally, ask yourself the following questions as you continue to develop your time line. If you're remodeling space, what is the projected time for completion? If remodeling or building is initiated in the winter or spring, how will weather affect your projected opening? When will you hire staff? How will the staff be paid before you generate revenue or receive funding? In anticipating responses to all of these questions, it is far better to be proactive than reactive; answers to these questions are necessary and must be represented on your time line.

EXERCISE 1
Establishing Your Time Line

Review your full program plan. Group the tasks to be completed according to the three phases included below. Following each, note what must occur.

1. Design and Planning Phase:

_____

_____

_____

_____

_____

2. Preparation and Implementation Phase:

_____

_____

_____

_____

_____

3. Program Review and Evaluation Phase:

_____

_____

_____

_____

_____

_____

_____

_____

If you are designing and planning a program as a student group, then your calendar will reflect the tasks that must be done to develop your *proposal* over the course of your academic semester or quarter; however, you will still develop the full time line for the remainder of the tasks even though you may not actually be implementing the program as part of your assignment.

4. When you have completed the above exercises and have defined all of the tasks that will be necessary to take your program from initial design through implementation to review and evaluation, transfer the specific tasks to a calendar of your choice.

SUMMARY

Regardless of the style, developing and following a time line is the key to accomplishing all of the tasks of program development in a timely and efficient manner. Several recommendations have been made for ways to develop your time line calendar, and Part III of this text includes additional examples. Organizing your time line around the three phases of program development has been identified as a preferred method of organization. These phases include 1) the design and planning phase, 2) the preparation and implementation phase, and 3) the program review and evaluation phase.

It will be important to make your calendar as functional as you can. Devising a method to note when a task has been completed (perhaps using a colored marker) can be encouraging and will keep you motivated during the months when things may slow down more than you would like. A wipe-off calendar that you can post on the wall is another option since you may have to frequently move things around (for example, acquisition of funding or a loan, staff hiring, arrival of equipment, and progress on developing a space). With the development of your time line, the proposal is now complete, and the real work can begin.

CHAPTER

15

Intervention and Support Programming in Day Camps, Sleep-Away Camps, and Adventures

Learning Objectives

1. To appreciate the importance of environments for intervention that support and encourage a "normalizing" experience for the participant
2. To explore potential program development within the structure of day camps and sleep-away camps
3. To identify programs that offer "adventure" as an opportunity for participants to explore meaningful challenge in their leisure occupations

Key Terms

1. Normalizing Environments
2. Day Camp
3. Sleep-Away Camp
4. Adventures

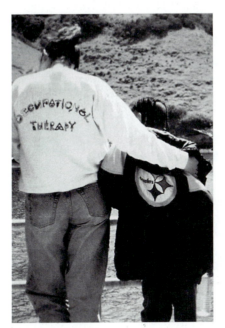

A hug on the deck of a boat, while returning home after a long day of fun, may be the best part of this "adventure."

INTRODUCTION

This chapter will offer some examples of what might be described as programming that showcases environment-centered occupations that provide significant meaning for all ages. Although certainly not restricted to one season, this type of programming does carry with it the flavor of summer with its games, crafts, fun, being outdoors, being with friends, and perhaps even nursing a sunburned nose, a few bug bites, and a bruised knee. Adults hold these moments of play/leisure in pockets of pleasurable memory, and children relish the time spent at play.

The selected environments for programming provide a comfort zone for children and adults with or without significant disability. They are user-friendly environments that offer all participants equal access and the opportunity for autonomy rather than dependency; in other words, they are **normalizing environments.** Day camps are probably the simplest to develop and program. Sleep-away camps, on the other hand, are more challenging and more costly but provide significant opportunities for building self-esteem and positive experiences for both the young and for those who are older.

What is meant by adventures, the third category of programming included in this chapter? Coming from the word *advent*, which means to begin or to commence, *adventure* is the undertaking of doing so (Random House, 1984). When participating in an adventure-oriented intervention program, it is not unusual for clients to exclaim "I'm alive again!" or "This is living!" The *adventures* of Christopher Robin at Pooh Corner, Alice in Wonderland, Robin Hood and his Merry Band, or Luke Skywalker in Star Wars conjure up exciting images of new places,

Whether in the ocean or a wading pool, water play is a significant activity for campers of all ages and abilities.

new events, mysteries, and maybe a little danger. These are the attributes that put the keen edge on "meaningful occupations" for many.

Dr. Elizabeth Yerxa (1999) describes the need for people to become "effective managers of their own environments" and notes that through this process there is undoubtedly an accompanying need to "search for novelty," perhaps the core of intrinsic motivation. Dr. Yerxa refers to *homo occupacio* to describe man's link with occupation: "occupation helps construct who I am" (1999). What better way to create this construct than through the novelty imbedded in an adventure? Whether these adventures come in the form of horseback riding, spending the night on a hiking trail high in the mountains, diving in the ocean, driving with the top down, spying an unseen species of bird, or another activity of equal challenge, they are all *adventures.*

Throughout this text, we have discussed that the prerequisite to programming for any population is to "know" that population on all levels. A thorough investigation of the developmental expectations along with the parameters of any disability or differing ability is of absolute necessity to provide programming that will be formative or preventative. Since day camps, sleep-away camps, and adventures are typically adjunct to other programming the clients are receiving, communications with other providers is important to maintain and support the goals for intervention that are already in place.

THE DAY CAMP

Day camps can be developed for clients of any age. They can be developed for the child alone, the child and a sibling, or the child and a parent; or they can be developed for the adult alone or the adult and a caregiver, depending on the goals of the program. Although not discussed at length here, day programs for adults, particularly those with cognitive dysfunction, are actually day camps. If you think of them in that way and incorporate many of the activities of a typical children's day camp in the adult treatment environment, goals can be attained while supporting the pleasurable attributes of camp. Most adult programs for clients with Alzheimer's Disease in fact do this by combining a routine of indoor and outdoor activity, rest, snacks, and celebration of life events (holidays, birthdays, and so on). Since the day programming offers some respite for the caregiver, much of the programming is for the client; however, selected shared adventures such as trips away from the treatment environment and the immediate community can provide an opportunity for the client and caregiver to enjoy positive experiences together. These shared experiences can assist in alleviating some of the daily stressors and often the accompanying guilt that may overpower the caregiver.

Supportive programming for children can occur anywhere; many after-school and Saturday day camp models are in the practice settings common to pediatrics. If at all possible, however, this kind of programming, particularly a day camp that occurs for a period of time (for example, daily for two-weeks), should be held at a camp site. This dissociation from the treatment environment provides a new arena for children to experience new challenges and opportunities to meet these challenges in different ways. Of course, some day camp programming can be for children who have no apparent cognitive, emotional, or physical disabilities. These day camps for children who may be considered to be at risk for losing out on what we might describe as "life's rewards" are excellent ways to provide supportive and preventative programming. The "club" models described in Chapter 16 highlight programming examples of this kind.

An Example of Programming for a Children's Day Camp

The Needs Assessment

The program we will examine in this section came to fruition when the City Recreation and Parks Department experienced numerous requests from parents and teachers to add children with emotional, cognitive, and physical disabilities to their summer camp programming. These requests were not new, and efforts had been made previously to mainstream these children into the existing structures but with limited success.

The 1997 mission of the City of Los Angeles Department of Recreation and Parks included the following sentence: "To unify Los Angeles by providing diverse recreational opportunities, beautiful facilities, and innovative leadership for the universal enjoyment of our residents and visitors by providing a broad range of recreational opportunities at various facilities to the general population, especially youth, and to *all special need segments of the population*" [italics added]. Thus, providing such a camp was well within the scope and interests of this department.

The department employed a recreation therapist (R.T.) and several adolescent assistants from the surrounding community to operate the summer day camp programs. The adolescents were thought to be at risk and had been selected to participate in an "opportunity for success" employment program operated under the auspices of the police department. The recreation therapist recognized that the potential campers identified with special needs were of sufficient number and variability, to require several small groups with different programming for any meaningful outcomes to occur.

Since occupational therapy became involved late in the process and the time frame was fairly short, an occupational therapist along with other therapists who were or had been seeing the children for varying kinds of therapeutic programming volunteered time to further develop the needs assessment. The children ranged in age from 5 to 8 years old. Some were no longer receiving therapy, and some continued to receive therapy on a weekly basis. All available information regarding individual therapeutic goals for the children was gleaned from a variety of services, and individual objectives were developed for each of the fifteen children who were expected to attend. The children were then grouped according to their objectives rather than by age or disability status.

A goal was developed for the camp and was shared by all of the children. "Camp for Friends" was designed to help each child increase his or her interpersonal and general social skills. The collective responses to the assessment of need provided assurance that the goal and objectives for the program were on target for all of the participants.

Thus, this example actually was initiated with the first expressed *need.* It would appear that the initial planning steps outlined in Part II were bypassed; however, it is important to note that an enterprising and experienced programmer carries all of the process in his or her head. The therapist involved in this example recognized the trends toward inclusion of differently abled children but also recognized that inclusion requires cognizance of appropriate and meaningful goals. In addition, this therapist knew how to expand the needs assessment so that programming ensures that the goal or goals are met and resources are not wasted.

The programmer should also know that with skillful task analysis and appropriate adaptations and modifications, a full round of camp activities can be enjoyed by every child in the program. This programmer will also be able to successfully market the uniqueness of occupation-centered intervention coupled with program evaluation methods so that a future for occupational therapy practitioners is assured in this particular community-based practice environment. When the programmer works cooperatively with the recreation therapist and other staff, a full round of therapeutic and supportive activities can be developed by this team and the concept of community can be strengthened and maintained.

Programming

Daily programming for the campers in our example was not unlike what other summer day camps were utilizing. Programming was held Monday through Thursday from 10:00 A.M. to 4:00 P.M. and lasted for one month. Transportation to

Adolescents and adults from many different cultures and with differing abilities learn to cooperate in a day camp parachute game.

and from camp was provided by Parks and Recreation Department vehicles, which also accommodated the two children in wheelchairs.

Daily programming consisted of arts and crafts, field trips, swimming, games, and pet care combined with snacks/lunch and a short rest period. Arts and crafts were similar to those enjoyed by all summer campers (including t-shirts sponge painted with the camp logo, lanyards for ID badges, leathercraft, and an assortment of other ideas all task analyzed and adapted to ensure full participation and successful outcome).

Cooking was also a favored activity, which was tailored to the out-of-doors camp environment (such as chocolate, graham cracker, and marshmallow S'mores, hot dogs on sticks, toasted marshmallows, and so on). Field trips included an amusement park, the local children's museum, the beach, and the zoo. The children collected an assortment of objects from the beach for a collage to be constructed later, and the wet sand provided an interesting tactile challenge for bare feet and bodies. Swimming also offered opportunities to practice dressing in and out of swimsuits, grooming wet hair, and toweling dry.

A task-analysis pre-visit by the therapist and/or students to all of the field trip sites paved the way for successful access and the "just-right" challenge with regard to managing the terrain and crowds and to avoiding potential exhaustion with resulting temper tantrums. Bathrooms and lunch areas were also mapped so that children would not experience any potentially embarrassing accidents or be unintentionally the brunt of discrimination.

Most games were played out-of-doors with the favored ones involving the parachute and variations of the parachute with foam balls that were large enough for all to grasp and throw. Pet care was actually serendipitous with the discovery

A field trip to an aquarium touch-tank transforms this camp activity into an *adventure!*

of a frog, which was later joined by a duck that happened to enjoy the swimming pool and rabbits that were adopted. One of the premises supporting pet care by children is that of offering the opportunity for experiencing responsibility—relentless as it is when it comes to feeding and taking care of an animal. But more important to our community was the normalizing process of caring for a pet that most children can access and many take for granted. The campers had more often been the recipient of caretaking rather than the provider of care.

You will find a number of resources at the close of this chapter to help you with camp programming. One of these resources, *Backyards and Butterflies: Ways to Include Children with Disabilities in Outdoor Activities,* includes descriptions of several adaptations to assist with pet care (Greenstein, Miner, Kudela, & Bloom, 1993).

Space, Staffing, and Cost

Space for this camp was in a city park with an adjoining secured building. The building provided some office space, a large gymnasium, a kitchen, and rooms for small-group activities. A playground with newly designed equipment, a swimming pool, and child-sized picnic tables and benches were adjacent to the building. All of the facilities were fenced away from other public park activities.

Since there were other camp activities scheduled at the same time as these camps, it was necessary to coordinate not only these groups through daily programming but also to coordinate with other groups as well for the use of the swimming pool, vehicles for field trips, and the use of the gymnasium. Several times each month there were opportunities for some shared activities, and many of the children had siblings in the other camps.

Since the budget had already been established before the camps were conceptualized and developed, the first summer of the program the occupational therapy personnel were largely volunteer or minimum wage employees. There were also four paid adolescent assistants assigned through a separate agency. Following the first summer, an occupational therapist, a certified occupational therapy assistant, additional adolescent assistants, and two Level II occupational therapy and/or occupational therapy assistant students were expected to be added to the budget. It was also anticipated there would be additional campers following further marketing efforts.

Costs for the activities were subsumed under the regular camp costs. The cost of supplies for one month of programming was approximately $120 per child. These were budgeted items for craft and activity supplies and did not include transportation, field trip admissions, or lunch; nor did they include the cost of salaries or use of space. These items were part of the larger Parks and Recreation Department budget obtained from individual fees, city funds, and donations. Some of the per-child tuition was funded through therapy services, and those who were not able to pay received tuition assistance through gifts from businesses and individuals.

Keep in mind that many day camp sites make use of donated or minimal cost lease sites with summer availability, including school buildings and grounds, community buildings, or churches. While having access to a swimming pool or beach is ideal, if these are not available, then wading pools can be substituted to satisfy some of the water-related programming. It must be remembered that some or all staff must be responsible for the appropriate credentials to ensure safety and liability (such as water safety and instruction).

Because normalizing environments can be dangerous ones, programming efforts must provide a median, or safe, zone between risk and safety. A sufficient number of personnel is critical, and one staff member per child is not excessive. Never permit yourself to be maneuvered into enrolling too many children for your available staff; if you have a greater need than you can safely manage, then run more and shorter-duration camps (for example, one-week or two-week rotations).

Marketing

Because the need and requests for services initiated the programming in this example, marketing was an afterthought. However, a brochure describing the occupational therapy services was sent to all recipients of Parks and Recreation Department mailings, and these services were also highlighted in that organization's newsletter. Keeping occupation, occupation-centered intervention, and, in this case, *therapy* strongly linked to the camp was a critical part of continued involvement in this setting.

Summer day camps or Saturday camp programming are excellent private practices or extensions of existing therapy practices. These may be specialty camps utilizing specific frames of reference such as sensory-integration or behavioral models for a number of differently abled children, or they might be specific to a diagnosis such as asthma, muscular dystrophy, eating disorders, spinal injury, or severe emotional disorders (SED).

As in this day camp example, camps may be mixed, without particular attention to diagnosis. In all of these cases, marketing and the other processes of program development will be followed by conceiving (as a first step) and then developing a program. Marketing will be to parents, to other professionals, and perhaps to the owner of a building and to potential donors of a tuition scholarship.

In general, most of the supply costs can be covered by tuition and some donations. Tuition can be paid out-of-pocket by consumers or can be partially covered by therapy payment services and/or tuition donations. For such a free-standing camp, corporate giving can be an important contributor depending on the mission of the program and the clientele.

Evaluation

Evaluation is, of course, directly tied to the goal or goals and to the objectives of the program. If campers bring with them individual therapy goals established by another practitioner or by Individualized Education Plan (IEP) goals, then these must be integrated into the goals of the programming; if they are not integrated directly, then the program goals must complement individual goals. For these children, progress will be measured by the programmer or, in some cases, by the occupational therapy practitioner who is seeing the client external to the camp. Camp experiences are excellent venues to maintain the goals and objectives of school-based therapies, for these goals otherwise may be abandoned over the course of a summer without continued programming. For goals supporting social skills development (appropriate for most participants regardless of diagnosis or functional abilities), an observer checklist provides a marker for daily observations of those behaviors determined to be appropriate to social skills goals and objectives.

For instance, for some children making eye contact with a therapist or another child is indicative of an objective at least partially achieved; for another, giving up a toy or receiving one would merit a mark. The person recording the observer checklist can be someone who is not directly involved in programming such as a volunteer. You could also consider the employment of a minimally cognitively impaired adult, which would be an excellent way to utilize the skills of therapy "alumni" who may be transitioning to a work environment. With some assistance and practice, they can make a significant contribution to this task that cannot be done by someone who is directly involved in activities with the children. There are other measures of social skills, but for the limited exposure of a summer camp, we are assuming that individual evaluations will occur at the primary therapy site and that our programming will enhance goal performance or at least assist in maintaining stability.

SLEEP-AWAY CAMPS

Anyone who has ever participated in a **sleep-away camp** knows what a life-changing experience being away from daily support systems can be for a child. There is probably no experience more frightening or more freeing for a child—abled or differently abled. Unfortunately, the differently abled child is most often restricted from such experiences. First of all, few opportunities exist, and for those that do, marketing such

For some an adventure means fishing for Marlin; for others it's the possibility of hooking a sunfish off the dock. *Adventures* are in the "eye of the beholder"!

a camp to protective and concerned parents would be quite a task. The cost of the additional and professional personnel could be expensive, and ensuring accessability and comfort in existing away-camp structures would be difficult.

Although not carried to fruition (more because of time constraints than anything else), a pilot plan for a sleep-away camp was developed as a programming proposal by graduate students. This camp was designed to accommodate 8- to 10-year-old children with mild to moderate cognitive and physical disabilities but of such significance that they would not likely be permitted to join most sleep-away camp groups. Programming was developed for the pilot group of ten children to be at the camp for a period of one week.

Goals

The broad goals for this occupation-centered program included 1) team building, 2) positive interaction with others, 3) exploration of new interests, 4) development of new skills, 5) accepting and meeting responsibilities, and 6) having *fun*.

Programming

Programming would provide a set of activities that would be as normalizing as possible. A typical daily routine might include the following:

Wake-up call at group tents (three children and a counselor)
Get ready for the day (morning routines and dressing)
Breakfast in the dining tent
Animal care/pet therapy
Morning exercise according to individual abilities and needs

Activities to include hiking (also wheelchair hiking trails), water sports, paddle
    boating, and burro trail riding

Lunch in the dining tent

Kitchen cleanup and help routines

Rest, sleep, and/or story telling

Preparation for Family Day skits/mini plays

Camp craft, gardening, pet care, and games

Dinner in dining tent

Campfire stories and activities

Preparation for bed and "good night"

Staffing

Staffing for a program such as this is best when overlaid on an existing camp structure with staff such as employed cooks, kitchen help, horse/burro wranglers, and
life guards. In fact, many organizations such as the Young Men's Christian Association (YMCA) and the 4-H Clubs have such camp facilities. There are also similar
camp facilities located in national parks and forests and in some state and city
parks and recreation facilities.

Overlaying occupation-centered programming on such existing structures is far easier than trying to do the whole thing yourself. If you would like
to develop a pilot camp such as this, first do a thorough two-phase needs assessment to other care providers in the community and to potential par-
ents/caregivers, then locate a suitable existing camp facility and market your
proposed program there.

The facility's administrators may be able to offer you funding or at least support funding for their services if you can obtain tuition for your attendees and perhaps some matching funding for the programming you are suggesting and for the
additional personnel you will require.

You will likely need one-to-one counselors (preferably students) under the supervision of an occupational therapist (OTR) or an occupational therapist and a
certified occupational therapy assistant (COTA). In addition, prerequisites include
any specialized staff to ensure safety and personnel with the therapeutic skills to
be sure that each child is meeting the goals and objectives of the camp experience.
The credentials and experience of your professional staff will be of extreme importance in your marketing efforts to parents.

Supplies and Cost

Assuming you are able to get the support services to offer the sleep-away experience, supplies and materials will not be unlike those described for day camp programming. Many parents would pay tuition out-of-pocket for such a camp
experience for their child; for those who could not, corporate sponsorship could
probably be obtained through your marketing efforts.

For an ongoing camp such as the one described here, the primary cost would
be in the professional personnel and perhaps for some initial physical alterations
in camp structures that may be required to ensure accessibility (for example,

ramps, bathrooms, and wheelchair-accessible trails). Volunteer groups, parents, and patient advocacy groups are generally more than willing to assist with meeting these requirements, and Wilderness Adventure organizations and conservation groups can assist with cutting wheelchair-accessible trails and trails adapted for others (such as emphasis on scents and sounds for the vision-impaired camper).

A camp such as this offers an excellent Level II fieldwork opportunity for student involvement at all levels of development and marketing as well as in actual programming.

ADVENTURES

Of course, camps are adventures in the making, but we will also explore ideas for **adventures** programming geared toward young adults and "not so young" adults. Most likely the *adventure* is identified and defined by the participants themselves. As was mentioned earlier, the client and the client's family are the best advocates for services. In these circumstances, the occupational therapy practitioner is the "coach" who provides information, access, and strategies for success. It is the practitioner who orchestrates the "just right challenge," or that set of circumstances where challenge and skills are exquisitely matched (Csikszentmihalyi, 1982).

Disabled Divers

Disabled Divers is a program that combines the services and expertise of the Office of University Disability Services and Programs, the Handicapped Scuba Association (HSA), associated fund-raising organizations and programs for University handicapped athletes, and the Student Occupational Therapy Association (SOTA). Strongly motivated by the athletes with disabilities themselves, the purpose of this program is to encourage and develop students with disabilities who have an interest in water sports to become certified scuba divers. Although strongly supported by spinal-injury participants in her California coastal occupational therapy practice, Dowd (1993) has also reported scuba diving interest from not only paraplegics and quadriplegics but amputees and the vision impaired as well. Water, at least for those who can swim, is truly a normalizing and equalizing environment. A certified scuba instructor herself, Dowd represents a common link among occupational therapy practitioners to mobilize the meaningful occupations they have selected in their own lives to motivate and encourage their clients.

In many universities, colleges, and YMCAs, there is strong participant support for the differently abled to access sports such as wheelchair basketball, rugby, skiing, and snowboarding. Recent interest on a national and international level in the Paralympic Games has offered further support for the model of adventures through sports and, in many cases, competitive sports.

The Disabled Divers program has provided an incentive to many men and women with disabilities whose opportunities for engagement in their choice of meaningful occupations seemingly have been obliterated or at least threatened. Remember that occasionally you may have to exceed your own occupational boundaries in

Anticipating a day of whale-watching is an adventure for campers of all ages and abilities.

considering the world of your clients. Do not limit their engagement in adventure and their pursuit of meaningful occupations by not being aware of the opportunities that exist for them. For example, although you may not want to go near the water, if your client does, then you should find the best avenues possible to assist him or her in reaching that goal. Of course, safety must be a primary consideration, and for programs such as the one just described, every precaution is taken to protect the participant. Certified and quality instruction is critical, and your task and that of your client is often to educate the instructor with regard to the disability so that he or she can be prepared for the additional precautions that may be required.

In your investigation of potential *adventures* with your patient or client, also consider such venues as wilderness outings, kayaking, sailing, or boating. Look to align yourself with organizations that offer such programming to the general public in your community. Also consider the activities of organizations such as the Sierra Club or Elderhostel for those still seeking adventure but perhaps less gregariously. Although Elderhostel and Sierra Club activities are not specifically designed for populations with disability, careful choice of programming can help your clients achieve goals directed toward the accomplishment of a camera safari, wild flower viewings, and numerous other activities with these organizations. Adventure, after all, is in the eye of the beholder!

SUMMARY

The opportunity for a child, adolescent or adult to participate in what has been described as normalizing experiences is considered to be significant in providing meaningful engagement in occupation. These experiences may consist of the conventional model for day camp that might include weekly, after-school, or weekend programming. The day camp example provided demonstrates the relationship between the assessment of need; the programming; space, staffing, and cost; marketing; and evaluation. Although sleep-away camps are more challenging for the planner, they are recommended as a way to provide opportunities for the achievement of autonomy and skill-building for the camper.

"Adventures" are novel, challenging experiences and are defined as such by the participant. For some, adventures might involve diving in the ocean as our "Disabled Divers" program describes, or perhaps it's kayaking or a camera safari. For others it may be viewing wildflowers from a wheelchair-adapted hiking trail.

The opportunity to play, have fun, find challenge and freedom defines the occupations highlighted in this chapter; in this regard they are those experiences that promote "normal" engagement in life—experiences that are of importance for the abled and the differently abled child, adolescent, and adult.

References

City of Los Angeles. (1997). *Mission Statement.* Department of Recreation and Parks.

Csikszentmihalyi, M. (1982). Toward a psychology of optimal experience. In L. Wheeler (Ed.), *Review of personality and social psychology, Vol. 2.* Beverly Hills, CA: Sage.

Dowd, D. (1993, Sept.–Oct.). Aquatic heaven. *California Active: The Guide to Health, Sports, and Fitness, 1,* 32–33.

The Random House Thesaurus (College Edition). (1984). New York: Random House.

Yerxa, E. (1999, April 9). Confessions of an occupational therapist who became a detective. Lecture. University of Southern California.

You will find the following references helpful in designing and implementing camp programming:

Ashton, M., & Varga, L. (1995). *101 games for groups.* Tucson, AZ: Communication Skill Builders.

Breines, E. C. (1995). *Occupational therapy: Activities from clay to computers.* Philadelphia: F. A. Davis.

Brown, O. (1983). *The metropolitan museum of art activity book.* New York: The Metropolitan Museum of Art and Harry N. Abrams.

Campbell, J. (1993) *Creative art in groupwork.* Bicester, Oxon, United Kingdom: Winslow Press.

Carlson, L. (1993). *EcoArt: Earth-friendly art and craft experiences for 3- to 9-year olds.* Charlotte, VT: Williamson.

Cohen, J. G., & Wannamaker, M. (1996). *Expressive arts for the very disabled and handicapped for all ages.* Springfield, IL: Charles Thomas.

Crist, J. (1996). *ADHD—A teenager's guide.* King of Prussia, PA: The Center for Applied Psychology.

Dikengil, A. T., & Kaye, M. E. (1992). *Building functional social skills: Group activities for adults.* Tucson, AZ: Therapy Skill Builders.

Drake, M. (1992). *Crafts in therapy and rehabilitation.* Thorofare, NJ: Slack.

Ettinger, J. (1995, July 27). Scuba diving surfaces. *O.T. Week,* 22–23.

Furrer, P. J. (1982). *Art therapy activities and lesson plans for individuals and groups.* Springfield, IL: Charles Thomas.

Goldstein, S., & Goldstein, M. (1991). *It's just attention disorder. User's manual, study guide, and video.* Salt Lake City, UT: Neurology, Learning and Behavior Center Publishers.

Gomez, A. (1992). *Crafts of many cultures.* New York: Scholastic.

Gray, L. (1990). *Something special: Seasonal and festive art and craft for children.* Twickenham, England: Belair Publishers. (Distributed by Incentive Publications, Nashville, TN)

Greenstein, D., Miner, N., Kudela, E., & Bloom, S. (1993). *Backyards and butterflies: Ways to include children with disabilities in outdoor activities.* Ithaca, NY: New York State Rural Health and Safety Council.

Harwell, J. (1989). *Complete learning disabilities handbook: Ready-to-use techniques for teaching learning-handicapped students.* West Nyack, NY: The Center for Applied Research in Education.

Henkes, R., & Smith, D. (1991). *Art projects around the calendar.* Portland, ME: J. Weston Walch.

Jones, C. B. (1994). *Attention deficit disorder: Strategies for school-age children.* Tucson, AZ: Communication Skill Builders.

Kamiya, A. (1985). *Elementary teacher's handbook of indoor and outdoor games.* West Nyack, NY: Parker.

Kay, J. G. (1977). *Crafts for the very disabled and handicapped for all ages.* Springfield, IL: Charles Thomas.

Knoth, M. (1995). *Activity planning at your fingertips.* Lafayette, IN: Valley Press.

Korb-Khalsa, K., Azok, S., & Leutenberg, E. (1991). *Life management skills I (II, III, and IV).* Beachwood, OH: Wellness Reproductions.

Korb-Khalsa, K., Azok, S., & Leutenberg, E. (1995). *Self-esteem and life skills (S.E.A.L.S. +PLUS).* Beachwood, OH: Wellness Reproductions.

Korb-Khalsa, K., Azok, S., & Leutenberg, E. (1996). *Self-esteem and life skills, Too! (S.E.A.L.S. II).* Beachwood, OH: Wellness Reproductions.

Lamport, K., Coffey, M., & Hersch, G. (1993). *Task analysis handbook.* Thorofare, NJ: Slack.

Morris, L. R., & Schulz, L. (1989). *Creative play activities for children with disabilities: A resource book for teachers and parents.* Champaign, IL: Human Kinetics Books.

Nelson-Jones, R. (1993). *Lifeskills helping: Helping others through a systematic people-centered approach.* Pacific Grove, CA: Brooks/Cole.

Nelson-Jones, R. (1993). *Student manual for lifeskills helping.* Pacific Grove, CA: Brooks/Cole.

Orlick, T. (1982). *The cooperative sports and games book: Challenge without competition.* New York: Pantheon Books.

Parker, H. C. (1988). *The ADD hyperactivity workbook for parents, teachers, and kids.* Plantation, FL: Impact Publications.

Rider, B. B., & Gramblin, J. (1987). *The activity card file.* Kansas City, KS: Rider and Rider.

Rider, B. B., & Scharfenberg, C. (1999). *The book of activity cards for D D adults: Designed for groups.* Kansas City, KS: Rider and Rider.

Rodriguez, A. (1984). *The special artist's handbook: Art activities and adaptive aids for handicapped students.* Palo Alto, CA: Dale Seymour.

Rohnke, K. (1984). *Silver bullets: A guide to initiative problems, adventure games and trust activities.* Dubuque, IA: Kendall/Hunt.

Rowland, A. (1995). *How I learned to make friends: A workbook of activities to help children make friends.* King of Prussia, PA: The Center for Applied Psychology.

Sattler, H. R. (1987). *Recipes for art and craft materials.* New York: Beech Tree Productions, William Morrow and Company.

Sayne, J. T. (1996). Ability awareness day: Summer day camp disability-education program. *Parks and Recreation, 31,* 24.

Sher, B. (1995). *Popular games for positive play: Activities for self-awareness.* Tucson, AZ: Therapy Skill Builders.

Smead, R. (1995). *Skills and techniques for group work with children and adolescents.* Champaign, IL: Research Press.

Sobel, J. (1983). *Everybody wins: 393 Non-competitive games for young children.* New York: Walker.

Tedrick, T., & Green, E. (1995). *Activity experiences and programming within long-term care.* State College, PA: Venture.

Terzian, A. M. (1993). *The kids' multicultural art book: Art and craft experiences from around the world.* Charlotte, VT: Williamson.

Tobin, L. (1991). *62 Ways to create change in the lives of troubled children.* Duluth, MN: Whole Person Associates.

Wankelman, W. F., & Wigg, P. (1993). *A handbook of arts and crafts.* Dubuque, IA: William C. Brown.

Watson, D. (1997). *Task analysis: An occupational performance approach.* Bethesda, MD: American Occupational Therapy Association.

Witoski, M. L. (1992). *It's not just a parachute: Integrative activities for children of all abilities.* Tucson, AZ: Therapy Skill Builders.

Wnek, B. (1992). *Holiday games and activities.* Champaign, IL: Human Kinetics Books.

Internet Sites

Elderhostel, United States and Internationally:
www.elderhostel.org

Sierra Club:
www.sierraclub.org

CHAPTER 16

Prevention and Wellness Programming Within Existing or Newly Formed Clubs

Learning Objectives

1. To understand the significance of the "club" as a structure within which to place occupation-centered programs
2. To appreciate how the structure of a "club" is defined by the developmental age and resulting needs of the child or adolescent
3. To identify examples of existing clubs and associations whose mission and goals are compatible with occupation-centered programs
4. To consider the importance of gender in developing the goals and structure of club-based programs

Key Terms

1. Clubs
2. Jane Goodall "Roots and Shoots" Clubs
3. 4-H Club
4. Boys and Girl's Clubs of America
5. YMCA/YWCA
6. Middle-Childhood
7. Adolescence
8. Gender-Specific Clubs

The "Roots and Shoots"/4-H Club members and student planners share a moment of pride!

INTRODUCTION

Chapters 16 and 17 will focus on the concept of *club* as a community within a community and will describe new and existing structures appropriate for the placement of occupation-centered programs. Chapter 17 provides program examples that offer a combination of preventative and restorative goals appropriate to the children and adults involved, and one—the "Jazz/Blues" club—demonstrates the specific intention of strengthening and reaffirming *community* for the members.

This chapter will provide a foundation for understanding why the concept of club is appropriate for occupation-centered programming and will describe the characteristics and goals of several organizational structures based on the concept of club. Examples of programs for children, adolescents, and adults will be provided that have been incorporated into existing clubs with missions and goals that are compatible with our own occupation-based views of effective programming. Two examples will be provided where a new club was established to support the proposed programming.

The first example for children and adolescents is occupation-centered programming that utilizes the Roots and Shoots project sponsored by Jane Goodall, which is then placed within an urban 4-H Club. Secondly, a program that exists within the structure of a Boys and Girls Club will be described, which is followed by two brief examples of programming under the umbrella structures of the Young Men's Christian Association (YMCA) and the Young Women's Christian Association (YWCA). The first is a program for adult Parkinson's patients and their spouses, and the second is a "Mommy and Me" program for adolescent mothers. The last two examples are of clubs created for the purposes of enhancing the goals and objectives of the developing occupation-centered programming. One is the middle-school "Ice Cream Cart" club, and the second is the "Jazz/Blues" club.

WHY CLUBS?

Think back to when you were a child. You most likely sought membership in both formal and informal **clubs.** Why are *clubs* so appealing to children? Perhaps some of the answers to this question can be found by exploring what is known of the social, behavioral, and cognitive development of children and adolescents that for each group would permit the *club* to be such a powerful motivator and, in that regard, a powerful agent for positive change. Florey (1998) and Florey and Greene (1997) discuss the occupation of play in middle childhood (ages 6 to 12) and the transition in social groups toward increasing structure and elaboration of membership requirements. Citing Boy Scouts and Girl Scouts as examples, Florey recommends that occupational therapy programming for children—particularly for children in middle childhood—include an emphasis on clubs to meet the inclusion needs of this age group.

Middle Childhood

In particular, the earlier years of **middle childhood** (ages 6 to 7) in most cultures appear to be the time that both adults (parents and caregivers) and peer groups alike place fairly stringent demands on children for new and more sophisticated social behaviors. This is particularly so in societies where formal schooling is a central occupation for this age group. Even more than the often stringent parental expectations for more *grown-up* behaviors, the peer group moves into position as perhaps the major context for continued development—particularly in the social and behavioral domain—during these years. Although adult control may appear to be absent in these peer groups, covert parental/adult sanctions are realized through the rules attached to games and, perhaps more specifically for our examples, through memberships in clubs or organizations. These club/organizational selections are often more formal in nature and are supported by the parent or adult caregiver. The peer-selected and peer-organized clubs are of a more informal nature but nevertheless have a tremendous impact on the child's social development.

Why do the child and adult parent both gravitate toward the idea of *club*? The work of Jean Piaget (1960) would suggest that cognitive changes—particularly those that serve to mediate social and behavioral learning—are occurring in middle childhood. These changes permit children to appreciate actions and views of others that may be in disagreement with their own, and through this awareness they may learn to mediate their actions to get along with adults and peers. The demands of this developmental "window" can best be realized through play, most likely through such forms of organized play as soccer, hockey, and baseball and the clubs organized around these sports. Membership and participation in such clubs have a set of prescribed rules/expected behaviors accompanying membership, and the rules for sports clubs might support cooperation, fairness, participation, spirit, and team building.

Adolescence

Many developmental theorists, including Piaget (1960), Inhelder and Piaget (1958), Erikson (1968), Havighurst (1972), Kohlberg (1984), Keating (1980), Siegler (1981), Gilligan (1982), and Sigelman and Shaffer (1995), have proposed numerous ways to define and understand development from childhood to older adulthood and, of course, including **adolescence.** Their varying theoretical perspectives describe development from an organismic view (biological, psychoanalytic, or cognitive-developmental) or an environmental view (sociological-anthropological or social learning-behavioral). Although agreeing on the general parameters, the developmental theorists differ in the emphasis they place on the influences that biology, cognition, social factors, environment, and culture have on the phases of development and on the psychological characteristics attached to it. As you review these theorists and others, you will likely find that you will be more influenced by some views than by others, and your programming goals and objectives will reflect this.

If middle childhood seems to hold the most opportunity and challenge for social behavior/rule development and seems to offer the strongest support for clubs, then the period of later childhood or adolescence, which begins at around age 12 and continues to age 20 and is accompanied by expectations for adult responsibility, is likely one of even greater potential social change. Numerous theorists, including those mentioned previously, have applied their knowledge to the period following middle childhood. This is the period that we have come to know as adolescence, which is derived from the Latin verb *adolescere* and means "to grow to maturity." Most agree that it is a developmental passage of fairly dramatic changes in all of the domains (physical, cognitive, psychological, and social). Expanding cognitive availabilities often invite the adolescent to think about worlds he or she does not yet have the physical and social development to master. The adolescent is not quite an adult but also is no longer a child. The potential frustration and impatience prompted by this discrepancy coupled with the "adult" desire for independence and the "child's" need to self-validate through belonging offer support of carefully structured club programming for the adolescent as well as for the child.

According to Keating (1980), adolescents are developing ways of thinking that are different than those of middle childhood, and these ways of thinking must be considered and encouraged as we write programming. Adolescents are capable of 1) thinking about possibilities, 2) thinking ahead, 3) thinking about hypotheses, 4) thinking about thought (that is, thinking about one's own thought processes or meta-cognitive thinking and second-order thinking such as developing rules about rules), and 5) thinking beyond conventional limits (Keating, 1980, p. 609; Piaget, 1960), and these characteristics must be considered.

These characteristics are in contrast to the middle childhood years, when much thought in response to choices and circumstances may be spontaneous and more self-centered. This is not to say that all adolescents have achieved the same level of thought or social/behavioral responsiveness, nor does this suggest that all younger children have not. Rather, it is always necessary to know the child regardless of chronological age expectations, for there may be broad ranges of variation between developmental and chronological expressions of age.

Another developmental factor that may influence programming for adolescents is their generalized ability to consider questions regarding the social order, values, and ethics (Kohlberg, 1984). For example, a club membership may have an entirely different meaning for an adolescent than it might for a younger child. The opportunity to meet with peers in a club format for projects and discussions dealing with issues of moral responsibility and global concerns might not only engage the adolescent in positive peer interactions but also might assist in the achievement of the underpinnings necessary for choosing all present and future occupations holding meaning and personal fulfillment. For example, the Roots and Shoots club may be equally appealing for younger children and for adolescents, but programming within the goals of the club would take on quite different features to hold the interest of the two age groups. Csikszentmihalyi and Larson (1984) have researched the lives of adolescents in order to provide a picture from the "inside-out," or the adolescent's internal dimensions of experience. They explore many areas that can assist us in organizing programming for this age group, but much of the adolescent experiences appear to be ones of conflict between instinctual choices (perhaps more similar to middle childhood) and emerging values. This transition reinforces the use of activity experiences to assist in clarifying thinking with regard to daily and long-term occupational choices and to value systems that may be in the process of development.

Whether one supports the view of adolescence as a generally unpleasant and stormy period of transition or not, it is surely recognized as one of considerable potential stress and responsibility as the child prepares for new roles requiring independence. This is a time when intervention in the form of education, information, skill building, and supportive coaching/mentoring is needed to encourage self-efficacy and a smooth transition toward positive choices. You should review the developmental theories of childhood and adolescence in depth as you prepare to work with these groups and as you select your conceptual framework or "window" through which to view your community group. When we consider the ideas for community programming with adolescent populations—whether these populations are thought to be at risk (note that some theorists believe this is such a difficult period that *all* adolescents may be *at risk*) or whether we are working with adolescents who have recognized psychopathology—we must utilize what is known developmentally about these children to build the goals for our programs.

If you are designing programming for children with known psychosocial dysfunction or children with delayed cognitive and social development, then you must be familiar with the literature on seriously emotionally disturbed (SED), autism, attention deficit disorder, and cognitive disabilities. Although it will not tell us much about the individual child's problems, the *Diagnostic and Statistical Manual for Mental Disorders, IV* (American Psychiatric Association, 1994) is widely used to describe the clinical manifestations of these disorders. Florey (1998) and Florey and Greene (1997) have noted that there is confusion in identifying children with emotional problems. The reasons for this dilemma may include fear of stigma, financial constraints, and lack of identification, which generally results in children being inappropriately labeled as "learning disabled."

The school system, which is where the child's primary occupation is enacted, is likely the "community" where much of your child-adolescent programming will take place (if not directly in the school, then in environments adjacent to the school). Alternative schools and detention centers are also excellent sites for programming; these are sites where children and adolescents may be placed following engagement in risk factors (such as substance abuse, delinquent behavior, and youth pregnancies) that may accompany SED or learning disability.

Gender-Specific Clubs

When considering the structure of a *club* or "community within a community," one must consider how much the structure/organization should mirror the so-called "real world" or expected environment of the child and how much it should be adapted to provide opportunities for learning and preparation for a reality not yet attained. Young (1992) and Batsleer (1996) support the idea of community programming as a way to support young girls' and women's concerns separate from those of young men, and they offer an agenda to challenge what they describe as sexism in community work—at least from a social service perspective. Although their particular examples are from England, there is likely cross-cultural validity in their findings. Hooks (1984) proposes the use of the forum of community programming to assist in advocating for women and their emancipation and to assist in obtaining justice. In her view, community programming can support feminism in its effort to end oppression. In fact, community work with young women who have been abused, are pregnant in childhood, are young single mothers, or have been accustomed to becoming sexually and emotionally support to or codependent with young male gang members may have such an awareness and intention as an obvious or, more likely, covert agenda.

Women and men as "communities" may share some but not all social experiences. Mixing same sex but different ages and cultures may offer new interpretations of experience and new identities. Taking risks and acknowledging differences and similarities may result in creativity in problem solving and resultant strength (Batsleer, 1996). Batsleer goes on to support offering young women relevant information in an environment where they feel comfortable and secure. The comfortable and secure environment may be the strongest support for **gender-specific clubs.** Beetham (1991) and Arendt (1986) refer to these community groups as "empowering," which is triggered by acting in concert. Arendt notes that "power is never the property of an individual; it belongs to a group and remains in existence only so long as the group keeps together" (1986, p. 64). Arendt goes on to say that same-sex groups (women in her examples) can exercise power by rules of exclusion. This exclusion of not only the opposite sex but also members of the same sex by arbitrarily changing "passwords" for entry or other such exclusionary rules is, in fact, part of the appeal of informal clubs in middle childhood.

Safe houses and other examples of community programming for abused women and their children are examples of what Arendt (1986, p. 64) might describe as "empowering practice." These are intended to be safe places to teach and support strategies for resisting or avoiding violence but perhaps more importantly to establish links to the legal and social systems and to other women.

With any community, group empowerment seems to be a desirable agenda even if it is not the primary or even visible one. Programming that includes informed choices, self-reflection through the telling of life stories, and survival techniques offers empowering opportunities. The "Mommy and Me" Story Quilt Club program described in Chapter 17 is an example. One should also note that empowerment is certainly not only for the young, for older adults are often disenfranchised when it comes to issues of power and efficacy as well. An important feature of the study on aging performed by Clark and associates (1997) was that wellness was supported in part by knowing how to access the occupations in which one wanted to engage. In this way, the occupational therapists offered information and opportunity with regard to access not only to such things as public transportation but more importantly to power and efficacy.

If these arguments seem too political for you, consider the work of several developmental theorists concerning gender and minority-group development. A number of researchers have studied identity formation as a critical stage of adolescent development, and several of these studies have focused specifically on gender differences (Abraham, Feldman, & Nash, 1978; Markstrom-Adams, 1992; Markus & Kitayama, 1991). Others have focused on minority differences where there appears to be much stronger evidence than for gender-based differences. Spencer and Markstrom-Adams (1990), for example, have researched identity formation among minority-group children in the United States. For these children the progression through childhood and adolescence is further complicated by negative social stereotyping by their majority peers and often by lower incomes that push them to a social status lower than their majority peers. If you consider these factors alongside James Marcia's stages of identity formation, then the children in this group may be at risk for altering their development through what he describes as foreclosure, or adopting an externally-based identity and prematurely committing to roles rather than to goals and values (1966, p. 556).

Earlier theorists, including Freud (1935/1953) and Erikson (1968), believed there were significant sex differences in the process of forming an identity. More recent research offers mixed support for this earlier contention. In their work on identity development, role-taking skills, occupational knowledge, and career development in adolescence, Grotevant, Cooper, and Kramer (1986) and Grotevant and Durrett (1980) reported that adolescent girls scored higher levels of identity achievement than boys with regard to friendship. Their work was supported by Archer (1982, 1992), who found that girls score higher in areas of choice with regard to combining career and family. Based on this somewhat limited research, support for gender-based clubs is not as compelling as support might be for minority-based programming. If one considers other measurements of development in addition to identity formation, however, then perhaps a stronger case can be made. Certainly gender-based and minority-based programming will likely have a different mission, goals, and objectives than those where the population is more diverse. Neville-Jan and colleagues (1997) offer a description of a middle school program that focuses on transition. The programming interweaves the developmentally related needs of these children along with minority-based concerns that extend into the family and the community.

THE CLUBS

Although this is certainly not an exclusive listing, there are many opportunities for programming across the country offered in conjunction with the following five organizations or clubs: the 4-H Club, the Jane Goodall Roots and Shoots Program, the Boys and Girls Clubs of America, the Young Men's Christian Association (YMCA), and the Young Women's Christian Association (YWCA). These organizations have been selected specifically because of the compatibility of their missions with our interests as occupation-centered practitioners. The following descriptions will provide you with some general background information on these four groups; as you read about the organizations, think about compatible occupation-centered programming that you might develop.

The 4-H Club

> I pledge my HEAD to clearer thinking, my HEART to greater loyalty, my HANDS to larger service and my HEALTH to better living.

Perhaps you recognize this as the motto, or pledge, of the **4-H club.** The beginnings of the twentieth century also witnessed the beginnings of what might be described as the demise of the rural American lifestyle, which was represented through a sense of "rugged individualism" coupled with a concern and kindness translated as "neighborliness." The young people of rural America were rapidly leaving for the cities and perceived brighter futures in industry. Beginning as early as the late 1800s, several factors brought about the beginnings of the 4-H club. These included a growing concern for the quality of rural education and the relevance of the public schools to country life and a concern for advancing agricultural technology that was being developed by land-grant universities but was not gaining rapid favor in most agricultural communities (www.4h-usa.org).

4-H appears not to be the idea of any one person; rather, it was developed as a widespread grass-roots movement to encourage rural youth to "stay on the farm" but to do so while embracing new ideas for productivity as well as sound values and behaviors. By 1904 clubs were formed to teach life skills and learning-by-doing projects. Community service projects were developed to capture the joint efforts of adults and youth, first by appealing to boys through activities such as rewarding the best corn crop and then to girls by fostering sewing, canning of vegetables, and baking projects. Interest spread throughout the midwest and Texas, and in 1906 Thomas M. Campbell, an assistant of George Washington Carver, organized clubs with similar goals for Black farmers and their children in the south. These so-called "corn" and "sewing" clubs came under the sponsorship of the Cooperative Extension System established by the Smith-Lever Act in 1914, and 4-H clubs soon were started in nearly every state. The clubs for boys and girls tended to be organized separately. While boys were being encouraged to adopt new agricultural techniques and methods to increase production, the girls' groups were evolving to examine the roles of women in the rural home and community. Self confidence and a commitment to community became goals.

Clubs were not only in rural areas but in cities as well. Many of the city-based clubs were organized to encourage activities between rural and city youth, and by 1948 the exchanges were matched by those between American and European club members through the International Farm Youth Exchange.

Today the 4-H club movement continues to be strong and is more centered on the personal growth of the child. 4-H boys and girls clubs are most often combined under similar interests. Projects continue to be utilized in the development of life-long skills, and efforts are rewarded. It is intended that participants become contributing, productive, self-directed members of society. Making decisions, learning to communicate, learning the characteristics of leadership, and learning how to cope with change are goals of today's clubs.

The 4-H club remains a largely federally organized group with county and states retaining control over its programs. International programs are presently active in more than 80 countries. A wide and diverse range of interests was represented in the listing of the National Training and Events Activities of Clubs in 1997–1998; these included such topics as Partnerships for Preventing Violence; Habitat Evaluation; Engineering, Science, and Leadership; Dairy Conference; Safety Council Congress and Exposition; and the Poultry and Egg Conference (www.4H-usa.org/history.htm; world.htm).

Today's clubs, which have expanded to become some of the most successful youth clubs in existence, range from the community club model to urban interest groups, community resource development, special interest groups, school enrichment, camping, and interagency learning experiences. It is not difficult to recognize the similarities between the purposes and goals of 4-H and those of occupational therapy. An occupation-based program focused on health promotion, social skills enhancement, and emotional risk reduction can be comfortably placed within the existing structures of 4-H club programming while retaining the vitality of both. Opportunities for creative programming based on the principles of occupation are boundless.

Roots and Shoots

Roots and Shoots was established in the summer of 1960 by the internationally recognized ethologist Jane Goodall. Dr. Goodall is best known for her research on chimpanzee behavior in Tanzania, but she is becoming equally recognized for her substantial interests in conservation, education, and animal welfare. Roots and Shoots is an international environmental education and humanitarian program for young people. The program encourages and empowers children and young adults to coordinate constructive activities that promote care and concern for the environment, for animals, and for the human community. Roots and Shoots was the name selected to recognize that "children are the fertile ground in which seeds are planted" (The Jane Goodall Institute for Wildlife Research, Education, and Conservation, 1995).

Once seeds germinate, of course, their roots spread in all directions and establish a firm foundation. Important work can be accomplished when each child is recognized as important to the future of all children. Clubs currently exist in 38 states and more than 30 countries around the world. The fundamental concepts and philosophy of Roots and Shoots include "care and concern for the environment; care and concern for animals; and community enrichment through constructive service projects" (The Jane Goodall Institute for Wildlife Research, Education, and Conservation, 1995).

The example we will explore in Chapter 17 is one of a club within a club, that is, Roots and Shoots within the structure of a 4-H club. Although the interests of the occupational therapy providers/occupation-based practitioners were in the enrichment of and concern for the individual child, all of the concepts and philosophies of both the 4-H club and the Roots and Shoots organization were utilized as tools in the development of programming.

Boys and Girls Clubs of America

The Boys and Girls Club movement is a nationwide affiliation of local autonomous nonprofit organizations. The mission of the Boys and Girls Clubs of America is "working to help youth from all backgrounds, with special concern for those from disadvantaged circumstances, develop the qualities needed to become responsible citizens and leaders" (www.ncnatural.com/UCYOUTH/youthweb.htm).

It is important to note that the Boys and Girls Club has a physical location, usually a neighborhood-based building where local community youth may congregate to participate in organized programs and activities. This is an important concept, for the intention is to keep children off the street and preferably not at home when adult supervision is absent. The clubs are open every day after school and on weekends. Every club has paid, full-time, trained youth-development professionals who are selected to be mentors and positive role models. Volunteers are relied on for key supplementary support. Children pay a small amount of dues per year, but supportive moneys are provided through campaigned gift donations based on the club's proven delinquency-prevention programs.

There are currently approximately 2,013 club facilities located in all fifty states, Puerto Rico, the Virgin Islands, and domestic and international military bases. In 1996 operating budgets for all clubs amounted to approximately $432,000,000 (www.bgca.org/html/numbers/html).

It is interesting to note that of the 2,800,000 boys and girls served in 1996, 71 percent lived in urban/inner-city areas, 53 percent were from single-parent families,

51 percent were from families of three or more children, 56 percent were from minority families, and 42 percent were from families with annual incomes below $22,000. Ages of members range from 7 years and younger (16 percent) up to 18 years of age (21 percent are between the ages of 14 and 18), with the largest group (34 percent) between 8 and 10 years of age. Boys make up 62 percent of the children and girls the remaining 38 percent.

Boys and Girls Clubs are another excellent site for occupation-based programming with general goals supportive of the prevention of behaviors leading to patterns of crime and delinquency.

The Young Men's Christian Association (YMCA)

The **YMCA** was founded in London in 1844 by Sir George Williams (knighted in 1894 for his lifelong service to boys). Impetus for the establishment of the organization was the unhealthy social conditions of the times apparent in the large urban cities at the end of the Industrial Revolution. The founding young business men wished to help young workers avoid the social "dangers" of idleness (such as gambling and drinking) through Bible studies and prayer meetings. The organization quickly gained popularity and spread to the industrial centers of North America and throughout Europe. The first YMCA to be established in America was in Boston in 1851, and by 1854 there were 26 associations in the United States and Canada.

In 1862 the attention of the association was turned to the welfare of American Civil War prisoners. This was the first civilian volunteer organization dedicated to the welfare of war prisoners and other servicemen, and this work continued through World War I and World War II. The YMCA continued to work not only with prisoners of war but also with displaced persons, refugees, and soldiers. In 1941 the YMCA joined with five other organizations to form the United Service Organizations (USO).

The post-war YMCA continued to evolve by incorporating libraries, gymnasiums, summer camps, colleges, night schools, swimming pools, mass swimming instruction, and hotel-type rooms. It is of interest that to meet the need for a "vigorous recreation suitable for indoor winter play," an instructor at the Springfield, Massachusetts YMCA, Mr. James Naismith, invented basketball in 1891 (www.tased.edu.au/tasonline/ymca/history1.htm). At this YMCA, which is now Springfield College, volleyball was invented in 1895 by Mr. William G. Morgan, the physical education director of the YMCA in Holyoke, Massachusetts. The YMCA also assisted in the development of other groups such as the Red Cross, Boy Scouts, the Student Christian Movement, World Council of Churches, and CampFire. The years between the 1930s and the 1960s were marked by diminished interest in the activities of the YMCA and difficult financial times. In the late 1970s, however, there was renewed interest in health and fitness, and child care was added to meet the demands and needs of young mothers.

Presently the YMCA serves approximately fourteen million people a year. Local YMCAs are independent and autonomous and are dedicated to *local community needs and service* and have as their goal the provision of *values-based experiences that nurture the healthy development of children and teens, support families, and strengthen communities.* Their mission is "to put Christian principles into practice through programs that build healthy spirit, mind, and body for all" (www.ymca.net/d/1/1.html). Each YMCA is a charitable, nonprofit organization.

The Young Women's Christian Association (YWCA)

The **YWCA** is the largest and oldest women's organization in the United States (www.ywca.org/). Its mission is to empower women and girls and to work to eliminate racism. The YWCA opened the first day nursery in the United States in 1864 and today continues to train child care providers and baby-sitters. Other child-related services are found in the forms of resource and referral agencies, child care for homeless children, services to family day care homes, and parenting education. Services for women include basic life skills training, GED courses, adult education, welfare-to-work programs, nontraditional employment, and other related services. It should be noted that women worked in the YMCA military canteens in World War I, but it was not until after World War II that they were admitted to full YMCA membership. The YWCA, however, establishes specific goals to meet the general needs of women.

Globally the YWCA represents more than 25 million women throughout 101 countries. The YWCA provides shelter, child care, employment training, racial justice, physical fitness, youth development, leadership training, and world relations. Each year more than 650,000 people come to the YWCA for services and support to overcome violence (www.ywca.org/mission/world_relations.html).

Two examples of occupation-centered programming will be described in Chapter 17. One program was established with the YMCA for older adults with Parkinson's disease and their spouses, and another was established for young, single, inner-city mothers under the umbrella of the YWCA. Both are quite different but are well within the mission of the YMCA and YWCA.

SUMMARY

Clubs are examples of a community within a community. They offer the child, the adolescent, and the adult structures that support and encourage their cognitive and social development. In this way they provide the potential for powerful interventions. The cognitive and social development of middle-childhood and adolescence has been discussed to provide a foundation for understanding how the structure of clubs can be utilized to support a program that is developmentally sensitive. Whether or not the program planner wishes to encourage gender-specific clubs or to mix participants has also been considered. Understanding the developmental period of the participant will assist the planner who wishes to place a program within a club in selecting an appropriate club structure from existing ones or in the creation of rules and structures for a new club.

Existing club structures have been described such as the 4-H clubs, Jane Goodall's Roots and Shoots clubs, Boys and Girls Clubs of America, and the YMCA/YWCA. All of these club structures can be compatible with developmentally appropriate occupation-centered program goals.

REFERENCES

Abraham, B., Feldman, S. S., & Nash, S. C. (1978). Sex role self-concept and sex role attitudes: Enduring personality characteristics or adaptations to changing life situations? *Developmental Psychology, 14,* 393–400.

American Psychiatric Association. (1994). *Diagnostic and statistical manual of mental disorders* (4th ed.). Washington, DC: Author.

Archer, S. L. (1982). The lower age boundaries of identity development. *Child Development, 53,* 1,551–1,556.

Archer, S. L. (1992). A feminist's approach to identity research. In G. R. Adams, T. P. Gulotta, & R. Montemayor (Eds.), *Adolescent identity formation* (Advances in Adolescent Development, Vol. 4). Newbury Park, CA: Sage.

Arendt, H. (1986). Communicative power. In S. Lukes (Ed.), *Power* (p. 64). Oxford: Basil Blackwell.

Batsleer, J. (1996). *Working with girls and young women in community settings.* London: Arena.

Beetham, D. (1991). *The legitimation of power.* London: MacMillan.

Clark, F., Azen, S., Zemke, R., Jackson, J., Carlson, M., Mandel, D., Hay, J., Josephson, K., Cherry, B., Hessel, C., Palmer, J., & Lipson, L. (1997). Occupational therapy for independent-living older adults. *Journal of the American Medical Association, 278*(16), 1,321–1,326.

Csikszentmihalyi, M., & Larson, R. (1984). *Being adolescent.* New York: Basic Books, Harper and Row.

Erikson, E. (1968). *Identity: Youth in crisis.* New York: Norton.

Florey, L. (1998). Psychosocial dysfunction in childhood and adolescence. In M. Neistadt & E. Crepeau (Eds.), *Willard and Spackman's occupational therapy* (pp. 622–635). Philadelphia: Lippincott.

Florey, L., & Greene, S. (1997). Play in middle childhood: A focus on children with behavior and emotional disorders. In L. D. Parham & L. S. Fazio (Eds.), *Play in occupational therapy for children* (pp. 126–143). St. Louis, MO: Mosby.

Freud, S. (1935/1953). *A general introduction to psychoanalysis.* (J. Riviere, Translator). New York: Permabooks.

Gilligan, C. (1982). *In a different voice: Psychological theory and women's development.* Cambridge, MA: Harvard University Press.

Grotevant, H. D., Cooper, C. R., & Kramer, K. (1986). Exploration as a predictor of congruence in adolescents' career choices. *Journal of Vocational Behavior, 29,* 201–215.

Grotevant, H. D., & Durrett, M. (1980). Occupational knowledge and career development in adolescence. *Journal of Vocational Behavior, 17,* 171–182.

Havighurst, R. (1972). *Developmental tasks of education* (3rd ed.). New York: David McKay.

Hooks, B. (1984). *Feminist theory: From margin to center.* Boston: South End Press.

Inhelder, B., & Piaget, J. (1958). *The growth of logical thinking from childhood to adolescence.* New York: Basic Books.

The Jane Goodall Institute for Wildlife Research, Education and Conservation. (1995). Roots and Shoots Fact Sheet. Ridgefield, Connecticut.

Keating, D. P. (1980). Thinking processes in adolescence. In J. Adelson (Ed.), *Handbook of adolescent psychology.* New York: Wiley.

Kohlberg, L. (1984). *The psychology of moral development: The nature and validity of moral stages.* New York: Harper and Row.

Marcia, J. (1966). Development and validation of ego identity status. *Journal of Personality and Social Psychology, 3,* 551–558.

Markstrom-Adams, C. (1992). A consideration of intervening factors in adolescent identity formation. In G. R. Adams, T. P. Gullotta, and R. Montemayor (Eds.), *Adolescent identity formation (advances in adolescent development)* (vol. 4). Newbury Park, CA: Sage.

Markus, H. R., & Kitayama, S. (1991). Culture and the self: Implications for cognition, emotion, and motivation. *Psychological Review, 98,* 224–253.

Neville-Jan, A., Fazio, L. S., Kennedy, B., & Snyder, C. (1997). Elementary to middle school transition: Using multicultural play activities to develop life skills. In L. D. Parham & L. S. Fazio (Eds.), *Play in occupational therapy for children* (pp. 144–157). St. Louis, MO: Mosby.

Piaget, J. (1960). *The psychology of intelligence.* Patterson, NJ: Littlefield, Adams.

Siegler, R. S. (1981). Developmental sequences within and between concepts. *Monographs of the Society for Research in Child Development, 46*(2, Serial No. 189).

Sigelman, C., & Shaffer, D. (1995). *Life-span human development* (2nd ed.). Pacific Grove, CA: Brooks/Cole.

Spencer, M., & Markstrom-Adams, C. (1990). Identity processes among racial and ethnic minority children in America. *Child Development, 61,* 290–310.

Young, K. (1992, April). Work with girls and young women: Losing the purpose? *Youth Clubs, 67,* 17.

Internet Sites

4-H	http://www.4h-usa.org
YMCA	http://www.tased.edu.au/tasonline/ymca/history1.htm
YWCA	http://www.ywca.org
	http://www.ywca.org/mission/shelter_services_victims.html

Boys and Girls Clubs http://www.ncnatural.com/UCYOUTH/youthweb.htm
http://www.bgca.org/html/numbers.html

CHAPTER 17

Programming Examples Within the Community of Clubs

Learning Objectives

1. To explore program examples housed in existing club structures and associations
2. To examine the design and development of free-standing club structures to meet the occupation-centered program needs of children, adolescents, and adults

Key Terms

1. 4-H Club
2. Boys and Girls Clubs of America
3. Jane Goodall's Roots and Shoots Clubs
4. YMCA/YWCA
5. Free-Standing Clubs

JANE GOODALL'S ROOTS AND SHOOTS CLUB

This example of Roots and Shoots programming was developed at two sites—in the **4-H club** after-school enrichment program established through the partial support of the Los Angeles Housing Authority and the County Parks and Recreation Department and at a Los Angeles **Boys and Girls Club.** Both sites serviced similar populations, which included Hispanic boys and girls between the ages of 7 and 11 who were from low-income families. The community profiles presented similar pictures of apparent neighborhood neglect as evidenced by graffiti, numerous gang signs, and garbage. More optimistically, it was noted that two parks were in the process of being repaired and landscaped by the city.

The two occupation-centered programs were identical in their after-school structure and in their affiliation with existing clubs. The Phase I needs assessment at both sites demonstrated an interest in programming that would support the existing goals of both the 4-H club and the Boys and Girls Club. Both groups expressed interest in improving their community and suggested several ways they might do so that ranged from picking up trash, to planting flowers, to helping older residents run errands in the neighborhood. Because of its supportive structure for understanding and building *community* through attention to one's habitat (that is, neighborhood) and its already-developed programming ideas along those lines, the **Jane Goodall Roots and Shoots** structure was selected as a vehicle for the occupation-centered intervention. The success of the after-school 4-H club at the Housing Authority site and the Boys and Girls Club as well as the chronological and developmental ages of the children involved supported the choice of a club format embedded within the existing programming.

Although not necessarily articulated, the combined message of all of the clubs was *empowerment to affect change* first in one's community and secondly in oneself. In addition, building a community of caring and concerned children whose example would encourage those around them to also build rather than destroy was equally important. A review of the purposes of both organizations as defined in Chapter 16 demonstrates that the goal of "empowerment through positive change" and the objectives to demonstrate care and concern for the community through such enabling activities as conducting a community celebration of "Earth Day" are appropriate. The specific activities of researching the habitats of butterflies and birds through field surveys, planting butterfly gardens on windowsills of nursing care facilities and in backyards of public housing, trash patrols, and "acts of kindness" patrols all targeted care for the community and were visible enough to encourage the participation of other children and adults in the activities.

The Jane Goodall Roots and Shoots clubs frequently form a liaison with local zoos, which offers additional programming opportunities. In this example, the zoo provided an opportunity to study and assist with the design of a chimpanzee habitat for the zoo and to attend the "official" opening. What does that have to do with an inner-city Los Angeles community? It is very applicable if the programmer makes good use of the opportunity to demonstrate "community" as a common and global concern. In addition, if the club can be visited by Jane Goodall or by the local media news team or has the opportunity to join in world-wide conservation-environmental activities with children from other cultures, then our goal of empowerment is enhanced through recognition and group consensus.

These clubs also developed programming slogans around the idea that humans—or at least the quality of life many enjoy or would like to enjoy—may be endangered. The similarities in the way that other endangered or extinct species used or abused their habitats was food for research and for planning.

Roots and Shoots club members learn how their conservation projects in the inner-city positively impact life in the ocean.

For both programs the low-budget activities were subsumed under existing resources in bimonthly programming. Existing space was utilized with all regular after-school club participants who were also participating in the Roots and Shoots activities. The personnel consisted of occupational therapy students who received service learning course credit for their contributions. At the Boys and Girls Club, older participants (teens) were paid by the club to assist with programming. At the 4-H club, paid staff also was involved with programming. In both of these cases, the consistency in programming was maintained by the paid staff when students were not available. This is a critical adjunct whenever students are involved in community-based programming so that continuity is maintained when students are not enrolled. Equally important is the presence of a consistent faculty or clinical advisor/supervisor to provide direction as goals, objectives, and programming are revised and developed. This person is the "keeper of occupation," which easily can be lost when programming is turned over to others less invested.

In order to accurately evaluate the effectiveness of the program, it would likely need a more consistent format and perhaps some way to distinguish it from the value of the 4-H programming. A measure of the effectiveness of the combined programming, however, might be acceptable since the goals and objectives are so compatible. Evaluation of these two programs consisted of two levels: 1) information and skill building in protecting and building community and 2) personal empowerment. Pretests and posttests of questions to determine what the children knew before and after each programming session were used to obtain immediate factual information. For example, an activity named "Take a Closer Look" was designed to sharpen their observation skills and to serve as a reminder of individual differences

(1998, p. 26). The pretest asked the children to carefully view color photos of the chimpanzees at the zoo (also identified by name), and the posttest consisted of matching the distinguishing characteristics of each and the names to the actual chimps at the zoo. This lesson was coupled with other activities supporting the importance of distinguishing ourselves as individuals while supporting the functions and roles of a group/community.

Teasing out the meaning associated with "empowerment" is much more complicated. In these instances the Nowicki-Strickland Locus of Control Scale for Children (1973) was used at the beginning and end of the programming cycle to attempt to distinguish each students' sense of internal personal control over his or her life and actions. This link between perceived control and empowerment is supported by the research of Gibson (1993) and by Chamberlin (1997), who broadened the link to include community involvement and group participation. The use of the instrument appeared to produce positive outcomes, but the population was too small and the programming too inconsistent in the earlier phases to provide a sound measure. However, continued work with the instrument seems advantageous as a potentially effective measure of the program's objectives. In work on self-concept formation, Harter (1982, 1985, 1990a, 1990b) developed the Perceived Competence Scale for Children, which also would be an appropriate measure of the goals for the children in these programs, as would the work of Battle (1981), Battle and Blowers (1982), Bruininks (1978), and Bryan and Pearl (1979). As an additional measure to further define the factors that contribute to community-building, empowerment, and personal control, one of the programs was videotaped to be qualitatively coded for further investigation.

Another consideration to keep in mind is that whenever you select a group as recipients of your programming (in the examples here, children), you must be very aware of the meaningful occupations those recipients (children) engage in during their normal round of activities. These children were primarily engaged in a combination of schoolwork and play during their week—not an uncommon combination for any child in early and middle childhood. The task of these programs was to support the goals of schoolwork and the developmental need for play through activities that supported and enhanced "community." All of the selected programming did this, although not without some trial and error. If you would like to learn more about the use of "play" in occupational therapy, review Parham and Primeau's discussion of play (1997) and Florey and Greene's discussion of play in middle childhood (1997).

At the Boys and Girls Club site, continued programming for older participants that is external to the 4-H club structure included the development of a Newsletter Project as well as other similar group projects to produce one shared outcome. These projects were designed to meet the goals of developing skills in the realm of leadership, communication, vocational choice, and writing and organization—all within and in support of the basic parameters of community.

As you develop your own programming, if you elect to support occupation-based goals for children to encourage the enhancement of normal development, support of school-room performance, or as a deterrent to negative-outcome

Parents work with their children in learning first-hand about the life of sea creatures as they participate in a "Heal the Bay" project.

"clubs" in the form of gangs, you may wish to more carefully examine the goals of 4-H, Boys and Girls Clubs, and, specifically, Roots and Shoots. As the Roots and Shoots programming was developed, planners discovered a number of conservation-concerned groups that provided volunteers and dollars to enhance programming. These groups included Wildlife on Wheels, Seeds of Simplicity, Heal the Bay, Tree People, and numerous parks, gardens, zoos, and museums. You will likely find similar organizations in your area.

THE YOUNG MEN'S CHRISTIAN ASSOCIATION (YMCA) AND THE YOUNG WOMEN'S CHRISTIAN ASSOCIATION (YWCA)

Programs can be developed within the mission of an umbrella organization but also can be very different in their goals and objectives and in the population that they service. There is no "recipe" for programs within the 4-H club, the Boys and Girls Club, or the **YMCA/YWCA.** The ability to see opportunities for creative expression of an organization's mission through the exercise of occupation is entirely the pleasure of the programmer.

A Shared Exercise Program for Patients with Parkinson's Disease and Their Spouses

We will now briefly contrast two programs, each carefully articulated with the mission and goals of the YMCA/YWCA. The first, an exercise program for patients with Parkinson's disease and their spouses, was initiated in a fairly common way—at the request of a participant in an out-patient occupational therapy program. This participant was also a member of a YMCA in an affluent neighborhood where he had long been a strong advocate for his community in many ways. He expressed to his occupational therapist a concern that he would like to return to his YMCA for an exercise group. At the time there was no such group that took into consideration the specific needs of people with Parkinson's disease. But there was another agenda as well; "meaning" for this patient was not only a wish to resume what for him had been a fairly normalizing activity ("adult play at the YMCA"), but also there was a need to continue or perhaps to encourage the expression of bonding and support by including the spouse. As a skillful and intuitive occupational therapist elicited this patient's story, he or she would recognize other meanings being expressed as well. Perhaps the patient wanted to not only engage in exercise and spend time with his spouse but also and more importantly wanted to return to a more proactive role in his life and his community (to be an advocate and someone who can still get things done). Perhaps he also wanted to return to a more normalizing spousal role in which he could engage in an activity with his spouse where she was not the caregiver but the partner.

With some guidance the patient (or in this case, a better term might be the community-member) developed an advocacy plan to encourage the initiation of a couples exercise/dance program for himself, his spouse, and others with similar needs. The program was developed much like what has been described in this text. When a needs assessment discovered that there was enough interest to start with several classes a week, the YMCA added the classes for a fee in a similar structure to other programming and took care of the promotion and marketing. The occupational therapist, who was also an aerobics instructor and an avid "line-dancer," was hired to develop the programming along with the assistance of the participants. This program demonstrates a nice bridge between the treatment setting (one of the arenas of occupational therapy) and the community (one of the arenas of the occupation-centered practitioner). It also demonstrates the true art of the practitioner—that of recognizing and enabling the strengths of the patients/clients to once again put them in control of their own lives.

The "Mommy and Me" Story Quilt Club

Another example appropriate to our discussion is that of a "Mommy and Me" program established in a YWCA in a far less affluent neighborhood than the one described previously. Affluence does not have much to do with these two stories, except that it does seem to go hand-in-hand with one's perceived sense of control over one's destiny, which makes for some difference in the selection of goals and objectives for a successful program. Following its own somewhat informal needs assessment, this program was initiated at the request of the YWCA. The YWCA was interested in two programs—one for young mothers (13 to 16 years old) and another for these mothers as well as the fathers. The program for the mothers was designed to also actively include the babies. The format also consisted of classes, which was similar to other programming at this facility but fees were not charged directly to the participants. The mother and baby classes involved the shared and enmeshed occupations surrounding the physical care of the baby and also the "learning how to play together" emotional care of both mother (an adolescent) and baby.

Perhaps the most successful activity associated with this program (as reported by the mothers) was one that focused on meaningful occupation and self-advocacy, which was a theme in the previous example as well. The activity consisted of making an over-sized quilt block that was large enough to function as a baby coverlet. The design of the block was developed as the mother's "story" that she wished to give her baby as her legacy or gift. The story was an expression of the mother's meaningful occupations, her values, her interests, and the things about life she most wanted her baby to know and remember. An important piece of the block also carried the theme of what the mother still wished to do with her life. Although the blocks were constructed individually, the activity was carried out as a group—the "quilting club"—and this community of storytellers shared and validated their experiences and came away with a tangible record. This class, which was a significant piece of work, was also conducted by occupational therapy students.

Free-Standing Clubs

The last two examples we will explore are again quite different from each other in terms of population, intention, and geography and are both examples of **free-standing clubs.** The Ice Cream Cart Club was a rural, midwestern venture, while the Jazz/Blues Club was an inner-city urban experiment.

The Ice Cream Cart Club

The Ice Cream Cart Club was developed in response to a need, which was expressed primarily by teachers in the beginning, to better integrate learning disabled and SED children into the student life activities of the middle school environment. All of the students identified first by the teachers were described as "socially isolated." The program was developed as a club in consideration of the developmental needs of this group (ages 11 to 14), but this idea was also strongly supported in the second level of needs assessment accomplished with the children who wished to be involved. All of the children first identified by the teachers were invited to be members but none were forced. By consensus the children elected to start a lunch-time ice cream cart business. The programming involved multiple skill development in sales, marketing/promotion, accounting, and personnel management. Although significant in helping the students to focus on future goals and staying in school, the more important goals of the program were centered again around empowerment, advocacy, and self-esteem—a theme that continues to resurface in much of our programming. Weekly club meetings were facilitated by a school-based occupational therapist who helped develop individual goals for each child as well as goals for the collective club. The club meetings were often indistinguishable from the goal-directed adolescent psychosocial group model (the goal being the business to be accomplished for the week). Continued plans for the programming include the addition of several high school mentors for the group to assist in the transition from middle school as well as mentors from local businesses.

The Dunbar Hotel Jazz Club

The second example of the development of a club model—in this case to create community—is that of the Jazz Club. The Dunbar Hotel is located in downtown Los Angeles and is part of the Dunbar Economic Development Corporation. In 1975 the Dunbar Hotel Black Cultural Historical Museum was established to save the Dunbar Hotel. Through these efforts, the Hotel was designated as a city and national historical landmark (The Dunbar Economic Development Corporation, 1996).

In recognition of low-income housing needs, in 1988 the hotel was financed for mixed use to include housing (73 units of low-income senior housing), commercial facilities, and cultural facilities. The intent of the occupation-based programming that was developed was to create a sense of shared "community" for these residents. In order to identify the characteristics of "community" and the meaning these residents assigned to their lives and their history, it seemed appropriate to investigate the history of the hotel. Oftentimes a building or a neighborhood has forgotten history that when resurrected can structure the goals and objectives of a program. In this case, the history was jazz. In its original 1920s state, the hotel was a first-class hotel for Blacks. It was surrounded by jazz clubs and became the hub of the Los Angeles Black night life. As integration grew into the 1950s and Black entertainers and club goers were no longer restricted to downtown, the hotel and the neighborhood drifted into decay. One of the occupational therapy students, a jazz historian, took an interest in the hotel and in the residents. Upon closer investigation and a cursory needs assessment accomplished with the assistance of the social service coordinator, it was determined that the general health and well-being of the residents could likely be enhanced if they could be encouraged to become less isolated and share in some kind of activity programming. Although there was a space designed for activities, no one frequented the room and attempts at programming had not been successful.

Upon further investigation it was discovered that many of the residents had been participants in the vibrant neighborhood of the jazz era, and a number were musicians themselves. Although we cannot assume that everyone continues to assign meaning to their own histories, with the kind of shared interests evident at the Dunbar it was a fair guess that jazz and blues, in some way, continued to have meaning for many of the residents. With the resources of the museum, a Jazz/Blues Appreciation Club was organized first to plan and celebrate birthdays of Black jazz and blues performers and then to organize jam sessions and mini-concerts. Residents were first involved as the audience, but those who were able quickly became more active participants. With small encouragement, many contemporary Black musicians and entertainers became participants and/or contributors.

Again, this example includes the theme of "meaning" as the significant indicator of well-being and therapy. In this example, the meaning is assessed through linkages with history, and those linkages weave the fabric of community.

Students and residents decorate cookies to celebrate a "jazz artist's" birthday.

SUMMARY

Examples have been provided for occupation-centered clubs within existing structures such as the 4-H Club, Jane Goodall's Roots and Shoots Clubs, Boys and Girls Clubs of America; the YMCA, and the YWCA. In addition the development of two free-standing clubs, the Ice Cream Cart Club and the Jazz/Blues club, have been described. The concept of "club" within developmentally appropriate contexts and rule-bound structures can provide a frame for the placement of successful occupation-centered programs for all ages.

REFERENCES

Battle, J. (1981). *Culture free self esteem inventory, self esteem inventory for children and adults.* Seattle, WA: Special Child Publications.

Battle, J., & Blowers, T. (1982). A longitudinal comparative study of the self-esteem of students in regular and special education classes. *Journal of Learning Disabilities, 15,* 100–102.

Bruininks, V. L. (1978). Actual and perceived peer status of learning disabled students in mainstream programs. *Journal of Special Education, 12,* 51–58.

Bryan, T. H., & Pearl, R. (1979). Self-concept and locus of control of learning disabled children. *Journal of Clinical Child Psychology, 8,* 223–226.

Chamberlin, J. (1997). A working definition of empowerment. *Psychiatric Rehabilitation Journal, 20*(4), 43–46.

The Dunbar Economic Development Corporation. (1996). *Organizational history.* Los Angeles: The Dunbar Economic Dev. Corp.

Florey, L., & Greene, S. (1997). Play in middle childhood: A focus on children with behavior and emotional disorders. In L. D. Parham & L. S. Fazio (Eds.), *Play in occupational therapy for children* (pp. 126–143). St. Louis, MO: Mosby.

Gibson, C. M. (1993). Empowerment theory and practice with adolescents of color in the child welfare system. *Families in Society, 74*(7), 387–396.

Harter, S. (1982). The perceived competence scale for children. *Child Development, 53,* 87–97.

Harter, S. (1985). *Manual for the self-perception profile for children.* Denver, CO: University of Denver Press.

Harter, S. (1990a). Issues in the assessment of the self-concept of children and adolescents. In A. M. LaGreca (Ed.), *Through the eyes of the child: Obtaining self-reports from children and adolescents.* Boston: Allyn and Bacon.

Harter, S. (1990b). Processes underlying adolescent self-concept formation. In R. Montemayor, G. R. Adams, & T. P. Gullotta (Eds.), *From childhood to adolescence: A transitional period?* Newbury Park, CA: Sage.

Nowicki, S., & Strickland, B. R. (1973). A locus of control scale for children. *Journal of Consulting and Clinical Psychology, 40,* 148–154.

Parham, L. D., & Primeau, L. (1997). Introduction to play and occupational therapy. In L. D. Parham & L. S. Fazio (Eds.), *Play in occupational therapy for children* (pp. 2–21). St. Louis, MO: Mosby.

"Take a Closer Look." (1998). *Roots and Shoots Los Angeles: A Curriculum Packet to Connect Community, Environment and Wildlife.* (Limited publication supported by The Los Angeles Roots and Shoots Steering Committee, The Los Angeles Zoo, and The University of Southern California Department of Occupational Science and Occupational Therapy)

CHAPTER 18

Programming to Support Meaningful Occupation and Balance for the Disenfranchised and Homeless

Learning Objectives

1. To appreciate the condition of homelessness
2. To understand the impact of homelessness on the program participants' choices and on their participation in occupation
3. To appreciate the impact of severe and persistent mental illness on the occupations of homeless persons
4. To identify how a shelter may be utilized as a site for occupation-centered programs

Key Terms

1. Disenfranchised
2. Homelessness
3. Homelessness and Severe/Persistent Mental Illness
4. Shelter

INTRODUCTION

According to *Webster's Dictionary* (1975), the definition of **disenfranchised** is "to deprive of the right to vote or some other right of citizenship." Therefore, the use of the word in connection to the homeless population is not entirely accurate, although it does carry with it an assumption as to the *rights of a citizen.* If the citizen has obligations to the community (such as governance, taxation, and so on), does not the community have obligations to the citizen? Having access to **shelter** is the foundation for any attention to meaningful occupation and must be attended to for the achievement of purpose.

Approximately 7 million people (men, women, and children) experienced **homelessness** in the latter half of the 1980s (Burt & Cohen, 1989; Interagency Council on the Homeless, 1994; National Coalition for the Homeless; 1997), and approximately 20 percent to 25 percent of the single, adult homeless population are considered to be experiencing some form of **severe and persistent mental illness** (Koegel, 1996). The general deinstitutionalization of the mentally ill during the 1950s and 1960s may have initiated some of the developing increase in homelessness; however, the vast increases in homelessness did not occur until the 1980s (Federal Task Force on Homelessness and Severe Mental Illness, 1992). Why did this occur? Koegel (1996), Kaufman (1997), and the report of the Federal Task Force on Homelessness and Severe Mental Illness (1992) attribute the cause, among other things, to the general decrease in incomes and to the loss of housing options for the marginalized populations. The mentally ill experience these causes as well as those associated with debilitating illness and frequently the inability to access or receive therapy services. They are also likely to remain homeless for longer periods of time and have less contact with family and friends than others who are homeless. Their opportunities for employment are fewer, and they tend to be in poorer physical health than their homeless peers (Federal Task Force on Homelessness and Severe Mental Illness, 1992). Although it has been a widely accepted belief that the homeless mentally ill refuse rehabilitative services, Oakley and Dennis (1996) reported that homeless individuals with serious mental illness are willing to use services that are easily accessible and that meet their perceived needs. Of course, there are others who are homeless and have debilitating illness such as drug and alcohol abuse and Human Immunodeficiency Virus (HIV). These persons require similar access to services as do the mentally ill. When rehabilitation includes active case management, therapy, housing options, and long-term follow-up and support services coupled with *meaningful daily activity in the community* (including work), homelessness can come to an end (Oakley and Dennis, 1996).

According to the Federal Task Force on Homelessness and Severe Mental Illness (1992), only 5 percent to 7 percent of homeless persons with mental illness need to be institutionalized; most can live successfully in the community but not without supportive services that include housing options. Unfortunately, there currently are not enough of either in any of the large urban areas of the United States. We are not without options, however; such programs as the Projects for Assistance in Transition from Homelessness, or PATH (Wells, 1996), and the many community-based programs across the country of which occupational therapists are an active part can make a difference.

There are also homeless who are living with Acquired Immunodeficiency Syndrome (AIDS) and other illnesses caused by HIV. These persons, an estimated 36 percent of whom have been homeless since learning that they had HIV or AIDS, experience many of the same problems of avoidance and stigma as do those who are mentally ill (O'Connell, Lozier, & Gingles, 1997; Robbins & Nelson, 1996). In many ways there may be less public support for this population than for the seriously mentally ill, particularly when it comes to employment and supportive housing. A related problem is experienced by homeless adolescents who often engage in sex in exchange for food, clothing, and shelter, for they are at great risk for contracting HIV-related illnesses. Robertson (1996) reported on the results of a series of studies performed in four cities across the United States in which a median HIV-positive rate of 2.3 percent for homeless persons under age 25 was found.

We have identified some of the problems of the homeless who are ill, but who are the homeless who are not ill? And do they share common characteristics whether they are found in urban areas or in rural ones? Do the homeless populations in the East, Midwest, South, or West have common characteristics? Even though we are able to make estimates of the numbers of homeless persons, based on the numbers of people in shelters and on the street, those estimates are undoubtedly below the actual numbers. Many people who lack a stable, permanent residence and, for example, are living from friend to friend or in a car have fewer shelter options and remain uncounted. In fact, in a recent study of homelessness in 50 U.S. cities, the estimated number of homeless people greatly exceeded the number of emergency shelter and transitional housing spaces (National Law Center on Homelessness and Poverty, 1996). As reported by Waxman & Trupin (1997), there is a nationwide shortage of emergency shelters. In addition, Aron and Fitchen (1996) reported that although there are significant numbers of homeless in rural areas of the United States, there are virtually no shelters; where there are few shelters, it is also likely that there are fewer support programs.

Most of the adults who are homeless, particularly the families, have experienced loss of employment. This loss coupled with little formal education or vocational training often prompts moves across the country in search of opportunities, which often results in becoming homeless in a strange city. Women with children may also become a part of this scenario when they are abandoned or divorced and have no resources or employment skills. Loss of employment is certainly not the only contributor to homelessness, but it is a significant one.

Programming for the homeless or near homeless can take many forms ranging from those that are conducted within shelters that provide the basics of comfort and safety to day shelter programs that provide temporary housing and a balance of occupations for at least the waking hours. Dear (1996) noted that the homeless are sometimes referred to as the service dependent. By intention or neglect those services that are accessed by the homeless, including health care, social welfare, emergency shelter, and job training, are most often localized to those areas of the city known as skid row or a similar term. This area, which becomes the *community*

Planting seedlings to bring "spring" into a shelter for homeless women is an activity designed to meet the goals of an occupation-centered program.

of the homeless, is where they live, eat, talk to friends, and oftentimes work. According to Dear, it is a well-defined time-space prism, and it is a coping mechanism for the homeless (1996, p. 109). Perhaps this *community* is a sanctuary just as your home may be after a long work week. Most likely any occupation-centered programming, as an extension of this service network, will also be part of this *community*. Any effort to move programming outside of the location where homeless people are congregated is often met with resistance from those living in the outside neighborhood or community. Whether this resistance is merited or not, if programming is to occur outside and a new community is to be created, we would expect that there are related goals to make this the most desirable circumstance. If this is the case, we must consider accessibility and motivation, and a transitional program might be the best way to initiate services.

Programs can be provided for children and adolescents within various educational formats (formal or shelter schools), but attention must be focused on the needs and concerns of these children who have lived without homes and the safety of a stable shelter. Neville-Jan and associates describe one such program that included some foster care children who had experienced homelessness (1997, pp. 144–157). Although this program included a broad range of children with varying needs, during the course of the programming it was noted that the children who had experienced what might be described as the culture of homelessness were more likely to engage in protective negative social behaviors such as hoarding of supplies, lying, and petty theft—attributes that were likely extremely adaptive on the street. Certainly these characteristics challenge the practitioner beyond what might be expected when programming focuses on the development of social skills and behaviors that enhance and support learning.

Chapters 18, 19, and 20 will describe several programs that were designed for and conducted with homeless and near homeless persons. The first example is an in-depth description of student-designed programming for a homeless women's shelter. This example will provide you with a step-by-step description, from the first examination of the site and the population to the final steps of evaluation. This fairly lengthy description will be followed by less inclusive examples of several other programs targeting persons in varying situations of homelessness and illness. All of these should provide you with ideas you can use for programming with similar populations in your area.

PROGRAMMING FOR A HOMELESS WOMEN'S SHELTER

The Site

Founded in 1941 by radio evangelist Sister Essie Binkey West, the Sunshine Mission began to offer shelter to homeless women in downtown Los Angeles. In later years the city condemned the downtown facility and another was purchased just north of the University of Southern California campus. Functioning first as a school, followed by a hotel, and then a USO facility, this building, Casa de Rosas, enjoyed a colorful history. In 1951 Sister West moved her entire Old Time Faith programs, including her radio broadcasts, publications, and services to the homeless and needy, to this site, and she remained there until her death in 1976. The Old Time Faith operated with donations from Sister West's followers, and some of them continue to support the Sunshine Mission with donations today.

In 1989 the organization ended its religious affiliation and reorganized itself into Casa de Rosas, Inc., a tax-exempt California corporation. The volunteer board of directors and management team initiated numerous programs to restore the agency both physically and financially. Support presently includes a range of government contracts, corporate charitable grants, fund-raising events, and regular individual donations. The physical structure was recently renovated by the city and the state as a historical residential project. The building now is an example of the community's architectural history and an example of modern, safe housing for its homeless and low-income citizens.

Today the Sunshine Mission provides housing, food, and life necessities to adult single women for periods of thirty to sixty days. The Mission can comfortably house 20 women per night, and each woman is expected to work with the shelter manager to develop and implement a plan to assist her in returning to independent living.

Adjoining the Sunshine Mission is the Casa de Rosas Hotel, which provides single-occupancy accommodations for the near homeless. Residents include senior citizens, the disabled, people in recovery, and working people of low income. The hotel can house 45 tenants who pay low monthly rents.

The above information incorporates the mission statement of Casa de Rosas, Inc. (1996), portions of the Agency Effectiveness Report, and Phase I needs assessment interview material provided by the manager.

The Community Profile

The Sunshine Mission is one of several connected buildings surrounding a central plaza and is secured from outside entry. It is located in South Central Los Angeles, approximately seven miles from downtown. The area is diverse with a mixed population of African American and Hispanic low-income families. There are several gangs occupying territory in the adjacent neighborhoods, and although the Mission is secured, it is considered to be in a high-crime area. According to 1996 Los Angeles Police Department (LAPD) statistics, nearly 50 percent of all crimes committed in Los Angeles County are perpetrated in the South Central area where the Mission is located.

The Target Population

From our earlier discussion, it would appear that there are multiple factors that contribute to and sustain the problem of homelessness. Many of these are no different in Southern California than in the larger United States. According to a 1993 Report of the Glendale, California Task Force on Homelessness, some of these factors include illiteracy, lack of competitive job skills, substance abuse, emotional trauma from histories of child abuse, extensive employment layoffs, deinstitutionalization of the mentally ill, working poverty, and lack of affordable housing. Much of the reported information deals with the male homeless population, but it is not difficult to draw the assumption that women fare far less successfully when measured against the above list of factors.

Recent statistics provided by the Mission show that 60 percent of the women in residence were African American, 20 percent were Caucasian, and 20 percent were from various other cultural groups. The typical age range was from 26 to 45 years of age. Fifteen percent of the women reported a background of domestic violence, and 12 percent had a history of alcohol and/or drug abuse. The average educational level was completion of elementary school, and some had differing amounts of vocational training. Most of the women had held previous jobs.

The Needs Assessment

The shelter manager was contacted by student representatives to gain a perspective on what programs were currently being offered and what needs the residents might continue to have that could be considered in designing a useful and meaningful occupation-centered program. The manager was also questioned regarding past, present, and future trends concerning homeless women at the Mission.

The students then did further research to develop the service profile and determined that in 1995 the homeless population in Los Angeles was estimated to be approximately 83,900. The Shelter Partnership of Los Angeles (1995) estimated this population to be even larger. This information coupled with a review of national as well as local community statistics seemed to indicate that the numbers of homeless would only increase and that their needs would become greater over time. In addition, women were becoming more proactive in seeking services and were advocates for other women. All of this information pointed to an increased demand for information and services tailored to the needs of women and was useful when resources were required.

According to the manager during the Phase I assessment to obtain a sense of the individual needs of the residents, the residents would be most interested in programs to prepare them for the job-search process. After researching the needs of shelter populations in general and women's shelters in particular, brain storming to generate ideas for programming that might be useful adjuncts to the present programs, and considering the manager's perspectives, a Phase II needs assessment was developed for distribution to the current residents.

Following a trial distribution, it was soon discovered that the Phase II assessment instrument was too broad and open-ended; residents requested services that the students were not prepared to provide or were beyond the scope of the program being considered. Thus, a second version of the Phase II needs assessment survey instrument (shown in Figure 18–1) was designed and distributed to residents in the dining hall. The students distributed the assessment personally, answered questions, and collected the assessments before leaving the site. Distributing the needs assessment at a time when the majority of residents were available, answering questions, and collecting the completed assessments before leaving the site were all ways to ensure a maximum number of responses.

This second assessment instrument was aimed at identifying what realistically could be provided in a mission environment with very little financial support. This instrument incorporated the ideas of the students and the concerns of the manager. The students wanted to ensure that the programs could be utilized and were also cognizant of the need to design programs that could be conducted by volunteers from the community and perhaps by occupational therapy students without loss of the goal structure.

Results of this second questionnaire indicated that the largest percentage of residents selected the *self-care* category as being of primary interest, and the separate categories were fairly even in distribution. This category was followed closely by the *Learning-About-the-Community* category, again with fairly equal distribution. Third was *Arts and Crafts* with a higher interest in holiday crafts. *Home Skills* and *Employment Skills* ranked next, with more interest expressed for job-search skills and interviewing skills. *Money Management* ranked at the bottom, perhaps with little surprise (as one of the respondents reminded the student group) since the women responding to the questionnaire had little or no money to manage at the time!

Drafting Goals and Objectives

Following careful review of the results of the needs assessment, the mission statement, characteristics of the facility, and the characteristics of the population, two goals for the program were drafted and were followed by measurable objectives, as shown by the following examples.

FIGURE 18–1   Needs Assessment Survey

Sunshine Mission Survey

We are interested in providing programming that will assist you in preparing for your return to the community. To do this we would like to know what activities you would find most useful. Please fill out this survey to help us identify your needs and interests. **Check all that apply:**
I am most interested in activities that will help me:
(Rate 1 through 6, with 1 being the area you are most interested in and 6 the area you are least interested in)
_____ learn how to get a new or better job
_____ meet people I can do things with
_____ learn about free or low-cost services in Los Angeles
_____ take better care of myself
_____ relax and enjoy life more
_____ develop new interests and/or skills
Things I would be interested in trying:
_____ arts and crafts
          anything in particular _____
_____ home skills
          _____ apartment hunting: how and what to expect
          _____ cooking/baking
          _____ nutrition/healthy meal planning
          _____ shopping/how to find coupons and discounts
          _____ small plot (or) community gardening
          _____ budget decorating
          _____ sewing
          _____ other (please describe): _____
_____ learning about the community
          _____ seeing Los Angeles on a budget
          _____ the Los Angeles library services
          _____ riding public transportation
          _____ activities of 'singles' organizations
          _____ assisting others in need of help
          _____ Los Angeles community social services
          _____ religious outings
          _____ other (please describe): _____
_____ pre-employment skills
          _____ how to 'job search'
          _____ developing a resume
          _____ how to fill out a job application
          _____ how to interview well
          _____ other (please describe): _____
_____ self-care
          _____ exercise classes
          _____ how to relax and manage stress
          _____ safety education/women's self-defense
          _____ grooming and hygiene
          _____ other (please describe): _____

Thanks for your time; you'll be seeing programs posted by the end of the month.
See you there!

Program Focus: Attention to Healthy Living

Goals:

1. *To be healthy* by increasing awareness of healthy living strategies to include nutrition, personal care, exercise, job search, self-defense, and safety
2. *To control one's destiny* by increasing the individual's sense of personal causation, self-esteem, and self-efficacy

Objectives:

1. (a) Fifty percent of the residents at the Sunshine Mission will attend four out of the six sessions (nutrition, personal care, exercise, job search, self-defense, or safety).
   (b) Of the women attending each session, 80 percent will demonstrate knowledge of information and techniques provided in that session.
2. (a) Of those women attending all of the sessions, 80 percent will demonstrate increased self-efficacy, self-esteem, and personal causation.

The Program

Single-session workshops that each lasted approximately 1 1/2 to 2 hours were developed in each of the above-identified areas (nutrition, personal care, exercise, job search, self-defense, and safety).

Nutrition

The session on nutrition was initiated with a verbal survey of how and what the residents preferred to eat and what, if any, problems they were experiencing that they thought might have a relationship to their nutritional likes and dislikes. Most of the residents preferred "fast food" when they were not receiving Mission meals, and many were either under or over their preferred weight.

From earlier discussion with the manager and some of the residents, the students were prepared with materials gleaned from the fast-food restaurants regarding their own statistics for calorie, fat, and salt content. This information was coupled with some suggestions for balancing fast-food meals and some hints for ways to reduce cholesterol and calories. Meeting the residents' basic needs was important to the success of this session and provided a good foundation from which other nutritional sessions such as healthy meal planning and cooking could develop.

Personal Care and Exercise

Personal care in the forms of personal hygiene and makeup were important as a segue to job searches. Enthusiastic volunteers were solicited from neighborhood shops to provide demonstrations of manicure and pedicure techniques and application of makeup. A local beauty school provided no-cost hair cuts and styling techniques.

A group walking program was established, and an aerobics dance class was initiated. Both quickly came under the direction of residents.

Job Search

Job-search skills consisted of exercises in learning how to read the classified section of the newspaper, how and where to access other job announcements, how to develop a skills-based resume that would not negatively highlight periods of unemployment, and how to write a cover letter. Videotaped role-playing provided practice in interviewing.

Self-Defense and Safety

A community martial arts studio volunteered the time and expertise of a female instructor to provide instruction in physical self-defense techniques. Small-group discussions followed the self-defense instruction to assist in the emotional buffering necessary for some women who had histories of physical abuse.

Representatives of the Los Angeles Police Department and the University Crime Prevention and Rape Awareness Group provided information verbally and in the form of handouts to assist the residents in being safe on the street and in the neighborhood, including safety precautions to follow if they were living on the street.

Since the residents frequently rotate, a set of programs can be repeated. This is positive in that the students have time to develop and enhance existing materials; but it can be something of a disadvantage when relying on volunteers from local shops and agencies.

Staffing

As noted previously, staffing for the sessions/workshops was provided by neighborhood volunteers in the form of representatives from local shops and agencies. Residents were trained to become facilitators whenever possible—not only to assist in providing "womanpower" but, more importantly, to provide as many residents as possible with leadership opportunities.

Another important source of assistance for the ongoing success of the program was the linkage to the Student Occupational Therapy Association and the O.T. Student Residence. Both of these organizations "adopted" the Mission as a service project. Occupational therapy graduate students may also obtain service-learning credit for participation in and expansion of the programs and activities. The on-site manager supports student involvement and acts as a liaison between the occupational therapy student programs and the needs of the residents.

Space

When the students first went on-site to conduct the tentative needs assessment, they explored the space (including storage) and materials/supplies that would be available to them. As shown in Figure 18–2, two rooms provided the space and work tables necessary for the planned programming—the existing dining room and a conference room. In addition, the outside courtyard and kitchen could be used for some activities.

FIGURE 18–2   Space Plan for Meeting Room and Conference Room

All space was used for multiple purposes and had to be scheduled at the convenience of the Mission. For the convenience of all concerned, it was determined that following the evening meal was the preferred time for activities (although it was a competitive time with television). Weekend times offered additional possibilities.

Tables could be moved aside for activities that required floor space. There was one file cabinet where some space could be provided, but secured storage was limited and could not be relied upon. The rooms contained electrical outlets that could accommodate a radio, VCR, and/or CD player, and the adjoining kitchen was well supplied with utensils. A small storage area contained rulers, pencils, and paper, and a typewriter and personal computer were available for the residents' use (donations). Secured parking for volunteers was limited.

Supplies and Equipment

Efforts were made to design activities requiring minimal equipment and supplies and little, if any, requirement for storage. All activities utilized the existing tables and chairs in the dining area and/or conference room, the kitchen, and the floor space in the dining area.

Cost

Even though most of the activities relied on donated supplies, a cost breakdown of supplies and equipment was done in order to anticipate replacement costs (if required) and to assist those who wished to donate by establishing a cost/value for items.

Funding

Since residents of the Mission were provided services and information free of charge to assist them as they prepared for independent living, this was clearly a service program. The program required the Mission to absorb minimal cost, if any, for supplies, and these costs were incorporated into the existing budget.

The occupational therapy students explored the processes of fund-raising, including those activities already in existence through the Mission. Successful efforts were made to build bridges with local shops and agencies for ongoing relationships to provide volunteer staff and donated supplies. A sense of *community* and *community responsibility* was created between the University, the local residents, and the local businesses and agencies.

In addition to the above efforts, the creation and maintenance of *community* was of equal importance to the occupational science and occupational therapy academic programs that assumed some fiscal responsibility for the student-related Mission activities as part of their Occupational Therapy-Los Angeles (OT-LA) community service and community service-learning programs and projects.

Marketing

There is some marketing to be done, even with community service programs. The first marketing, of course, was to the Mission manager who, in turn, brought the ideas to the board of directors. This first effort was accomplished in the initial on-site meeting. The students were prepared with appropriate and relevant questions and could offer a brief scenario of their interests in working with the residents. This was also an excellent opportunity for the students to market some of the basic tenets of occupation, meaningful engagement in activity, and occupational therapy. In addition, they were able to link their interest in occupation with the work of the Mission.

Secondly, the residents needed to be informed of the program's activities. This was done initially through the needs assessment and the verbal/visual introduction to the students who would be involved. When plans for programming were finalized, the students prepared colorful flyers advertising the full program and giving information about the activities as well as how residents could benefit. These were supplemented by weekly flyers highlighting the "program of the week." Programming was offered whether there was one participant or twenty participants.

The next phase of marketing required some substantial networking as well as leg work. The purpose of the Mission's activities and the goals and objectives of the students' programming was taken to the shops and agencies that the students' had targeted as providing services that would benefit the residents of the Mission. The idea of volunteering time and, in some cases, supplies had to be "sold" to the shop owners and employees. The students found this to be the most disconcerting aspect of marketing the program, but in many ways it turned out to be the easiest.

It should not be lost that this third phase of marketing strongly involved the encouragement of responsibility—and perhaps obligation—to the *community*. This was made even stronger through the residence of the programmers within the neighborhood where the Mission existed. Certainly students are transients, but the responsibility that is created by an investment in the shared premise of *community* can become a legacy handed from one student group to another through the investment of the institution (the University) and the department.

Outcomes

Taking time to work and rework program goals and objectives is worthwhile when it comes to determining how effective the program has been and continues to be. Of course, to really know long-term effectiveness, it would be necessary to follow the residents' progress in obtaining employment and acquiring suitable housing. Although today this follow-up is attempted by the Mission, for numerous reasons it is difficult to accomplish. As the occupational therapy student's programming continues to attract residents and if that programming is effective, then we would expect to see this reflected in any data the Mission is able to obtain.

The goals and objectives of the student's programming can be measured for short-term effectiveness in the following ways:

Goal:

1. *To be healthy* by increasing awareness of healthy living strategies to include nutrition, personal care, exercise, job search, self-defense, and safety

Objective:

1. (a) Fifty percent of the residents at the Sunshine Mission will attend four out of six sessions.

Measurement

This objective is measured simply by an organized system of attendance marking and is compared to the number of women who are in residency during the programming. The relationship of the objective to the goal carries the assumption that being present during the session does, in fact, increase awareness. Since awareness is a fairly superficial goal, the objective is likely being measured adequately. Measurement of this objective could be strengthened with the use of an observer checklist similar to the one shown in Figure 18–3, which is used to note the level of each participant's engagement in the session.

Objective:

1. (b) Of the women attending each session, 80 percent will demonstrate knowledge of information and techniques provided in that session.

Measurement

This objective is best measured in two ways. A brief questionnaire can be distributed following each session to focus on the information that the facilitator wishes to convey, or a brief structured interview can be utilized for participants in a small group. It is important that the facilitators think carefully about the content and reflect the main ideas in their questionnaire/interview. Always ask the following question: What is really important to assist the participants in meeting the goal? See Figure 18–4 for an example of a content questionnaire.

If there are demonstrated techniques, as there were with the sessions on personal care, exercise, job search, and self-defense, then an observer checklist is again appropriate. The facilitator must determine the level of competency that is desired to assess achievement of the objective and measure at that level. An actual resume was required as part of the session(s) on job search—either this was accomplished or it was not. If a particular level of quality is expected when something is actually produced, then this must be reflected in the checklist.

Pretests and posttests could be utilized to get a truer measure of information the participants bring to a session as opposed to new information they acquire in a session. For the purposes of this program, it was thought that a pretest was most useful to determine at what level to introduce information; however, planners were able to accomplish their objective without benefit of a pretest.

FIGURE 18–3 Observer Check-Sheet for Participation Level

Client Attendance and Performance Rating Form

Name	Session 1	Session 2	Session 3	Session 4	Session 5

Key:

Rating	Performance
0	Did not attend
1	Attended session but did not participate in activity
2	Quietly participated but not interactive with others
3	Engaged, active participation, interaction with others

FIGURE 18–4 Safety Self-Assessment Check-Sheet

SAFETY SELF-ASSESSMENT

Please read the following statements carefully. Rate each statement using the following scale:

    1 = **strongly agree**
    2 = **agree**
    3 = **doesn't apply/don't care**
    4 = **disagree**
    5 = **strongly disagree**

1) I feel that I can protect myself.   _____
2) I feel that I DON'T give up easily when faced with problems.   _____
3) I feel safe when walking to the store.   _____
4) I feel comfortable saying "No."   _____
5) I understand the difference between verbal abuse and physical abuse.   _____
6) I feel comfortable when a stranger approaches me.   _____
7) I feel that I know how to deal with confrontation.   _____
8) I feel that I can rely on myself.   _____
9) I feel confident that I would survive an attack.   _____
10) I know when to use my words and when to use my fists to protect myself.   _____
11) I feel that I have control over my life.   _____
12) When I want something, I work hard to get it.   _____

Goal:

2. *To control one's destiny* by increasing the individual's sense of personal causation, self-esteem, and self-efficacy

Objective:

2. (a) Of those women attending all of the sessions, 80 percent will demonstrate increased self-efficacy, self-esteem, and personal causation.

Measurement

An important aspect of this objective is the requisite that all of the sessions be attended. The selection of content, or enabling activities, was made with the belief that mastery would, in fact, increase the participant's self-esteem, self-efficacy, and sense of control over her environment or personal causation. Further, it was assumed that the participants were deficit in these characteristics and that this could be the area that could make a difference in their future successes.

In this case, pretest and posttest measurements were selected. The Generalized Expectancy for Success Scale, or GESS (Fibel and Hale, 1978; Asher, 1996), and the Self-Efficacy Scale, or SES (Asher, 1996; Sherer, Maddox, Mercandante, Prentice-Dunn, Jacobs & Rogers, 1982), were given to all participants at the first session in the series, and individual scores were calculated. The measures again were given to all participants (those who had attended all of the sessions) at the last session of the series.

Differences in individual scores were calculated. Although the numbers attending all sessions were small, there was improvement in each set of scores. Of course, there may have been many factors affecting the increased scores, and if the objective were a research project, they would have investigated further to find answers to the following questions: Why did some residents attend one session and not another? How did the women who attended all sessions differ from those who did not? How did their initial scores compare? Did the content of some sessions affect the scores more than others (for example, self-defense or personal care)? These are all legitimate questions that would strengthen the measures; however, since the objective was satisfied, for some of the residents the goal was satisfied.

Time Frame

The programs were prepared over the course of an academic semester (15 weeks), with student groups meeting one time each week for 2-hour periods. The initial program, healthy living, was conducted in 2-hour sessions, one time per week, over a 6-week period.

Minimal supplies were required, and there was no substantial lag time for acquisition. The most difficult aspect of the time line was the substantial marketing effort to those organizations who would provide volunteer time and the scheduling of sessions for their convenience and for the convenience of the residents. Since their initiation, the programs have continued to be conducted with new ideas and new participants.

SUMMARY

The disenfranchised and homeless include children, adolescents, and adults; the numbers are growing daily. Homelessness is sometimes by choice, but most often it is a product of the individual's loss of control over his or her life. Matters of economics and loss of income are integrated with loss of meaningful occupations and hope. One program has been described to provide an example of services for the homeless and/or those in shelter environments. This was an in-depth description of a program provided for homeless women living in a shelter. The goals for this program included the pursuit of "health" and the development of knowledge and skills to "control ones' destiny." To support the goals and to meet the objective, programming focused on self-care, community awareness, holiday arts and crafts, home skills, and pre-employment skills.

REFERENCES

Aron, L. Y., & Fitchen, J. (1996). Rural homelessness: A synopsis. *Homelessness in America.* (The "series" of pamphlets/reports.) Washington, DC: Oryx Press/National Coalition for the Homeless.

Asher, E. (1996) Occupational Therapy Assessment Tools: An Annotated Index (2nd ed.). 2nd edition. Bethesda, MD: AOTA publ.

Burt, M., & Cohen, B. (1989). *America's homeless: Numbers, characteristics, and programs that serve them.* Washington, DC: The Urban Institute.

Dear, M. (1996). Time, space, and the geography of everyday life of people who are homeless. In R. Zemke & F. Clark (Eds.), *Occupational science: The evolving discipline* (pp. 107–114). Philadelphia: F. A. Davis.

Federal Task Force on Homelessness and Severe Mental Illness. (1992). *Outcasts on main street: A report of the federal task force on homelessness and severe mental illness.* Delmar, NY: National Resource Center on Homelessness and Mental Illness.

Fibel, B., & Hale, W. D. (1978). The generalized expectancy for success scale—A new measure. *Journal of Consulting and Clinical Psychology, 46,* 924–931.

Interagency Council on the Homeless, U.S. Department of Housing and Urban Development. (1994). *Priority: Home! The federal plan to break the cycle of homelessness.* Gaithersburg, MD: Community Connections.

Kaufman, T. (1997). *Out of reach: Rental housing at what cost?* Washington, DC: National Low Income Housing Coalition.

Koegel, P. (1996). The causes of homelessness. In *Homelessness in America.* Washington, DC: Oryx Press, National Coalition for the Homeless.

Los Angeles Police Department (LAPD). (1996). *Los Angeles county crime report.* Los Angeles, CA: Author.

National Coalition for the Homeless. (1997). *Homelessness in America: Unabated and increasing.* Washington, DC: National Coalition for the Homeless.

National Law Center on Homelessness and Poverty. (1996). *Mean sweeps: A report on anti-homelessness laws, litigation and alternatives in 50 United States cities.* Washington, DC: National Law Center on Homelessness and Poverty.

Neville-Jan, A., Fazio, L. S., Kennedy, B., & Snyder, C. (1997). Elementary to middle school transition: Using multicultural play activities to develop life skills. In L. D. Parham & L. S. Fazio (Eds.), *Play in occupational therapy for children* (pp. 144–157). St. Louis, MO: Mosby.

Oakley, D., & Dennis, D. (1996). Responding to the needs of homeless people with alcohol, drug, and/or mental disorders. In *Homelessness in America.* Washington, DC: Oryx Press, National Coalition for the Homeless.

O'Connell, J., Lozier, J. & Gingles, K. (1997). *Increased demand and decreased capacity: Challenges to the McKinney Act's health care for the homeless program.* Nashville, TN: National Health Care for the Homeless Council.

Report of the Glendale, California Task Force on Homelessness. (1993). Glendale, CA: City of Glendale, California.

Robbins, G., & Nelson, F. (1996). *Looking for a place to be: A report on AIDS housing in America.* Seattle, WA: AIDS Housing of Washington.

Robertson, M. (1996). *Homeless youth on their own.* Berkeley, CA: Alcohol Research Group.

Shelter Partnership of Los Angeles. (1995). *Annual Report.* Los Angeles, CA: Author.

Sherer, M., Maddox, J. E., Mercandante, B., Prentice-Dunn, S., Jacobs, B., & Rogers, R. W. (1982). The self-efficacy scale: Construction and validation. *Psychological Reports, 51*, 663–671.

Sunshine Mission/Casa de Rosas, Inc. (1996). *Mission statement: Agency effectiveness report.* Los Angeles, CA: Author.

UNAIDS: (1997, December). *Report on the Global HIV/AIDS Epidemic.* New York: Author.

The International Webster New Encyclopedia Dictionary of the English Language. (1975). Chicago: The English Language Institute of America.

Wells, S. M. (1996). *Projects for assistance in transition from homelessness: A summary of fiscal year 1994 state implementation reports.* Washington, DC: National Coalition for the Homeless.

Internet Sites

HIV/AIDS and Homelessness:
http://nch.ari.net/hivaids.html
HIV/AIDS Statistics:
http://www.ama-assn.org/special/hiv/support/aidstat.htm
Mental Illness and Homelessness:
http://nch.ari.net/mental.html
National Resource Center on Homelessness and Mental Illness:
email:nrc@prainc.com.

Shelter Programming for Persons with HIV/AIDS and Mental Illness

Learning Objectives

1. To appreciate the complexity of programming necessary to meet the multiple needs of those homeless persons with HIV/AIDS who may be mentally ill
2. To examine the development of a sample program to meet the goals and multiple objectives of a selected group of homeless persons with HIV/AIDS and mental illness
3. To understand the contributions of task analysis to the success of an occupation-centered program designed to meet multiple objectives

Key Terms

1. HIV/AIDS and Homelessness
2. Mental Illness and Homelessness
3. Shelter
4. Community
5. Occupational Balance
6. Prevocational and Vocational

The population introduced in the title of this chapter appears to be cumbersome in description, but it is, in fact, quite common in today's shelter and mission system to find **HIV/AIDS, mental illness,** substance abuse, and physical illness existing simultaneously in one individual who is **homeless.** This truly challenges the skills of the occupational therapy practitioner to bring to the forefront all of the academic information and experience he or she can accumulate while maintaining a focus on meaningful occupation and the self-assigned needs of the person.

Of course, successful programs can be conducted in the community for all of the aforementioned groups, individually, with entirely different objectives; however, when working in the community, it can be more beneficial to combine groups whenever possible and to remember that the presence of a diagnosis or disease entity has little bearing on your programming. Rather, it is your challenge to design meaningful programming for the individual and to remember that your intervention occurs within and is strongly influenced by the orientation of **community.**

You must also remember that even though a population may share the condition of homelessness, this is by no means perceived in the same way by each individual. For some it may be disabling; for others it is desirable and enabling. The condition or circumstance of homelessness represents a *community* of individuals who must be treated as such.

THE POPULATION CHARACTERISTICS OF OUR PROGRAM EXAMPLE

Schizophrenics make up a large portion of the population of the mentally ill who are homeless, and this was true for the program we will describe. Chronicity with acute episodes is a frequent pattern, and failure to obtain and/or maintain medications is a common occurrence (albeit a result of neglect, misinformation, fear, or lack of availability). Self-medicating behaviors through street drugs or alcohol complicate and exacerbate already unpleasant symptoms such as hallucinations and delusions. In addition, depression is a common factor and is even more likely to prompt self-medicating behaviors than perhaps the symptoms of schizophrenia. In combination with mental illness or existing alone, HIV/AIDS must also be considered.

There are approximately 30.6 million people worldwide living with HIV/AIDS, and the Centers for Disease Control and Prevention, or CDC (1997), noted 612,078 reported cases in the United States (Centers for Disease Control and Prevention, 1997; Karon, 1996; UNAIDS, 1997). Assuming that all cases are not recognized or reported, it is difficult to obtain an accurate estimate, and the official estimates are probably low. This population also is often homeless and may use street drugs and alcohol to mediate their symptoms. On a more optimistic chord, according to 1997 statistics provided by the Los Angeles County Department of Health Services, the fatality rate in Los Angeles County has dropped from 95 percent in 1983 for advanced HIV disease to 11 percent in 1996. These statistics are encouraging for those with HIV disease and AIDS and for those who care for them.

THE SITE OF OUR PROGRAM EXAMPLE

The site/location of the "papermaking for profit" program was within a **shelter** system consisting of seven houses each supporting the combined mission to provide residential care and supportive housing to assist those in transition to independent living. There were from five to seven residents in each home, and all were considered to be homeless before coming into the residential system. To receive funded services in this particular system, residents were first required to be HIV positive and symptomatic. Other illness as described previously (alcoholism/substance abuse, mental illness) was secondary to the HIV/AIDS diagnosis. In addition, a small number of HIV/AIDS persons came to the system on a daily basis for food, showers, medications, and activities but remained living on the street. It should be considered that for many, remaining homeless was the desirable option.

The seven houses were located within a geographic region with similar community characteristics. All were surrounded by small, single-family homes with a few scattered apartment structures. Other residents of the community were largely Black, Hispanic, and Asian and would generally be considered low-income/poverty level. The seven residences easily could be linked through public transportation and on foot. This was an important characteristic that permitted programming to be established at one site while meeting the needs of all residents of the system.

ASSESSING NEED AND PLANNING THE PAPER-MAKING FOR PROFIT PROGRAM

Planning for the residents was not unlike other programs described in this text. The sponsoring system was engaged to provide the mission and purpose and to elicit the goals each residential advisor had for his or her residents. The goals were examined in light of the mission and purpose of the full system, and these were utilized to structure a needs assessment for the individual residents. Resources available from regional and county social services and private donations were examined.

Information received from these combined efforts stimulated the establishment of goals and objectives that were deemed appropriate to the needs of the shelter system and to the needs of the individuals who would be involved in the program. Shared goals were drafted around several central themes: (1) the establishment and strengthening of a *community* to incorporate all of the residents of the seven houses, (2) the creation of a balance of occupations demonstrated through a daily routine of independent living skills for each resident, and (3) the establishment of a venue for the testing and practice of **prevocational and vocational skills** appropriate for residents' transition to other communities of their choice.

Objectives were then drafted with each individual who wished to participate in programming, including those who wished to remain homeless. Regardless of individual interests, each participant was required to attend one *community* meeting a week conducted in each house. The meetings were intended to provide the route for self-governance and self-empowerment, which may accompany the shared responsibility of achieving positive outcomes. When the paper-making business was initiated, this meeting also became the place where group business decisions were made.

Previous to this program, the second theme of **occupational balance** and daily routine of independent living skills had had little success with residents who spent much of their time watching television, smoking, and sleeping. Some previous residents had experienced success with the third theme of prevocational and vocational exploration, but the residential managers felt that something more was needed at a more achievable foundational level since many of the residents had never worked in what might be described as a socially acceptable system (for example, some had worked as prostitutes and some as drug dealers, and some had participated in petty thievery).

Following evaluation of all of the information collected in on-site interviews, through paper/pencil assessments and substantial library and Internet research of the population and the systems supporting the existing programs, it was time for some substantial brainstorming between the students assigned to this opportunity and the instructor. Through this process and a review of the basic tenets of occupation and occupational therapy, it was determined that all of the theme-goals of the program could be incorporated through the use of a carefully selected activity and could also meet the therapeutic objectives of individual residents through the employment of the *foundation skills of task analysis*. Further, the activity to be selected would have the potential to become a profit-producing mechanism.

In today's language of self-efficacy, empowerment, and personal advocacy, the above conclusion may seem too simplistic to some and may provide a bit of an enlightening experience for others. Whichever it is, it is important to remind ourselves to continue to cultivate our historical roots and to recognize that some of our most significant strengths reside in that soil. The mix of a well-understood and carefully selected occupation/activity, comprehensive and skillful task analysis, and the combination of clinical reasoning and a strong therapeutic self can be powerful in achieving occupation-centered outcomes, even within the most sophisticated paradigms.

THE SELECTION OF AN ACTIVITY
TO MEET THE PROGRAM GOALS

Following lengthy discussion, it was determined that the task ahead was to select an occupational activity that would (1) produce a relatively inexpensive but marketable product (2) with good or at least tolerable profit margin, and that the production of this product would be (3) broad and flexible enough to meet the shared goals and objectives of each resident while (4) offering a realistic example of the business characteristics appropriate to umbrella the development of prevocational and vocational skills.

Contiguous to the discussion was that the selected activity must be meaningful and relevant to the participants and to the potential market. Arts and crafts were considered because they can offer a certain mystique in today's mechanized and mass-produced environment. For these reasons and more, it was anticipated

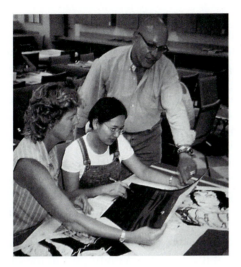

Silk-screen, paper-making, or both? Choosing the craft that will best meet the needs of members with HIV/AIDS and psychiatric disability is a task shared by all involved.

that they would be taken seriously by street-smart participants who likely had numerous agendas for being in the program but perhaps none of them were the ones expressed to the planners.

Some of the students had heard of similar projects with varying populations. Suggestions were made to include the packaging of dry ingredients for a favored soup recipe, selling produce and/or flowers from a community gardening venture (perhaps also packaging the seeds, assuming the garden was organic), making candles and soap, or collecting and mixing potpourri. Constructing small wooden toys and compiling books of poems, personal journal notes, or recipes were suggested as well.

All ideas were entertained with equal enthusiasm, but when these and numerous other suggestions were measured against the desired goals and objectives, the desired characteristics of the project, available space, and proposed cost, paper-making—or more accurately, paper-recycling—was selected. The first step was to research paper-making and paper-recycling, select an appropriate recipe, and obtain the necessary supplies and equipment. (Resources for task analysis and paper-making are included in the recommended reference list.)

The next step involved the actual experimentation with recycled-paper production so that all members of the student group could gain some experience with the media before attempting a task analysis of the steps involved. Finally, a step-by-step list of the tasks involved in the process was completed. Following some experimentation, it was determined that small packets of blank note paper would be packaged as well as sheets of wrapping paper that would be printed with natural object impressions (such as shells and flower petals). Following further experimentation and later consultations with the residents, it was decided to use pre-designed stamps to print the name of the program on attached cards and to use raffia to tie the packages. Plastic bags were the preferred product packaging, although equipment for shrink-wrapping could be a future consideration.

The most formidable task was the completion of the full task analysis of the process from the first step to the last, including preparing and maintaining supplies and equipment, actually making and drying the paper sheets, printing, packaging, obtaining retailers, marketing, and accounting. Several resources were used to assist in formatting the task analysis, and these are included in the reference list.

The next step of this first stage was to locate space and to obtain funding for start-up. Space was provided in an empty garage at one of the residential sites and was brought to functional use through donations from a local builder's supply and several residents, students, and volunteers with suitable carpentry skills. It was determined that several corporate groups were accustomed to offering assistance to charitable groups in need through volunteer days, and these were utilized as well. A small $3,000 start-up grant was received from a local philanthropic organization, which was a satisfactory sum to obtain the supplies and equipment to initiate the program.

The next phase involved a fairly lengthy evaluation period to determine the perceived and actual baseline skills of the residents with respect to the categories utilized in *Uniform Terminology for Occupational Therapy* (AOTA, 1994) and a matching of these to the steps of the activity. Following initiation, it was planned that the residential project would be able to support the work of a supervisory occupational therapist, one certified occupational therapy assistant, and one resident who would function as an aide. This group along with the community of participants and volunteer retired business entreprenuers would determine the future direction of the project. The occupational therapy staff would provide individual evaluation and recommendations to appropriate professionals regarding the prevocational and vocational readiness of participants and would also monitor the evaluation of the program in general.

This program provides an exciting model that easily can be tailored to the needs of many populations in the community and is one that challenges us to use all of our skills as occupation-centered practitioners. Survey your community, and you will find the challenges to which this model is responsive.

SUMMARY

This chapter has continued to provide discussion of those persons who are homeless with mental illness and has also provided a description of the complex needs of those with HIV/AIDS who are homeless. The problems of both groups may be further complicated by the presence of self-medicating behaviors in the form of substance abuse and often physical illness. A multi-shelter program has been described that is structured around goals to establish and strengthen "community," to balance individual occupations, and to create a venue for the testing and practice of prevocational and vocational skills. The program example emphasizes the importance of task analysis to ensure that the selected activity/project matches the individual needs of the participants while meeting the goals of the program for all participants.

REFERENCES

American Occupational Therapy Association, Inc. (1994). "Uniform Terminology for Occupational Therapy, 3rd edition." American Journal of Occupational Therapy. 48, p. 1047–1054).

Centers for Disease Control and Prevention (CDC). (1997). Update: Trends in AIDS incidence—United States. *Morbidity and Mortality Weekly Report, 46*(37), 861–867.

Centers for Disease Control and Prevention (CDC). (1997). *HIV/AIDS Surveillance Report, 9*(1), 1–37.

Karon, J. M. (1996). Prevalence of HIV Infection in the United States, 1984 to 1992. Journal of the American Medical Association 276(2): 126–131.

Los Angeles County Department of Health Services. (1997). *Advanced HIV disease surveillance summary.* Los Angeles, CA: HIV Epidemiology Program.

UNAIDS. (1997, December). *Report on the global HIV/AIDS epidemic.* New York: Author.

Recommended Reading

Lamport, N., Coffey, M., & Hersch, G. (1996). *Activity analysis and application* (3rd ed.). Thorofare, NJ: Slack.

Toale, B. (1983). The Art of Papermaking. Worcester, MA: Davis.

Watson, D. (1994). *Creative handmade paper.* Kent, Great Britain: Search Press.

Watson, D. (1998). *Task analysis: An occupational performance approach.* Bethesda, MD: American Occupational Therapy Association.

CHAPTER 20

Programming for the Homeless Adolescent in Transitional Shelter

Learning Objectives

1. To appreciate the conditions that prompt running away and resulting homelessness in children and adolescents
2. To understand the particular challenges experienced by children and adolescents when living on the street
3. To identify services offered to homeless children and adolescents
4. To review the example of the development of an occupation-centered program for an adolescent shelter population

Key Terms

1. Homeless Families
2. Family Shelters
3. Homeless Adolescents
4. Crisis Intervention
5. Transitional Living

Homelessness is a condition that not only cuts across cultures, socioeconomic considerations, and gender but also does not have much consideration for age or family structure. Although not nearly adequate, shelters and temporary housing are available across the country to individuals, families, and teens. In Los Angeles County there were approximately 5,500 intact **homeless families** in 1995 (Los

Angeles County Families of Dependent Children Annual Report, 1995). Certainly many families disintegrate under the pressures of homelessness.

A trends analysis of the constant flux in the job market and of affordable housing in this urban area and others like it does not appear optimistic for families who are presently low income or who rely on vocational skills that may become obsolete. **Family shelters** are excellent communities for occupation-centered services, for they provide access to a family system within the protected environment of the shelter.

Programming in such shelters can include life skills for adults and teens, vocational assessment and prevocational training for adults, developmental screening and creative play opportunities for young children, and educational support services for school-aged children. Family shelters are generally nonprofit organizations with a mission to provide food, shelter, and other services to homeless families. They are often funded by city governments, foundations/corporations, and private donations. The residences may include a family bedroom, common dining room and bathrooms, a day care/play room for infants and toddlers, a tutoring/educational support room for school-aged children, and a playground. Occupation-centered services, therapeutic or formative, find a comfortable fit with this structure.

Although teens may be found as part of the homeless family, when they are alone and homeless, their problems and concerns are quite unique. The next program description will provide a view of the special concerns of **homeless adolescents.**

THE POPULATION CHARACTERISTICS OF OUR PROGRAM EXAMPLE

Homeless youth, which are most frequently runaways, dot the United States as they make their way to various perceived *utopias* around the country. According to The U.S. Department of Health and Human Services (1991) and the National Network of Runaway and Youth Services (1995), upwards of one million youth run away from home each year (2,740 of them every day). Shelters of many kinds may be found in virtually every city, urban or rural, in an effort to stop or at least postpone this exodus from home. Although there are many popular destinations for runaways, Hollywood, California, has the dubious distinction of being the "runaway capital" of this country, with an estimated 4,000 children and adolescents surviving on the streets and in the abandoned buildings (Covenant House Fact Sheet, 1994; Esperanza, 1997). Although runaway children and adolescents include all ethnicities, the Hollywood Covenant House, whose mission it is to serve runaway teens, reported that caucasian youths accounted for nearly half of all of their contacts in recent years (Covenant House Fact Sheet, 1994).

The largest population seems to be those between the ages of 18 and 21 who are too young for adult shelters and yet too old for the shelters and systems caring for minor children. Many of them "aged out" of the foster care system at age 18, and even though they were often ill-prepared for adult life, they were released to the street. According to a 1991 study by the U.S. Department of Health and Human Services, 45 percent of homeless youth in California were in foster care in the year before they took to the streets. Perhaps surprisingly, 42 percent of the homeless youth across the country were locked out by their parents, as was reported in a 1995 survey by the National Network of Runaway and Youth Services.

According to Esperanza (1997), 81 percent of Covenant House clients in Hollywood have been victims of some kind of abuse, which includes physical, sexual, and emotional abuse, neglect, and abandonment (1997). Approximately 11 percent of these children had sex before the age of 9, and 46 percent had sex before the age of 15. Other statistics that are significant in understanding this group include that 83 percent have a family history of substance abuse, and 74 percent have substance abuse problems themselves. An estimated 93 percent have an array of emotional disorders, which include depression, suicidal ideation, and psychosis. Most have not graduated from high school (92 percent) and have inadequate skills for any employment.

Wherever there are large numbers of homeless adolescents, there are those who victimize them with promises of notoriety, money, and affection. One out of three runaway children is lured into prostitution within 48 hours of leaving home, and it is estimated that nearly 30 percent of youths on the street have been paid for sex and 22 percent have traded sex for food or shelter (Covenant House Fact Sheet, 1994). Unfortunately, opportunities to become victims far exceed the available shelters and services.

When we review the developmental considerations of adolescence, it is not difficult to see how vulnerable they may be to those so-called temptations that are believed to accompany the perceived freedoms, attributes, and rights of adulthood. The community of homeless adolescents, wherever it exists, is a strong one with many of the *club* characteristics noted in the previous chapters. There are perhaps more covert rules than in the adult homeless community, and adolescents are more likely to group and support each other than homeless adults. Considering that they are all likely to be either "running away from" or "running to" something and considering that many are being searched for by families, they tend to be less trusting, more furtive, and more secretive than the communities of homeless adults.

THE SITE OF OUR PROGRAM EXAMPLE

A fairly common model for programs targeting homeless youth is a frontline crisis-intervention outreach program of some sort. Intervention counselors, often volunteers from the police departments or churches, go to the streets where homeless youth are likely to congregate. Crisis intervention often takes the form of assisting youth who are endangered by excessive drug use or a "bad drug trip" or those who are being pursued by pimps or pornographers. Although occupational therapy intervention is not likely to find a foothold in crisis intervention, it is an opportunity to observe and to begin to understand what this community is about, which is critical for those who wish to provide programming to this group. It is also an excellent way to become familiar with the other service providers and volunteer organizations and a way to become known to them, for they are your potential allies.

Beyond this front line is usually an emergency bed shelter that may also provide medical services as well as counseling. In addition, there may be a transitional living environment that offers support directed toward the skills necessary to live independently and to remain off the streets. Transitional living is generally reserved for those adolescents who have demonstrated the motivation, interest, and initiative to benefit from this opportunity. There are paid personnel who work in the transitional living environment who may be social workers, teachers/tutors, and occupational therapists, and there are many volunteers from the surrounding community to provide role-modeling and skill development.

ASSESSING NEED AND PLANNING THE PROGRAMMING

The mission of the selected transitional living unit provided in this example was developed by the Catholic church when the first such shelter was established in New York in 1967. The mission statement included directives for immediate needs and for sanctuary. The mission further offered structure, trust, respect, and choice. Following several evenings with the crisis-intervention teams, reading of the mission, and discussion with personnel as well as observation of existing programming (collectively constituting the Phase I needs assessment), it was determined that occupation-centered providers could best match their body of knowledge and expertise with the aspect of programming that was directed toward life skills development. It was the interest of the director to offer small, individualized opportunities for learning. These opportunities were preconceived as modules with a similar format and structure to what is expected in formal education, which was a large part of the residents' day.

A Phase II needs assessment to be given to residents was developed according to the structure and content requested by the director and in keeping with the mission and philosophy of the facility. This assessment included life skills development modules in the areas of communication, goal setting, time and task management, and sexuality. Through this assessment, which was conducted in personal interviews, specific concerns were elicited in each of the areas first noted by the director. Most of the residents were fairly disinterested in the idea of yet "another class" and were not as helpful in this stage of program development as might be desired.

Although the occupational therapy student group conducting the needs assessment was fairly disheartened by the response, after some discussion, it was thought that the respondents might be more motivated if they had a hand in selecting how the content of the modules would be disseminated or investigated. Another series of interviews gleaned an assortment of creative but often impractical (generally because of time and/or cost) ideas. It was clear though, as was mentioned in chapter 19, that street-smart clients offered a substantial challenge for the creation of stimulating and engaging programming.

THE SELECTED PROGRAM

Bringing together the larger program goals and objectives that incorporated the enhancement of communication, setting realistic and manageable life goals, managing time and tasks, and exploring developmentally appropriate and safe sexuality in an informative and captivating programming package was the challenge. The response came in the form of a series of documentary videos.

Through investigation of volunteer resources of persons and companies, it was discovered that one of the local movie studios had previously offered an internship program along with high school credit for the experience to residents of the transitional living unit. The occupational therapy students first prepared a proposal for the approval of the director of the shelter. Following this step, a similar proposal that outlined the program and the purpose was developed for the studio executives. Although it had different goals than the traditional internship had offered, the proposal was received positively and the studio agreed to offer the internship/high school credit format. In addition, the studio offered the services of other college film program interns to advise and assist and to be responsible for video equipment to be loaned to the program.

The film interns supplied the technical expertise and advice, and the occupational therapy students offered the structure to make sure that the content of the scripts and the process of residents' involvement met the goals of the program established from the earlier needs assessment. A time line was developed; tasks were determined, analyzed, and distributed; the product was developed; and the process was evaluated.

The goals of establishing realistic objectives—time and task management—were accomplished in the process of planning and scripting, filming, and editing. The goals of developing communication skills and learning about sexuality were accomplished through the group decision that the film would be a documentary of individual "life story" vignettes provided by each of the participants. Not only were individual goals met through this activity, but there also were numerous other positive outcomes related to prevocational and vocational exploration (for example, discovering talents for writing, directing, and acting).

The initial format for program evaluation was eventually discarded in favor of a qualitative analysis of the filmed vignettes for the five participants. Since numerous practice films were made, there was substantial footage available for analysis. This was conducted both by the occupational therapy students and by the participants with shared observations of progress and identification of areas still needing improvement.

Videotaping or film-making is an excellent tool for occupation-centered interventions. If there are film students in the community, they are most likely looking for practice opportunities and generally have access to equipment. If not, then perhaps the local television station can become involved, particularly if the programming can be developed to advance the station's public relations as well as benefit participants. If no television stations are available, then consider "oral histories" and radio as the medium.

Even if none of these external resources are available, the seemingly simple process of using a camcorder can still utilize the development of a script through the telling of personal stories or story-making, and review of the film can be a powerful evaluative tool for both respondents and for students in the classroom.

This review of programming for homeless adolescents has presented some of the advantages and potential dilemmas you may find working with this community. They are perhaps the most challenging of the homeless persons for which you may wish to develop programs. They offer all of the characteristics of the homeless alongside the particular characteristics of the developmental phase of adolescence. Frequently they are abused and neglected, and they are often the most disenfranchised of all—rejected from family systems while in many ways still children.

SUMMARY

The problems of homeless children and adolescents, whether part of a homeless family unit or alone, are complicated by their developmental characteristics and their lack of preparation for the adult roles that may be thrust upon them. Communities of homeless children and adolescents resemble the structure of clubs discussed in previous chapters. There are often more covert rules than in adult homeless communities, and adolescents as well as younger runaway children who may be present are more likely to group together and support each other.

Children and adolescents are more difficult to engage in programs because they are often being searched for by families or are engaging in law-breaking behavior and fear being found or identified. The program described in this chapter provided an example of how homeless adolescents might be engaged in an occupation-centered program targeting the development of age-appropriate life skills.

REFERENCES

Covenant House Fact Sheet. (1994). Hollywood, CA: Covenant House.

Esperanza, M. L. (1997). *Covenant house California: Service plan, 1996–97.* Hollywood, CA: Covenant House.

Los Angeles County Families of Dependent Children. (1995). *Annual Report.* Los Angeles, CA: Los Angeles County.

National Network of Runaway and Youth Services. (1995). *A report on anti-homeless laws, litigation and alternatives in 50 United States Cities.* Washington, DC: National Law Center on Homelessness and Poverty.

United States Department of Health and Human Services (HHS). (1991). *Runaway youth annual report.* Washington, DC: Author.

Sample Cost Sheet for a Day Camp

This particular day camp program is a variation of the one described in earlier chapters. It is an extension of a pediatric not-for-profit practice, but it also welcomes the siblings of clients. It is staffed by full-time employees of the practice during the three summer months. The following is the service provision formula: two four-day weeks (=) one camp session (×) 3 summer months (=) six sessions (×) ten day campers each session (=) a total of 60 children serviced. The following is a partial cost sheet for the program. *Items marked with an asterisk (*) indicate a partial list.*

1. STAFFING
   a. Full-time camp: occupational therapist (OTR) entry-level
      Yearly gross salary (=) $46,000
   b. Part-time camp, part-time practice: occupational therapist (OTR), six years experience, sensory-integration certification
      Yearly gross salary (=) $62,000
   c. Part-time camp, part-time practice: certified occupational therapy assistant (COTA), one year experience
      Yearly gross salary (=) $28,000
      Total yearly professional salaries (=) $136,000
      Approximate combined benefit packages (×) 20% (=) $27,200
      Total professional employee cost to company (=) $163,200
   d. Part-time camp, part-time practice: office assistant
      Yearly gross salary (=) $19,200
   Approximate benefit package (×) 20% (=) $3,840
   Total administrative staff cost to company (=) $23,040
2. MARKETING
   a. Computer-generated flyers hand-distributed by practice professional staff to parents of children already being seen in the practice and to Regional Center offices. Approximately 200 flyers distributed at a cost of $.02 per flyer (=) $4.
      Sixty registrations and deposits were received, and a waiting list was quickly generated that exceeded the capacity of the camp. Thus, no further marketing to obtain campers was required.
   b. Personal marketing to local businesses and companies to obtain donated equipment and supplies and tuition scholarships was part of the responsibility of the therapists who were 100% camp time. An end-of-summer "thank you" picnic lunch for donors and full-time campers was donated by a local caterer.
3. OVERHEAD
   a. Utilities: Water and trash pickup were the only requirements and were at an approximate cost of $52 for the summer (absorbed into the larger practice bills).
   b. Van rental (1 × each week of camp) (=) 12 (×) $17 (=) $204
4. EQUIPMENT (Capital)
   None Required

5. EQUIPMENT*(noncapital): Purchased locally, so no shipping charges.
    a. 4 picnic tables with attached benches (ea. $210) (=) $840
    b. 4 large inflatable wading pools (ea. $42) (=) $168
    c. 3 kinder chutes (ea. $49.95) (=) $149.85
    d. 3 soft ring toss games (ea. $18) (=) $54
    e. 1 parachute (=) $215
    f. 15 beach balls (ea. $1.99) (=) $29.85
       Total cost of equipment if purchased*: $1456.70
       Items 1, 2, and 5 Were Donated: −1223.00
       Actual cost of equipment to company: $ 233.70
6. NONEXPENDABLE SUPPLIES* (purchased for full summer)
    a. 1 class-pack scissors—included 36, left and right handed (ea. $32) (=) $32
    b. 1 class-pack paint brushes—100 assorted (ea. $28) (=) $28
    c. 3 packs printmaking sponges—35 assorted shapes (ea. $15) (=) $45
Total cost of expendable supplies for summer: $105
7. EXPENDABLE SUPPLIES* (figured for one two-week session (×) 6 sessions)
    a. 10 1.7 fl. oz. nontoxic, nonflammable glue sticks (×) .99 ea. (=) $9.90 (×) 6
       sessions (=) $59.94 (Note: bulk of 100 glue sticks at a cost of $.52 ea. offered a
       savings of $.47 per stick (=) total cost of $52.00.)
    b. 2 class-pack assorted construction paper—500 sheets (×) $4.72 ea. (=) $9.44 (bulk
       savings of approximately $.03 per sheet over smaller pkg.)
    c. Crayola washable paints nine colors: 1 gallon each (×) $15.95 gal. (=) $143.55
    d. 500 paper paint pans (=) $9
       Total cost of expendable supplies for summer* (six sessions) (=) $213.99
       Total cost of expendable supplies for summer * (divided by six sessions) (=)
       $35.67 approximate supply cost for each session (divided by 10 children per
       session) (=) $3.57 approximate supply cost per child.

Considerations for Establishing Fees and Funding Camp Tuitions

If we had generated a complete list of equipment and supplies for this example (as you will
for the program you are designing), we would be able to closely figure the cost of the program for each participant. Knowing this exact figure will help us establish tuition costs for
each camper in this program and would also help us estimate the costs of adding more sessions or more children per session. For programs such as this, some planners/managers also
figure a breakdown of salary/equipment/overhead charges per client along with supplies
in order to arrive at a per-person cost.

   If the campers require extremely close attention for effective intervention and for safety
(for example, children with behavior disorders or other special problems), then we might need
to hire more staff and perhaps additional time of specialized professional staff. The cost of
higher levels of staff expertise and more personal attention are generally figured into the
client's costs. We might also consider training volunteers for the program or adding students.
Both volunteers and students require professional time for supervision, and these costs must
be included in the financial mix but are not generally included in the client's costs.

   Funding options for a camp such as the one described in this example include the following:

1. Private pay (may be considered day care for tax purposes)
2. Regional centers or other avenues of pay already established for the child's therapy
3. Donated "scholarships" based on financial need

Index

Note: Page numbers followed by *f* denote figures.